PRIMAL NUTRITION

D0447710

"*Primal Nutrition* is a well-researched, comprehensive resource for achieving better health with the use of traditional foods and time-honored methods of preparation. Dr. Schmid clearly explains why understanding and implementing the ancestral dietary principles outlined by Dr. Weston A. Price in his worldwide travels is critical if we are to overcome many of the health challenges of our time. This essential book is especially useful for anyone who desires to adopt all or part of a 'paleo diet' but is confused by its various interpretations."

EDWARD BENNETT, PRESIDENT OF
THE PRICE-POTTENGER NUTRITION FOUNDATION AND
EDITOR OF THE *JOURNAL OF HEALTH & HEALING*

"In *Primal Nutrition,* Dr. Ron Schmid has done a superb job of integrating the work of Weston Price, D.D.S., and Francis Pottenger, Jr., M.D., with recent research and a variety of popular diets, such as the macrobiotic diet, the Atkins diet, and the Pritikin diet. This book will be of great value for all clinicians interested in healing their patients or clients. In my opinion, it should be required reading for all medical students, dental students, nutritionists, chiropractors, naturopaths, dentists, and others in the healing arts. It will also be valuable to anyone interested in improving his or her health. I recommend it without qualification."

MICHAEL B. SCHACHTER, M.D., CNS, DIRECTOR OF THE
SCHACHTER CENTER FOR COMPLEMENTARY MEDICINE AND
CERTIFIED IN PSYCHIATRY, NUTRITION, AND CHELATION THERAPY
BY THE AMERICAN COLLEGE FOR ADVANCEMENT IN MEDICINE

"Throughout my years of research and teaching food energetics, I am often asked to recommend books on the subject. Naturally and without hesitation my suggestions include Weston Price's seminal work, along with Sally Fallon's *Nourishing Traditions,* and a few other authors who extol the many benefits of traditional foods. Ron Schmid's *Primal Nutrition* is a welcome addition to my list.

With so many diet books available we are often confused with which direction to turn, whether it's for general health maintenance or more personal health issues. *Primal Nutrition* is a great book for helping you get past the confusion inherent in making these choices. Schmid has a great respect for all traditional primal foods and knows well their historical role in health and their nutritional benefits. He leaves few stones unturned when it comes to supporting you in making wise and sensible decisions with diet and traditional foods."

STEVE GAGNE, AUTHOR OF
FOOD ENERGETICS: THE SPIRITUAL, EMOTIONAL, AND NUTRITIONAL POWER OF WHAT WE EAT

"*Primal Nutrition* brings you back to the basics of a good and healthy diet. It is well grounded and invaluable."

CHRISTOPHER VASEY, N.D., AUTHOR OF
THE ACID–ALKALINE DIET FOR OPTIMUM HEALTH AND *NATURAL REMEDIES FOR INFLAMMATION*

PRIMAL
NUTRITION

Paleolithic and Ancestral Diets for Optimal Health

RON SCHMID, ND

Healing Arts Press
Rochester, Vermont • Toronto, Canada

Healing Arts Press
One Park Street
Rochester, Vermont 05767
www.HealingArtsPress.com

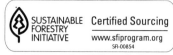

Text stock is SFI certified

Healing Arts Press is a division of Inner Traditions International

Copyright © 1987, 1988, 1994, 1997, 2015 by Ronald F. Schmid
Photographs by Weston Price, courtesy of the Price-Pottenger Nutrition Foundation

Originally published in 1987 by Ocean View Publications under the title *Traditional Foods Are Your Best Medicine: Health and Longevity with the Animal, Sea, and Vegetable Foods of Our Ancestors*
2nd edition published in 1988 edition published by Ballatine Books
3rd edition published in 1994 by Healing Arts Press under the title *Native Nutrition: Eating According to Ancestral Wisdom*
4th edition published in 1997 by Healing Arts Press under the title *Traditional Foods Are Your Best Medicine: Improving Health and Longevity with Native Nutrition*
5th edition published in 2015 by Healing Arts Press under the title *Primal Nutrition: Paleolithic and Ancestral Diets for Optimal Health*

All rights reserved. No part of this book may be reproduced or utilized in any form or by any means, electronic or mechanical, including photocopying, recording, or by any information storage and retrieval system, without permission in writing from the publisher.

Note to the reader: *This book is intended as an informational guide. The remedies, approaches, and techniques described herein are meant to supplement, and not to be a substitute for, professional medical care or treatment. They should not be used to treat a serious ailment without prior consultation with a qualified health care professional.*

Library of Congress Cataloging-in-Publication Data
Schmid, Ronald F., 1946-
  [Native nutrition]
  Primal nutrition : paleolithic and ancestral diets for optimal health / Ron Schmid, ND.
      pages cm
  Originally published in 1987 under the title: Traditional Foods Are Your Best Medicine : Health and Longevity with the Animal, Sea, and Vegetable Foods of Our Ancestors.
  Includes bibliographical references and index.
  ISBN 978-1-62055-519-4 (paperback) — ISBN 978-1-62055-520-0 (ebook)
  1. Nutrition. 2. Natural foods. 3. Health. 4. Food habits--Psychological aspects. I. Title.
  RA784.S3828 2015
  613.2—dc23   2015013554

Printed and bound in the United States by Lake Book Manufacturing, Inc.
The text stock is SFI certified. The Sustainable Forestry Initiative® program promotes sustainable forest management.

10 9 8 7 6 5 4 3 2 1

Text design by Virginia Scott Bowman and layout by Debbie Glogover
This book was typeset in Garamond Premier Pro with ITC Avant Garde Gothic Std and Gill Sans MT Pro as display fonts

To send correspondence to the author of this book, mail a first-class letter to the author c/o Inner Traditions • Bear & Company, One Park Street, Rochester, VT 05767, and we will forward the communication, or contact the author directly at **drron@drrons.com**.

Thanks to everyone for the second chances.

CONTENTS

ACKNOWLEDGMENTS

The people at Inner Traditions have kept the forerunners of this book in print for over two decades. Without them this new edition would not have been possible. Years ago, Sally Fallon Morell, president of the Weston A. Price Foundation, graciously went through this book's former incarnation, *Traditional Foods Are Your Best Medicine,* and made notes in the margins—suggestions, corrections, bits of information, and ideas for me to develop. She recently went through the manuscript of this book and did that all over again. I have incorporated nearly all of her work; any errors and omissions that remain are mine. Her constructive influence on this updated version of *Traditional Foods* cannot be overstated. I am so fortunate to have Sally in my corner, and I very much appreciate her writing a foreword to the volume you now hold in your hands.

I would also like to thank Nora Gedgaudas, author of *Primal Body, Primal Mind,* for her outstanding body of work, which has influenced mine. I would also like to thank her for writing a second foreword to this book.

The wonderful people on my staff who work with me every day make it possible for me to do the things I do. Special thanks go to my sister-in-law and brother-in-law, Elaine and Mike Stern, and my nephews Chris Stern and Nick Hughes. Our photographer and good friend Marcus Halevi hears all my ideas, good and bad, hopefully before they go anywhere and do damage. He's been there for us for just about longer than I can remember, and we love him.

"We" means my wonderful wife, Elly, and I. Her sweetness lights up my life every day. Her strengths balance my weaknesses in so many ways, influencing everything I do. May it always be Ron and El, El and Ron, devoted.

FOREWORD

SALLY FALLON MORELL

Paleo and ancestral diets are in the news these days, with dozens of books on the subject, plenty of media attention, blogs, and conferences, and even special paleo labels and paleo vitamin pills! But confusion reigns as to what actually constitutes a paleo diet or ancestral diet. Is it the lean-meat, low-fat diet proposed by authors Loren Cordain and Robb Wolf? Or is it a high-fat diet that embraces bacon, liver, and lard? Should grains be included in paleo or ancestral diets? And what about dairy products?

The first researcher to describe the diets of nonindustrialized peoples was Weston Price, D.D.S., in his groundbreaking book *Nutrition and Physical Degeneration*. He called these diets "primitive" diets. During the 1930s and early 1940s, Price traveled to remote corners of the globe to study the health and diets of isolated groups. His investigations took him to remote Swiss villages and a windswept island in the Outer Hebrides. He studied traditional Eskimos, Indian tribes in Canada and the Florida Everglades, islanders of the South Seas, Aborigines in Australia, Maoris in New Zealand, and Peruvian and Amazonian Indians and tribesmen in Africa.

He studied rates of tooth decay, which were invariably very low in isolated communities. He also described dental and facial structure, noting that primitive peoples universally had straight teeth and well-developed cheeks and jawbones. He noted the absence of chronic diseases such as tuberculosis, cancer, and heart disease, and he marveled at the reproductive health of the people who lived in these villages and tribes, where women easily gave birth to sturdy children. *Nutrition and Physical Degeneration* provides a fascinating record of his findings, and includes the photographs he took.

The difficulty has been in making Price's findings accessible to the public, for even those individuals who take the time to read his book come away with questions. All the primitive diets he described were so different from one another, they observed. How then could Price's discoveries be translated into practical dietary advice for modern people? Some groups, like the Eskimos and northern Indians, consumed a very high-fat diet containing almost no plant foods. African agriculturists, on the other hand, lived on a plant-based diet; the animal foods they ingested were limited to insects and small fish. Dairy foods and grain provided the bulk of calories in the diet of the Swiss villager; Gaelic fisherfolk of the Outer Hebrides ate mostly seafood and oats. The most varied diets were found in the South Seas, where an abundance of fruit, vegetables, and tubers thrived in the warm climate. Despite this, however, animal foods formed the basis of the diet of these people—everything from shellfish to shark to pig. Some groups had lots of fat in the diet, others had plenty of carbs.

From these cursory descriptions, can we come to any conclusions about how we should eat today in order to be healthy?

The way to answer this important question is to look at the basic underlying principles of healthy ancestral or traditional diets. In the concluding chapter of his book, Dr. Price formulated four basic precepts; additional principles can be gleaned from other researchers. With all of these principles in mind, we as individuals can create a diet that works for us—one containing foods that are available to us, that we can afford, that we have time to prepare, and, most importantly, one that we like to eat.

The first principle is obvious: the diets of isolated primitive or traditional peoples contained no refined or industrially processed food—no sugar or white flour, no industrial seed oils, no partially hydrogenated fats, no extruded breakfast cereals, no pasteurized or homogenized milk, no canned or irradiated food, no artificial sweeteners or additives. Thus, the first step that anyone wishing to improve his or her health needs to take is to remove these items from the diet. Price referred to these foods as the "displacing foods of modern commerce." They were devoid of nutrients—in fact they often *deplete* the body of nutrients—while displacing the kind of nutrient-dense foods the body needs to maintain good health.

The second principle was Dr. Price's greatest disappointment: all primitive diets contained animal foods. A few diets were 100 percent animal foods, a few contained low amounts of animal foods, but most were somewhere in the middle. Dr. Price had hoped to find a culture that was healthy and lived exclusively on plant foods, but no traditional culture practiced a purely vegan diet.

The third principle is the most important. Dr. Price took samples of traditional foods home to his laboratory in Cleveland, Ohio, and tested them for their vitamin and mineral content. The best way to summarize the main characteristic of traditional diets is "nutrient-dense." Price found that these diets contained at least four times more minerals (calcium, magnesium, copper, iron, etc.) compared to the American diet of his day, and high levels of the water-soluble vitamins—vitamin C and all the B vitamins.

The real surprise, however, was the very high levels of fat-soluble vitamins found in ancestral diets—at least ten times more true vitamin A, vitamin D, and vitamin K_2 compared to the American diet of his day. Which foods provide these vitamins? Not the foods that modern man is used to eating. Certain seafood, such as fish eggs, fish liver oils, shellfish, and oily fish are good sources. In land animals, we get these vitamins from egg yolks, butterfat, organ meats, and animal fats—especially when these animals have grazed outdoors on green grass.

Sunlight maximizes the level of vitamin D in our food, and green grass provides the precursors (carotenes and vitamin K_1) for animals to make true vitamin A and vitamin K_2. These three fat-soluble vitamins are key to every process that occurs in the body—from bone health to an optimistic outlook.

These vitamins are also germane to fertility and growth, which brings us to the fourth principle that Dr. Price described. Primitive peoples consumed special nutrient-dense "sacred" foods in preparation for pregnancy, during pregnancy and breastfeeding, and during the period of growth. These foods were particularly rich in the fat-soluble vitamins and included butter from cows eating rapidly growing grass in the spring (Switzerland), cod heads stuffed with oats and chopped cod liver (Outer Hebrides), fish eggs (consumed in many parts of the world, including Alaska and Peru), raw milk from cows eating rapidly growing green grass (Switzerland and Africa), shark-liver oil (South Seas), liver and other organ meats (wherever land animals are consumed), and fish-liver oils, such as cod-liver oil (Europe and America). These foods also support healing at any age.

Thus, according to Dr. Price, the key to good health is not just found by avoiding processed foods, but also by making an effort to include special nutrient-dense foods in the diet. That means overcoming the modern strictures against cholesterol and saturated fat, because most of the sacred foods are indeed high in these demonized substances. A politically correct low-fat diet will not confer good health, whatever the so-called experts may claim.

Additional fundamental principles can be gleaned from other researchers. One principle involves cooking. Should we cook our food? Some diet gurus claim we should only eat raw foods, but all human cultures cooked some or most of their food—especially plant foods like grains, legumes, tubers, and fibrous vegetables. It is also true that some traditional cultures ate some of their animal foods raw—as raw seafood, raw meat, and raw dairy. (Raw animal foods are our best source of vitamin B_6).

Furthermore, all diets contained "super raw" foods in the form of lacto-fermented vegetables, meats, fish, and dairy foods. Lacto-fermentation, a process of preserving foods, greatly increases vitamins, enzymes, and beneficial bacteria. One serving of genuine sauerkraut contains ten times more vitamin C than the equivalent amount of raw cabbage, and as many beneficial bacteria as a whole container of probiotic pills. Recent discoveries about human gut flora show us why lacto-fermented foods like sauerkraut, natural pickles, yoghurt, kefir, sour cream, and lacto-fermented beverages like kombucha are so important in the diet. They nourish our internal biology, thereby supporting good digestion, protecting against toxins and pathogens, and even enhancing mood and mental health.

What about grains and legumes? The paleo community insists that these have no place in the diet. But Price described several healthy cultures that consumed grains and legumes, and we now know that so-called primitive groups actually cultivated and harvested wild grains. Science tells us that grains and legumes are hard to digest. Primitive peoples knew this instinctively, which is why they subjected these foods to careful preparation methods involving soaking or souring. Soaking and souring are processes of fermentation that neutralize the nutrient-blocking and irritating qualities of these foods. Grains and legumes may best be avoided in those with compromised digestion, but foods like soaked and cooked oatmeal and rice, genuine sourdough bread, and soaked and long-cooked beans provide variety and nourishment to the modern diet.

Traditional communities that used milk and milk products—whether from cows, goats, sheep, water buffalo, reindeer, or camels—always consumed them raw, straight from the animal, or they fermented them into cheese, yoghurt, kefir, and similar products. These products came from healthy animals raised outdoors and fed on natural food—not confined to the indoors and an unnatural diet. These traditional milk products provide superb nutrition, and they are easily digested.

Traditional cultures also made good use of bones. The Eskimos ate the softened bones of fermented fish, and hunter-gatherers ground up the bones of small animals and added them to their food. But mostly, bones were cooked to make broth, which the American Indians considered superior to water. Today Asian cultures consume bone broth at every meal. Science validates the long tradition of broth as a healing food. Special amino acids and the components in broth help the body heal, support detoxification, contribute to good digestion, and provide the building blocks of cartilage and collagen.

Finally, all traditional cultures consumed salt—whether sea salt, mined salt, or the naturally salty blood and urine of their animals. Salt is crucial to digestion—the chloride component of salt is needed to make hydrochloride acid for protein digestion, and the sodium portion of salt activates enzymes needed for carbohydrate digestion. Salt is the basis of cellular metabolism, allowing us to have a different biochemistry on the inside and the outside of the cell. When traditional cultures could not find salt locally, they traded for it and/or travelled a long way for it.

Today, sixty years after the publication of *Nutrition and Physical Degeneration*, the name Weston Price has become better known. The first author to make his work accessible to the public was Dr. Ron Schmid, in an earlier edition of this book. Now enlarged and updated, *Primal Nutrition* presents the principles of healthy traditional diets along with Dr. Schmid's vast clinical experience. A diet based on these principles should be the main focus of any therapy. These diets have worked for millions of years, and they continue to work today.

SALLY FALLON MORELL is the president and treasurer of the Weston A. Price Foundation. She is also the president and owner of NewTrends Publishing, serving as editor and publisher of numerous books about healing and nutrition. Her lifelong interest in the subject of nutrition began in the early 1970s when she read *Nutrition and Physical Degeneration* by Weston Price. She is the coauthor of *Nourishing Traditions: The Cookbook that Challenges Politically Correct Nutrition and the Diet Dictocrats*. This well-researched, thought-provoking guide to traditional foods contains a startling message: Animal fats and cholesterol are not villains but vital and necessary factors in the diet. Morell is also the coauthor of *Eat Fat, Lose Fat: The Healthy Alternative to Trans Fats; The Nourishing Traditions Book of Baby & Child Care; The Nourishing Traditions Cookbook for Children*; and *Nourishing Broth: An Old-Fashioned Remedy for the Modern World*.

FOREWORD

NORA GEDGAUDAS, C.N.S., C.N.T.

My own passionate interest and background in nutritional science spans roughly thirty-five years, but it wasn't until about twenty-one years ago that I came across an earlier incarnation of the book you now hold in your hands. From the moment I first picked it up off the shelf, I almost literally couldn't put it down. Ron Schmid's unique, exciting, and illuminating treatise on diet and health served as my introduction to the work of Weston Price, as well as the (duh!) concept of ancestral nutrition. I was instantly hooked. It's as though nearly two decades of sorting through and attempting to piece nutritional information into a cohesive, foundational perspective suddenly came together with resounding, thundering clarity.

In short, I was gobsmacked and nothing has been the same ever since.

Drawing heavily from his dedicated research into traditional and ancestral diets, as well as his own extensive career as a naturopathic physician, Ron's book opened my eyes to a completely different way of looking at the field of nutritional science. What I read in those pages sparked a whole new level of passion in me about the origins of human dietary requirements and optimization, which continues to burn brightly in me to this very day. In short, it changed my life and the trajectory of my career as a nutritional consultant (not to mention the lives of clients I have managed to influence in a positive fashion along the way). It also eventually led me to become the author of my own bestselling book, *Primal Body, Primal Mind: Beyond the Paleo Diet for Total Health and a Longer Life*. The rest, as they say, is history. I owe Ron a debt of gratitude for that.

Three years before I picked up Ron's book for the first time, I had spent the summer living less than five hundred miles from the North Pole with a family of wild wolves. My purpose in the high Arctic was basically to perform behavioral research related to *Canis lupus arctos*—the Arctic wolf. While there, I was also able to freely indulge in my lifelong fascination with Inuit/Thule culture and history. Numerous archaeological sites—some thousands of years old—dotted the vast tundra like some forgotten dream. Many of the prehistoric sites at that time in this exceedingly remote and isolated location had yet to be studied or disturbed in any way. The "primal" nature of the landscape and terrain heralded back to the Ice Age permafrost-paved tundra of northern Europe during the great Cro-Magnon migrations there.

This Arctic environment captured my imagination and got me thinking in some new and somewhat startling ways. It was in this vast, remote, and distant place that I forged my first awareness of the primacy of dietary animal fat to our species, and realized how this blatantly conflicted with widespread assumptions universally promoted by mainstream authorities. When I picked up Ron's book, those cogs in my head were already turning.

Although over time my own perspective on this vast and complex subject has diverged slightly from Ron's, we clearly maintain some meaningful common ground. I respect him greatly, as well as the extraordinary integrity that he applies to his work as a researcher, medical practitioner, and a uniquely dedicated formulator of clean, effective, and unadulterated nutritional supplements that are in keeping with his philosophy.

To this very day, I know of no better introduction to the works of

Weston Price, or a better and more thoughtful discourse on the subject of Neolithic and traditional diets, than this book that you hold in your hands. Ron meticulously weaves his own threads of research into a comprehensive and compelling tapestry that is as warm and accessible as it is practical in its application. In this new edition, Ron has also proven his own capacity to question foundational assumptions—including his own. With grace, respect, and a rare open-mindedness, Ron has renewed his perspective in a way seldom revisited by established experts in any field, and he continually expresses a willingness to see the evidence he has uncovered in new ways. To his credit, I have noted the very same in our own personal conversations and exchanges over the years.

May the newest and best incarnation of this book rock your world even a fraction as much as its earlier predecessor rocked mine.

NORA GEDGAUDAS, C.N.S., C.N.T., a widely recognized expert on what is popularly referred to as the "paleo diet," is the author of the international bestselling book *Primal Body, Primal Mind: Beyond the Paleo Diet for Total Health and a Longer Life* as well as *Rethinking Fatigue: What Your Adrenals Are Really Telling You and What You Can Do about It*. She is also a highly successful experienced nutritional consultant, speaker, and educator, widely interviewed on national and international radio, popular podcasts, television, and film. Her own popular podcasts are widely listened to on iTunes and are available for free download, along with numerous articles and a location on the homepage, where anyone can subscribe to her newsletter. She maintains a private practice in Portland, Oregon, as both a board-certified nutritional consultant and a board-certified clinical neurofeedback specialist.

HEALING, HEALTH, AND WHOLENESS

In the mid-1980s I wrote the first edition of *Traditional Foods Are Your Best Medicine*, which was based on the belief that food was the essential element for healing to take place. That was how I began my own healing, and how I had helped many people recover from various diseases.

In *Traditional Foods Are Your Best Medicine*, I presented the details of my research on food and health, and my experience utilizing food as a healing agent. The research I had done up until that point was grounded in the work of Dr. Weston Price, the great dentist and anthropologist of the 1920s and 1930s who discovered fundamental laws of nature that indigenous cultures throughout the world had followed from time immemorial to ensure vibrant good health, the absence of disease, and the production of robust babies—generation after generation. The diet these indigenous people followed is referred to as a primal diet, which seeks to guide us to eat the way our ancestors did, with subsequent health benefits.

This book is the latest edition of *Traditional Foods Are Your Best Medicine*. We've changed the title to reflect the fact that Weston Price's work demonstrates the principles that should be at the heart of every primal healing diet. Subsequent editions of *Traditional Foods* retained most of the information of the original, but I added certain of my conclusions and recommendations in light of new experiences. I rewrote sections of the book to reflect my growing awareness of the importance of—to put it most simply—that which may not be perceived by the five senses, nor by the most sophisticated scientific instruments.

I've also corrected errors that I had made in previous editions. My chief error was understating the critical importance of substantial quantities of quality animal fats in the diets of the native—primal, if you will—people that Dr. Price studied. This is the same error most people advocating and attempting to follow "paleo" diets are making today, and it is the same error that many healers and their patients make in utilizing what are called paleo and sometimes primal diets.

Despite this popular misconception, I remain convinced that animal food of a certain quality, as well as seafood, are needed in the diet to support optimal health. This belief is supported by overwhelming evidence from diverse fields—anthropology, biochemistry, clinical nutrition among them—and the experience of a multitude of healers besides Dr. Price. Additionally, I find it fascinating that the foods considered "sacred" in native cultures—that is, the foods considered to have spiritual qualities and to be absolutely essential for a culture's people, the foods around which rituals and ceremonies evolved—to the best of my knowledge were mostly animal foods, (although occasionally corn and grains were included).

In some places, these sacred foods were also raw dairy products. What might the role of high-quality, grass-fed dairy food be in a primal diet today? For most people, these foods are a useful or even essential option in finding a path to health. And although primal diet advocates are generally more cognizant of the importance of high-quality fats derived from grass-fed animals, a thorough understanding of Price's work is absolutely essential to really get this right. Thus, I have sought to show why a modern primal diet is best built upon a thorough understanding of the Weston Price principles.

Much of this book describes how Price discovered those principles in his studies of indigenous—primal—peoples; how other researchers—

particularly physicians and anthropologists—confirmed and enlarged his work; and how my own clinical work utilizing those principles has enabled me to help thousands of patients heal from serious medical problems.

May you use this book wisely and well, and may it contribute to your own good health in the months and years ahead.

PRIMAL DIETS, WESTON PRICE, AND HEALING

THE CURATIVE POWER OF NATURE

The human body has an inherent ability to heal. Think of a cut, or a broken bone. Given time, the cut heals, the bone mends. What accomplishes these small miracles?

Nature. Nature cures. This is the basis of lasting healing and lasting health.

The same intrinsic force that mends a broken bone can heal arthritis; in both cases, the body reacts to disturbances in its natural balance in a way that restores that natural balance. The bone is more easily repaired than is the arthritis, for trauma caused the bone to break suddenly—no deep-seated underlying problem must be corrected in order for healing to occur. Arthritis is not so simple because it develops primarily as a result of years of faulty dietary habits. And although the broken bone usually heals *even with* what may be somewhat faulty nutrition, to heal arthritis, the underlying conditions that cause it must be changed.

But for nature to cure, one must first understand what nature is—what is natural—and live by it. Even when this is comprehended, a problem remains: few modern people understand what constitutes a natural diet.

1

This is no surprise. A systematic investigation of the issue takes years of study; research in a broad range of related fields is necessary. Relentless and constant experimentation with one's own diet is required. Clinical work adds valuable lessons based on professional experience. Other methods besides diet may be tried in attempts to enhance one's health and alleviate disease, but one soon learns that no other approach to healing holds the curative power and potential that food does.

In the field of biology, Charles Darwin's treatise on the evolution of life on Earth, *On the Origin of Species,* stands out as a classic. Darwin demonstrated that in nature there are no accidents; for every effect there is a cause. Darwin's work made me wonder: Could human evolution have been shaped by the diet of early man, with the result being that modern man is best suited to a certain kind of diet? Humans today are genetically very much the same as our ancestors were in preagricultural times, thousands of years ago. Perhaps the best diet for modern man is the primal diet that we were genetically adapted to back then. What I call the "modern primal diet" consists of foods generally available today that affect us in the same way that primal foods thousands of years ago affected our preagricultural ancestors—who were free of our modern diseases, the so-called diseases of civilization.

That an individualized modern primal diet is the best diet for mankind today is a reasonable possibility. We may expect that for each person there may be variations, of course, depending on the individual's biological and cultural history. But the same fundamental laws of human nutrition should apply to everyone.

These laws became clearer to me when I encountered a little-known but monumental work entitled *Nutrition and Physical Degeneration,* by Dr. Weston Price. Initially published in 1939, this work was based on Dr. Price's lifetime of research studying the nutrition and health of traditional native cultures around the world. Dr. Price's studies taught him the natural principles governing human nutrition and health. My studies and clinical experience have since confirmed for me the wisdom of Price's observations and conclusions, which will be elucidated in this book.

REBUILDING YOUR BIRTHRIGHT
OF GOOD HEALTH

Our genes and the structure of our enzymes have been passed down to us through thousands of generations. The building-block molecules of genes are identical in all living things. Biological laws unite all life-forms.

Laws of physics govern the movement of the planets, the changing of the seasons, the coming and going of the tides. Biological laws govern the ways in which the human body reacts to different foods. People once argued that Earth was flat, that blood did not circulate in the human body, that physicians need not wash their hands before assisting women in labor. Some now argue that our ills are not intimately connected with our food.

Illness weighs heavily, but those willing to give nature's methods an honest try are making a step in the right direction. The body needs primal foods—foods in their natural state, as nature provides them—in order to function well. Most of these foods are readily available, although some shopping in special places—markets selling fresh high-quality vegetables and fruits, natural food stores, seafood markets, farms, and co-ops—may be needed.

By making an effort to incorporate elements of a natural diet into your lifestyle, you may begin to rebuild your birthright of good health. This is not an all-or-nothing proposition. A foundation of commitment allows you to make gradual changes and enhance your health at your own pace.

If you have intuitively turned to nutrition as a means to better health, if you want to understand how and why foods affect you, and if you want to learn more about the role of food in the human story, this book may become very important to you. Embracing its wisdom may lead you to increased health and happiness, two conditions that are not the same but that certainly support one another.

When we think of the physical aspects of health, we think of the body and the brain functioning well. Happiness may be thought of as more a matter of the human spirit, perhaps as a lasting sense of spiritual wholeness and fulfillment. Is it possible to live a long and healthy life, one free of the degenerative diseases plaguing modern people? And can health and happiness be found by following the appropriate diet? If so, how does one begin to alter one's eating habits so that optimal health may be realized?

Dietary changes are best achieved gradually, as an understanding of food and your own needs deepen. Trying to change too much, too abruptly, may create physical and emotional difficulties. A reasonable middle course involves being flexible and realistic so that the new diet can ultimately take hold and work. A diet of simple whole foods becomes more palatable as one grows accustomed to it; eventually, one may lose all desire for the refined foods that once seemed irresistible. Changes in habits lead to changes in tastes and inclinations.

For people seeking to correct troubling conditions, the foundation of success is a commitment to personal growth. This commitment and a thorough understanding of our traditional foods may enable one to reach the simple but elusive goal of radiant and lasting health.

NATUROPATHIC MEDICINE AND THE "CAVE MAN DIET"

One of naturopathy's founding principles comes from the writings of Hippocrates: "Let your food be your medicine, and your medicine be your food." Given the proper conditions, the human body contains the power to heal itself. Making the right food choices helps set the stage for healing to occur.

Be that as it may, this orientation toward food as a source of healing has been somewhat eclipsed today, especially within the medical community. One reason is that the influence of pharmaceutical companies on medical-school curricula has made it difficult for medical students to learn the underlying causes of disease and the fundamental steps leading to health; the vast majority of present-day medical schools do not require courses in nutrition. Students learn to use drugs to alleviate symptoms and to perform surgery to remove diseased body parts, rather than learning to use a fundamental understanding of health as a basis for guiding people to natural recovery as is taught in naturopathic medical schools.

As an undergraduate I studied architecture at M.I.T., and several years after graduation I attended naturopathic medical school, from which I graduated in 1981. In my practice of medicine, I have worked with medical doctors as a staff nutritional consultant and independently as a naturopathic physician. A few words are in order here about the interwoven history of natural health care in America and naturopathic medicine.

Naturopathic medicine (pronounced *NA-ture-oh-pathic*) is a separate and distinct branch of the healing arts. From nineteenth-century European roots, the movement grew and became popular in America in the early part of the twentieth century. Most states then licensed naturopathic physicians, but under pressure from the American Medical Association, in the 1930s, state legislatures began repealing the licensing laws, limiting the practice to those already holding licenses. The influence of the medical monopoly that was subsequently established outlawed naturopathic medicine in most states.

But in recent years, new laws licensing the practice of naturopathic medicine have been passed, and naturopathic physicians now practice in over twenty states in America and most of the Canadian provinces. To become licensed, one must graduate from one of the naturopathic medical schools recognized by states granting licenses and pass the state licensing examination. Today there are four accredited naturopathic medical schools in this country: the National College of Natural Medicine in Portland, Oregon; John Bastyr University in Seattle, Washington; the Southwest College of Naturopathic Medicine in Scottsdale, Arizona; and the College of Naturopathic Medicine at the University of Bridgeport in Bridgeport, Connecticut.

All are four-year graduate programs granting the degree doctor of naturopathic medicine.

The training of naturopathic physicians is rigorous. The usual medical school core curriculum of anatomy, physiology, pathology, embryology, and various other sciences are studied intensively during the first two years. During the third and fourth years, students focus on natural therapeutics in a clinical setting.

Following my graduation from naturopathic medical school, I went to work at Mountainview Medical Associates, a large, alternative-medicine practice in my hometown of Nyack, New York. As mentioned earlier, I was greatly influenced in my work by the conclusions of Dr. Weston Price, which were derived from his lifetime of research studying the nutrition and health of traditional native cultures throughout the world.

The two medical doctors who were my colleagues in the medical practice in Nyack (David Schienken, deceased, and Michael Schachter, now at the Schachter Center for Complementary Medicine in Suffern, New York) used vitamin, mineral, and food supplements as part of their therapies, but they had no experience using the Weston Price dietary principles clinically. Indeed, they had not even heard of Weston Price. During my time at Mountainview I followed the precepts of Weston Price to successfully treat many patients. Witnessing this, my medical colleagues were rather amazed at the recoveries they saw, especially given the fact that many of these patients had been suffering from chronic diseases that were typically incurable.

Soon my colleagues were talking about "Ron Schmid's Cave Man Diet," and they asked me to write it up in a handout that they and other health-care professionals on the staff could use. I explained to them that because my healing protocol wasn't based on one diet, but rather on a set of principles that could be used to help each individual find his or her own best traditional diet, I couldn't write up the handout they were asking me for.

I used the word *traditional* to describe my approach because it evoked Price's studies of traditional indigenous peoples from which his dietary principles emerged. But to my colleagues at Mountainview, it was the Cave Man Diet—meat, vegetables, fruit, and little else—and they imagined one size fit all comers.

Their prompting and support eventually led to the publication of the first edition of this book that you now hold in your hands. Published in 1987, it was entitled *Traditional Foods Are Your Best Medicine*. Others in the medical community were, at the time, working in this area of dietary research as well. They included Leon Chaitow who, also in 1987, published his book *Stone Age Diet*—and S. Boyd Eaton, M.D., and Melvin Konner, Ph.D., who in 1985 published the seminal article: "Paleolithic Nutrition" in the *New England Journal of Medicine*. My Cave Man Diet was going mainstream. Now, twenty-nine years later, we find ourselves presented with a myriad of paleo and primal diets.

Many popular paleo diets today, in general, make the same big mistake that the authors of the Paleolithic nutrition article referenced above (and I, originally) made in vastly underestimating the amount and importance of animal fat in Paleolithic diets. Medical treatises on the primal diet that I have studied by and large don't make this error— they acknowledge the critical role of grass-fed animal foods in a diet designed to enhance one's health. Specifically, these foods provide the quantities of fat-soluble activators—vitamins A, D, K_2, essential fatty acids, and associated nutrients—that are essential for resistance to disease, physical development, and optimal health to occur.

This book demonstrates that the world's healthiest, strongest, and most disease-resistant cultures lived on whole, natural food—mostly seafood, wild game, or robust, well-exercised domestic animals, fresh wild or cultivated vegetables and fruits, and, for some cultures, properly prepared grains, as well as raw, unprocessed dairy products. How and why modern foods differ, the effects of those differences, and steps that may be taken to build health with superior foods will be explained in the following pages. The appendices contain additional, associated material for the interested reader.

THE ESSENCE OF HEALING

This book provides a roadmap to participating in one's own health and well-being through proper nutrition, however, this is no substitute for a physician's care if needed. Indeed, many doctors practicing medicine today are sympathetic to the idea that nature cures. That said, the greatest experts in health care often have *not* been physicians, but rather people possessed of a certain wisdom about the human body, a wisdom understood, lived, and taught to the next generation. Much of this book is about such wisdom.

This traditional wisdom can be researched, written down, and studied—yet it remains, paradoxically, beyond the reach of *any* book. References in this book provide evidence, but something outside of the proven must also play a role. Knowledge and understanding of health as part of the human condition may be grounded in observations, published information, and years of personal and clinical experience. Yet conclusions of lasting value must, when practiced, feel intuitively right; the body's response is the final arbiter.

And although food as medicine is clearly the topic of this book, I have come to believe the essence of healing lies beyond food. Many people today may believe that they're incapable of improving their diets and thus are reluctant to try. Only a reasonably healthy attitude toward life can support and maintain the discipline required to follow a healthy diet. Without this positive attitude—one that acknowledges that change *is* possible—most people are unable to maintain a new dietary regimen and instead are apt to slip back into faulty eating habits that exacerbate their medical conditions.

That said, I believe that healing begins and proceeds for each of us in a totally unique and mysterious way. Each of us may begin where it is easiest for us to make changes in our lives—whether that is in the physical, spiritual, or emotional realm. And although I have read cases where changes in emotional attitude and spiritual orientation have led to a dramatic recovery from a physical ailment or ailments, my experience with thousands of people tells me that, for the vast majority of individuals, it's only by making consistent efforts in *all* areas simultaneously that true emotional, physical, and spiritual health may be reached.

Most of this book is about the relationship between food and physical healing, an area in which I have considerable experience and expertise. When I write about emotional and spiritual well-being, however, my words may only reflect how far I have traveled on this path in my *own* search for wholeness—no healer can take another to places he has not traveled himself. Natural foods have played an important role in my journey and in the journeys of many of my patients. My hope is that by sharing some of these journeys, I may help my readers in their efforts to understand the role that food plays in one's path to wholeness.

EMOTIONAL, PHYSICAL, AND SPIRITUAL HEALTH

What do I mean by the emotional, physical, and spiritual health that constitutes wholeness?

Emotional health is more than, yet encompasses, what is generally referred to as mental health. It is a feeling of rightness about oneself and one's place in the flow of life. It is the capacity to feel healthy and appropriate emotions in any situation and to take appropriate actions. It is the capacity to accept and give unconditional love to everyone in one's life, within the framework of protective personal boundaries. It's an ability to be truly intimate and to share one's life with other human beings. It is loving and caring for oneself and others.

Physical health includes having a body and mind that function easily. Desires for a full life are strong, as is the ability to live a full life. No signs or symptoms of distress are present. There is a feeling of physical strength, endurance, and vigor, and a certain assumption that one's body should and does function perfectly and effortlessly.

My definition of spiritual health has little to do with churchgoing and conventional religiosity, though one may find comfort, companionship, and guidance in a church or religion. For me, spiritual health is internalized and doesn't depend upon belief in an external God who grants favors or rules our lives. Rather, spiritual health involves recognizing, awakening, and nourishing the spirit within—the universal Creative Energy, the Great Spirit—so that we may each light our own path. The healed soul shines from within.

Breaking free of physical and emotional addictions is, for many of us, the nuts-and-bolts work we must undertake in our quest to satisfy that drive of our soul to shine from within. Our dietary habits are integrally related and interwoven with our physical and emotional addictions and, as such, cannot be separated from considerations of spiritual growth and a sense of wholeness.

Each of us may choose to deal with a respective addiction as a first step of our growth. Some of us may be dependent upon alcohol, drugs, nicotine, caffeine, or other addictive substances, and choose to examine this. Others may choose to confront their blatantly addictive or more subtle behaviors involving food—or their inability to be emotionally intimate, wherein they exhibit isolationist or codependent behavior. Or they may exhibit sexually inappropriate behavior. Still others may deal successively with a whole *host* of addictive substances and behaviors.

Many of the things we take for granted—substances and behaviors that are a part of our everyday lives—can be used as painkillers, as ways to feel good temporarily while avoiding real growth and a search for wholeness. At some point, as we strip away the layers of our addictions, we find that we must deal with food. As we become more capable of making choices about the food we eat, as we seek to consciously eat in a healthy manner, many questions arise.

This book seeks to answer those questions and to provide a blueprint to the nutritional aspects of healing. It seeks, furthermore, to provide a notion of the integral role which that blueprint must play in a journey to wholeness. This guide of sorts is very different from any you may have seen elsewhere, for it's based on biological laws discovered—not by modern scientists—but rather by native cultures the world over.

PART 1

AN ANCESTRY OF PRIMAL NUTRITION

Diets of Traditional Societies and a Legacy of Health

Every popular diet book presents different theories and opinions about the food we eat. What should we eat and how much? What are the effects of cooked and raw vegetables, fruit, meat, and fish, cholesterol, fats and oils, eggs, dairy foods, and grains? Is sugar really harmful? What about refined flour? Which "experts" are right—those who say cholesterol is killing us, or those who tell us it is not the real culprit in heart disease? And which foods help prevent chronic disease? Which foods will enable us to enjoy the robust good health we sense has been partly lost to modern living and a modern diet?

These questions have no simple answers. My approach is to seek answers by first asking several other relevant and related questions: What was the health of people in traditional and so-called primitive cultures existing into the early twentieth century—people eating only traditional natural food? What about the health of isolated cultures that still survive, and the health of the few remaining hunter-gatherers living and eating primitively today?

If the health of such people is superior to ours, could this be directly related to their diet? If so, which foods did and do such people eat? What differences exist between their food and modern food? How do their vegetables, grains, meats, dairy products, fish, and fruits differ from ours? And do the differences help explain the existence of our modern diseases—diseases that anthropologists and researchers agree by and large did not exist in traditional cultures?

Might the concept of "sacred food," common in so many native cultures, provide important clues about what kinds of food are most important in maintaining physical and spiritual health? What about the effect of traditional, primal foods—seafood, for example—on people with chronic diseases? What evidence has been published in the medical literature? (Plenty, as we'll see.)

Although people of our modern world may appear jovial despite poor health, this is often a mask used in attempting to hide underlying unhappiness or denial of the fact that a problem exists. Others who are very ill truly do adapt, and lead emotionally fulfilling lives in the face of great pain and suffering. Perhaps they think one must accept one's lot in life, that they have no alternative. But such an attitude sadly relegates to fate a small part of the world you may control—your own body.

As we seek to understand what aspects of our health we can control and what aspects we cannot, we will, in this first part of *Primal Nutrition,* review the historical, anthropological, and evolutionary aspects of traditional primal foods. We will also detail the current and historical research into the health effects of these foods, and discuss my clinical experience relating to the use of these foods in the treatment of acute and chronic diseases.

Good health is your birthright and if you do not presently enjoy it, there is no better time than the present to set that aright.

1
SACRED PRACTICES OF ANCIENT ANCESTORS AND CONTEMPORARY HUNTER-GATHERERS

The history and evolution of the human diet is a subject rife with opinion and conjecture. Be that as it may, evidence exists, and anthropologists are generally in rough accord about, what our ancestors ate, if not precisely when they ate what. A consensus also exists about the fact that people who eat a traditional diet today—one similar to an ancestral diet—generally enjoy the same good health that their forebears did. An examination of the evidence, inferences, and conclusions of anthropologists and medical researchers sheds light on why contemporary cultures that follow a traditional diet tend to enjoy excellent health.

THE INTIMATE CONNECTION BETWEEN DIET AND DISEASE

Controversy surrounds the story of the evolution of early humans. What is clear, though, is that the diet of *all* humans contained substantial amounts of meat and other animal foods until roughly ten thousand years ago.

Whatever our beginnings, the agricultural revolution—the cultivation of plants and the domestication of animals—of the past ten thousand years is thought to have had little effect upon our genes. One exception is that, in some parts of the world, people have evolved the ability to digest milk as adults. As regards more recent trends (masses of people leaving the countryside to live in cities; the development of modern commercial agriculture; the refinement of much of our food), not enough time has elapsed for the effects of these trends to cause changes in our genes. Thus we are genetically equipped to eat foods our hunter-fisher-gatherer ancestors ate: the preagricultural-revolution diet.

Many of us are descendants of ancestors who settled into agricultural life less than two thousand years ago; for others, their agricultural roots go back some fifteen thousand years. Agriculture markedly affected human diets, with a shift to more vegetable foods (grains especially) and a decline in animal consumption (particularly wild animals). The effect on the size of humans was profound: European big-game hunters of thirty thousand years ago were an average of six inches taller than their farmer descendants. A similar change occurred in the Americas among Indians shifting to a more agricultural way of life in the period just before the Europeans arrived.

Over the past two hundred years, the larger amounts of animal-sourced foods in Western diets have resulted in an increase in average human height, so that we are now almost as tall as our big-game-hunting ancestors. Today, diseases that plagued neither the hunter-gatherers nor the agriculturalists have become major health problems. As mentioned in the introduction, writing in the January 31, 1985, issue of the *New England Journal of Medicine* under the title "Paleolithic Nutrition," S. Boyd Eaton, M.D. and Melvin Konner, Ph.D. reported that heart disease, high blood pressure, diabetes, chronic intestinal disease, and most types of cancer have been reported by medical authorities to be virtually unknown in hunter-gatherer cultures surviving today. Those cultures include the Hadza of Tanzania, the !Kung and Kade San (Bushmen) of the Kalahari, the Philippine Tasaday, the Aché of Paraguay, the Australian Aborigines of Arnhem Land, and the Arctic aboriginal Eskimos, among others.

The publication of this information in this particular professional journal, long a bastion of conservative medical opinion, was an important milestone. For many years other medical journals and professional publications had carried articles linking diet, health, and specific diseases, yet the U.S. medical establishment has steadfastly ignored the evidence. With the appearance of "Paleolithic Nutrition" and related articles in the *New England Journal of Medicine*, more American physicians became aware of the intimate connection between diet and disease.

It has been noted by the medical community that chronic diseases in America around the turn of this century were relatively rare. Paul Dudley White, who was President Dwight D. Eisenhower's personal physician during the years the former president suffered his two heart attacks, wrote in 1943 in his textbook, *Heart Disease*: "When I graduated from medical school in 1911, I had never heard of coronary thrombosis, which is one of the chief threats to life in the United States and Canada today. . . . It is now responsible for more than 50 percent of all deaths."

The refinement of grains; the production and consumption of excessive amounts of sugar, white flour, industrial vegetable oils, and alcohol; confinement farming; and the decline in the quality of food from both plant and animal sources are the major causes for the emergence of chronic disease as a major threat. Around 1900, new methods of milling flour were introduced that completely stripped out the very perishable wheat germ from the grain. By 1910, these methods were in general use, and as a result, many people lost their major source of vitamin E and an important source of other nutrients, including the B vitamins and several minerals. Trends since then have been toward the use of refined foods and more refined foods. Confinement animals have been injected with chemicals, drugs, and hormones, as the mechanization of agriculture has transformed them into meat, milk, and egg machines.

We turn now to evidence pertaining to the appearance of species that may have been ancestors of the human species, and to preagricultural humans who roamed the earth as hunter-gatherers for hundreds of thousands of years before the agricultural revolution began to end their way of life.

THE DIETS OF EARLY MAN AND CONTEMPORARY HUNTER-GATHERERS

Early relatives of humans lived in trees probably more than five million years ago, eating fruit, eggs, and nestlings. Changing climatic patterns in Africa near the equator are thought to have driven these creatures down from the trees in times of drought to forage for food in grasslands. Certain relatives of early humans, classified in the genus *Homo*, and other creatures of the genus *Australopithecus*, appear in the fossil records of two to nearly four million years ago.

Australopithecines were similar to our ancestors in many ways; both are thought to have descended from the same ancestral line, and both walked with feet nearly identical to those of modern humans. Though the head has undergone drastic changes, particularly in the size of the brain, they walked upright. We know this from the position of the foramen magnum, the hole in the base of the skull through which the spinal cord passes en route to the brain.

Australopithecus was first named by anatomist Raymond Dart when skeletal remains of the creature were discovered in 1924. For many years, it was thought to be the direct ancestor of humans. Recent discoveries, however, indicated *Australopithecus* was a vegetarian cousin of the genus *Homo*, the line believed to lead to modern humans. The jaw and teeth are heavier, more suited to chewing and grinding roots. The teeth of *Homo* species of the same period are smaller and lighter, more suited for tearing and chewing meat. While *Homo* developed, *Australopithecines* became extinct between five hundred thousand and one million years ago.

Almost two million years ago, *Homo erectus* appeared; it was believed to be the first human. Meat consumption increased during this time, as evidenced by the animal bones that litter the caves that *Homo erectus* inhabited. Additionally, they had tools for hunting and cleaning animals, and they lived in areas well populated with large game. These people spread far from central Africa, where they most likely had originated. A classic find of this species is Peking man, who lived approximately four hundred thousand years ago and was the first to use fire.

Further changes led to Neanderthal man, considered the first of the *Homo sapiens* (*Homo sapiens neanderthalensis*). These people ate a diet estimated to have been perhaps 50 percent meat. But as Cro-Magnon man and other modern humans (*Homo sapiens sapiens*) appeared, they improved their weapons and communications skills, and groups became more efficient at hunting big game. Meat assumed an even more dominant role in human nutrition.

This trend was reversed in the period shortly before the beginnings of agriculture. Need for fresh hunting grounds had spread humanity all over the globe, and by the eve of the agricultural revolution we numbered some three million people. Together with changes in animal populations and climate, this human population growth may be the reason why hunting large animals became less important for many cultures. Fish, shellfish, and small game assumed increasing importance, and a new pattern emerged. Tools for processing plant foods became more common at this time (some ten to twenty thousand years ago). Trace-mineral analysis of strontium levels in bones has shown vegetable consumption increasing as meat consumption was decreasing.

A mixed diet was typical of the estimated three hundred thousand contemporary hunter-fisher-gatherers who survived into the 1970s. Animal food was estimated to constitute, by weight, an average of 35 percent of the diet of several cultures studied. A similar range was found among cultures that Weston Price studied, though some used even more animal-sourced food much of the year.

THE SANCTITY OF FOOD TO
INDIGENOUS PEOPLE

The diet of the Australian Aborigines today is in many ways typical of both ancient and contemporary hunter-gatherers. Thought to be the oldest surviving culture on Earth, the Aborigines depend on plants, seeds, small reptiles, mammals, insects, fish, and birds. Although men spend much time hunting for larger animals, overall their diet is 70 to 80 percent vegetarian.

In Robert Lawlor's book, *Voices of the First Day,* the author discusses the spiritual aspects of food in Aboriginal life.

> For the Aborigines, eating is a sacred act; it represents humanity's deepest communication and kinship with the life-giving forces of the earth. . . . Hunting and gathering are considered the basis of developing the physical and spiritual potential of human nature. The great hunt is the means by which the spiritual powers of the earth and sky educate humanity. Animals and plants nourish the body, and the process of hunting, foraging, and preparing imparts dexterity, physical skills, and intellectual and spiritual knowledge. (p. 302)

I find this concept of "sacred food" fascinating, and it's interesting to note that half of aboriginal society—the men—spends its time securing 10 to 20 percent of the calories in the form of meat. Why? Though this is controversial, their culture has been said to be egalitarian—men and women function as equals in theory and in practice. Lawlor writes that "the natural male-female complementarity forms the basic unit of Aboriginal society. . . . Men and women as a group decide the clan's food-gathering strategy for the day, depending on weather conditions, locality, and the direction of their wanderings." Apparently they believe that meat is of sufficient importance that its procurement is worth a highly disproportionate amount of effort.

Native Americans also had a concept of "sacred food." In *Of Wolves and Men* Barry Hoistun Lopez writes that sacred food is "earned" by hunting in a very specific way, and it nourishes the soul along with the body. Without this kind of food, the body merely survives and the spirit suffers. Hunting tribes called meat "medicine" (and in the Pacific Northwest, salmon assumed this central role in the culture). This meant that it was sacred because it came from a sacred ceremony—the hunt and its aftermath (just as in the Aboriginal tribes). It also meant that the meat contained the power of the plants (that the animal had eaten) to cure and to soothe. This was one reason why Native Americans did not eat wolf meat: wolves primarily ate meat, not plants. Nor did Native Americans wish to eat cattle once the white man came—it was not sacred to hunt cattle.

It's clear that in these and other native cultures, the connection between food (particularly mammals and fish) and well-being was at least as much a spiritual connection as a physical one. The capture of wild animals, together with the procurement of plant foods, was at the very heart of the spiritual and physical lives of the people.

Lawlor also noted that "The spiritual dimension is also respected in cooking and food preparation."

Ideally, an animal is cooked and eaten as close as possible to the place where it was killed; all things, including food, are more sacred by virtue of being in place. When a kangaroo or other large animal is roasted whole on an open fire, it is first exposed to roaring flames for ten minutes, during which time the spirit of the animal escapes to the metaphysical abode of its species. After the initial roasting the carcass of the animal is removed from the fire, its fur is scraped off, and its intestines removed with a sharp stone. It is then returned to a bed of hot coals and cooked on each side for twenty minutes. The warm, partly cooked blood is thought to have magic properties; the men drink it in a post-hunt ritual and rub it on their spears for continued accuracy. . . . Other cooking methods, such as baking in ashes, steaming in ground ovens, or boiling in seawater and tortoise shells, all have ritual and Dreamtime connotations. (p. 310)

It is noteworthy that the meat was cooked. Clearly, a modern primal diet that reflects ancestral ways need not be entirely raw.

In the Kalahari Desert of Botswana, about two hundred members of a contemporary hunter-gatherer tribe, the !Kung, still carry on their ancient way of life. Like all remaining hunter-gatherers, they occupy a marginal area that modern civilization has not yet claimed. They have existed there for at least ten thousand years.

The !Kung are one of the groups that medical teams studied before concluding that contemporary hunter-gatherers do not develop the diseases of modern civilization. According to these studies, about 10 percent of the !Kung were more than sixty years old—approximately the same percentage found in contemporary populations that have been studied. They live quite a leisurely life. Men hunt two or three days a week, and women spend an equal amount of time gathering plant foods, which constitute about two-thirds of the diet. Much time is spent socializing, visiting, sharing food, and teaching children. Some anthropologists have called hunter-gatherers the original affluent societies; many definitely do not lead the hard and short lives of popular conception.

Richard Leakey writes in *Origins,* his excellent account of human evolution, that the sharing of food formed the strongest of bonds among early hunter-gatherers living in small groups. Many anthropologists believe this socialization led distinctly to our development into complex social beings. The sharing of meat—and for coastal peoples, fish—specifically formed social bonds around which the physical, social, and spiritual lives of early humans revolved, and helped make possible our subsequent evolution. Vegetarian cousins of early humans, the *Australopithecines,* were solitary feeders who did not share food with companions; they became extinct.

Among the !Kung, Leakey writes that the killing and sharing of meat is surrounded by great excitement and a sense of mysticism.

Customs dictate how and with whom animals will be shared (this is true in Aborigine tribes as well). The communal feasting is done with a great deal of fanfare and ritual that is not attendant to the sharing of plant foods. Leakey offers no explanation why meat rather than some other food is the center of such ceremony and holds such importance.

Consideration of historical evidence and recent research reviewed earlier suggests meat and fish were placed on a pedestal simply because native people everywhere recognized how essential animal food was in the diet. These foods were elevated to the status of "sacred" foods, with essential spiritual connotations. In coastal cultures fish was central; later, in some nomadic and agricultural societies, dairy products came to the fore. Hunter-gatherer societies were marvelously efficient. If they hadn't been, early prehumans wouldn't have proceeded to three million subsequent years of evolution.

The traditions, rituals, and mysticism of the !Kung surrounding the capture, sharing, and eating of meat are logical. Wild game might supply only one-third of the bulk of their food, but they recognized it as essential and behaved accordingly.

Analysis of some of these hunter-gatherer diets shows an average fiber content of forty-six grams, which is eight to ten times that found in the modern diet. The calcium content of sixteen hundred milligrams in the ancient diet is at least twice as great as is found in the modern diet. This figure is calculated from plant foods and animal flesh consumed, and does not reflect bones that have been ground up or cooked. Trace-mineral content in the ancient diet was high.

The composition of fats in a hunter-fisher-gatherer diet is different from that of fats eaten by most people today. As we'll see in later chapters, the fatty acids in vegetable oil are precursors of different prostaglandins than those that are derived from the fatty acids of free-ranging animals and in saltwater fish; evidence clearly indicates the latter fatty acids are inadequately supplied in the modern diet. Primitive diets are low in the fatty acids derived from today's vegetable oils, but high in those richly supplied in fish oils and in meat.

IMPLICATIONS FOR POST-AGRICULTURAL-REVOLUTION DIETS

These analyses of ancestral and contemporary native diets present a comparison of primal and modern foods. Whether weighted more toward plant foods or more toward game and fish, ancestral diets included more fiber, less vegetable oil, and more fat-soluble vitamins and minerals than modern diets do.

After the agricultural revolution, diets changed considerably, but many elements of hunter-gatherer diets stayed the same until recently. Fresh meat from free-ranging domestic animals, rich in saturated fats, was a staple that was used regularly almost everywhere. This meat has certain qualities of wild game. Raw milk and dairy products from these free-ranging animals are similarly rich in saturated fats; they too were regularly used until recently. Fish remained a staple for coastal and river people. Fresh raw vegetables and fruits remained a staple for rural people everywhere, as did whole grains (before modern milling techniques were employed).

Agricultural cultures ate these foods for thousands of years; their people were healthy and largely resistant to the diseases that are prevalent today. Whether one ate more like the hunter-fisher-gatherer or more like the agriculturist, a wide spectrum of healthy foods was available—the cornerstone to building healthy bodies.

If we are to look to our ancestral heritage for answers to our modern ills, we need to introduce an element of the mystical into our discussions of nutrition and disease. Can consuming organic vegetables and free-range domestic meat, organ meats, whole grains, seafood, vitamin supplements, and the purest water fully nourish us if we fail to maintain the spiritual connection between the earth and ourselves, which our ancestors placed at the core of their existence?

I think not. Ancestral wisdom tells us that feeding the soul is quite literally as important as feeding the body. As we learn how our ancestors fed their bodies, I believe we must pay equal attention to how they fed their souls. And if the few remaining native cultures are to survive—and I believe their survival is important not only for them but for everyone on the planet—we must work together to find ways to fully protect these indigenous people. They need space, they need their native habitats left intact, and they need to be left alone.

In the next chapter, which details the groundbreaking work of Dr. Weston Price, we will learn more about these native cultures so that we can better understand how we may apply the precepts that they live by to our own lives today.

2
DR. WESTON PRICE
AND HIS STUDIES OF
TRADITIONAL SOCIETIES

The name Weston Price has become more familiar in recent years, but is still not widely known. This is ironic in a world that is now—more than ever before—so much in need of the wisdom and knowledge he discovered before his death in 1948. It is heartening that *Nutritional and Physical Degeneration,* the text of his most important work, is widely available in bookstores and online.

Controversy surrounded the book when it was first published in 1939. Dr. Price was a dentist, and many in his profession viewed his work as profound and significant. So too did many anthropologists; for years, the book was required reading for Dr. Ernst Hooton's anthropology classes at Harvard University. But the majority of professionals ignored it, and some attacked it. Among the public, there was some enthusiastic acceptance, but the book is long and not an easy read. Not written with an eye to the public, it never became widely read. Nevertheless, it remains a classic. Let's take a closer look at Dr. Price's seminal work now.

DR. PRICE'S UNIQUE FINDINGS

Weston Price was born in Ontario in 1870 and raised on a farm. After receiving a degree in dentistry in 1893 and moving to the United States, he began practicing his profession and performing research. His many published articles brought him recognition, and his textbooks on the dangerous effects of root canals became world renowned (if little heeded).

During his years in dental practice, in the children of some of his patients, Dr. Price began noticing problems that the parents hadn't experienced. In addition to exhibiting more decay, the teeth of many children didn't fit properly into the dental arch and were, as a result, crowded and crooked. Price suspected that nutritional deficiencies were responsible for this. He also noticed that the condition of the teeth reflected the child's overall health, which further confirmed his suspicion. Anthropologists had long observed and written about the excellent teeth found in people of primitive cultures. While others in his profession continued looking for external causative factors in dental decay, Price decided to turn his attention to primitive people, and searched for a nutritional factor that might be protecting them from similar dental degradation.

His discoveries may genuinely surprise you. He found entire cultures that had no tooth decay. Nor did he find anyone with misshapen dental arches or crowded teeth. He interviewed an American medical doctor living among Eskimos and northern Indians who reported that in thirty-five years of observation, he had never seen a single case of cancer among the natives who subsisted on their traditional foods. When natives eating white man's foods developed tuberculosis, this doctor eventually took to sending them back to their villages where they resumed their native diet. Typically, they recovered. In every culture where the people were immune to dental and degenerative disease, biochemical analysis showed the diet to be rich in nutrients that were poorly supplied in modern diets.

Throughout the world in the 1930s, groups in the early stages of modernization were using foods imported from Western countries— sugar, white flour, canned foods, and condensed milk. Price visited and studied cultures where people following traditional ways and diets lived near kinsmen who were eating these foods of modern civilization.

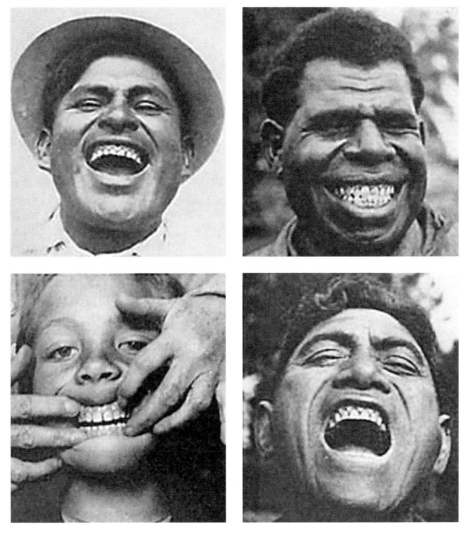

Figure 1.1. These photographs, typical of those taken throughout the world by Dr. Weston Price, are of native people living on traditional foods. Uniformly broad dental arches were found—with all thirty-two teeth present, little or no decay, and no crowding of teeth. (The photographs in this chapter were taken by Weston Price in the 1930s; most appear in his book *Nutrition and Physical Degeneration*. These prints were made by Marcus Halevi and appear here courtesy of the Price-Pottenger Nutrition Foundation.)

Upper left: Peruvian coastal fisherman

Upper right: Great Barrier Reef (Torres Strait) fisherman

Lower left: Swiss girl (Loetschental Valley)

Lower right: New Zealand Maori fisherman

His travels took him to the corners of the earth. He and his wife, Florence Price, R.N., lived with the Swiss in high alpine valleys; Gaels on islands of the Outer Hebrides; Eskimos in Alaska; Indians in the far northern, western, and central parts of Canada, and in the western United States and Florida; Melanesians and Polynesians in the southern Pacific; Africans in eastern and central Africa; Aborigines in Australia; Malay tribes on islands north of Australia; Maori in New Zealand; and descendants of ancient civilizations in Peru.

Skeletal remains of ancient people were studied by Price wherever they were available. He also studied dental health, keeping detailed records that included thousands of photographs. He analyzed native and modern foods for their calorie, mineral, and vitamin content, and he made extensive studies of the effects of different foods on the chemistry of saliva and its relation to dental decay. Scores of his articles were published, including a series in the *Journal of the American Dental Association*. He examined the general health of his subjects, and whenever possible, he interviewed medical personnel caring for the people he studied.

Dr. Price's observations were not limited to health and diet, for he sought to understand the nature and character of these thousands of people he encountered. He came to know many of them well, and his insights reveal the strength of character of many of them, a trait he found typical in native cultures. This chapter chronologically tours Weston Price's search for health among indigenous cultures all over the world.

EUROPE (1931)

The Swiss of the Loetschental Valley

The Loetschental Valley, nearly a mile above sea level in an isolated part of the Swiss Alps, had been for more than a dozen centuries the home of some two thousand people when the Prices first visited in 1931. The people lived in a series of small villages along a river that wound its way along the valley floor. The completion of an eleven-mile tunnel shortly before the Prices' visit had made the valley easily accessible for the first time.

The people lived as their forebears had. Wooden buildings, some centuries old, dotted the landscape, with mottoes expressive of spiritual values artistically carved in the timbers. Snowcapped mountains nearly enclosed the valley, making it relatively easy to defend. Though many attempts had been made, the people had never been conquered.

There was no physician, dentist, policeman, or jail. Sheep provided wool for homespun clothes, and the valley produced nearly everything needed for food.

Their crops, many of them on steep hillsides rising from the river, produced winter's hay for the cattle, and rye for the people. Most households kept goats and cows; the animals grazed in the summer on glacial slopes. Cheese and butter were made from fresh summer milk for use all year, and garden greens were grown in summer. Whole rye bread, made in large stone community baking ovens, was a staple all year, as was milk. Most families ate meat once a week, usually on Sunday when an animal was slaughtered. Bones and scraps were used to make soups that were eaten during the week.

Price examined the teeth of all the children in the valley between the ages of seven and sixteen. Those still eating the primitive diet were nearly free of cavities. On the average, one tooth showing evidence of decay was found for every three children seen.

Many young people examined had experienced a period of rampant tooth decay that suddenly ceased, often having first lost teeth. All the individuals who exhibited evidence of tooth decay had left the valley prior to this period and had spent a year or two in some city. Most had never had a decayed tooth before or since.

Tuberculosis at this time took more lives in Switzerland than any other disease. Yet Swiss government officials reported that a recent inspection of the valley hadn't revealed a single case of it. Astonishingly, a thorough study of records of death certificates demonstrated clearly that no deaths had occurred from tuberculosis in the history of the valley. This is evidence of profound natural forces at work.

Upon returning to America, Price had samples of the dairy products from this valley sent to him twice a month throughout the year. A pioneer in developing methods for measuring fat-soluble vitamins in foods in the early 1920s, he had written extensively on the subject and was a recognized authority on it. His analyses found these dairy-product samples higher in minerals and vitamins—particularly the fat-soluble D complex vitamins—than samples of commercial dairy products from the rest of Europe and North America.

The vitamin D complex helps regulate the utilization of calcium and other minerals. Price believed that the D complex and another unidentified nutrient he called "activator X" played crucial roles in the excellent general health, immunity to dental disease, and splendid physical development of the people of the Loetschental Valley. The quality of their food was apparently responsible for the presence of rich amounts of these nutrients.

The Swiss people Price studied recognized the crucial importance of their food. The clergymen told how they thanked God for the life-giving qualities of butter and cheese made in June when the cows ate grass near the snow line; their worship included lighting a wick in a bowl of the first butter made after the cows reached this summer pasturage. Price's analyses showed butter made then was highest in fat-soluble vitamins and minerals.

This late spring butter obviously had a special place in the culture; it was, in a sense, considered a sacred food. Weston Price tested more than ten thousand samples of butter and cheese over the course of many years. Consistently he found the content of fat-soluble vitamins was highest during the months when grass grew most rapidly. For much of North America, there are two such periods, one in late spring and the other in late summer. In more northern areas, the two periods occur more closely together than in southern areas, around midsummer. But for every area, Price's graph of the fat-soluble vitamin content of the dairy products of the area (plotted against the time of year) echoed a graph of that area's rate of plant growth (plotted against the time of year). I believe it is no coincidence that this butter contained the same fat-soluble nutrients, from an animal source, that were found in other sacred foods in other traditional and native hunter-gatherer cultures.

Statistics for mortality from heart disease and pneumonia for all districts in the United States and Canada were then plotted. Price found the rise and fall in mortality from these two diseases followed regular yearly cycles in each section of the country. These cycles were exactly opposite the curve for the vitamin content of the dairy products and the curve for the rate of plant growth for that section of the country. In more northern districts, where the twin peaks of the vitamin curve (and also the twin peaks of the plant-growth curve) tended to blend together into one midsummer peak, mortality rates tended to bottom in midsummer. In more southern districts, where distinct peaks occurred (one for late spring and one for late summer) in both vitamin and plant-growth curves, there were two low points on the mortality curve—one in late spring and one in late summer.

Price analyzed the incidence of children's diseases in Ontario, including chicken pox, measles, nephritis, and scarlet fever. For each disease, a graph of the number of cases was opposite the graph of vitamin levels in the dairy products of Ontario (both graphs were plotted against the time of year).

This is evidence of a direct relation between the quality of foods and the incidence of illness and death. All life depends upon the sun. Is it strange that the green life springing from the sun's rays, the fresh greens making higher life-forms possible, should prove so vital?

Spiritual values dominated life in this Swiss valley at this moment in time. Part of the national holiday celebration each August was a song expressing the feeling of "one for all and all for one." Price wrote: "One wonders if there is not something in the life-giving vitamins and minerals of the food that builds not only great physical structures within which their souls reside, but builds minds and hearts capable of a higher type of manhood in which the material values of life are made secondary to individual character."

He found other evidence of this throughout the world.

Health conditions in the Loetschental Valley were in stark contrast with those in the lower valleys and plains country in Switzerland—modernized areas where rampant dental decay, misshapen dental arches with crowding of the teeth, and a high incidence of tuberculosis and other chronic health problems were the norm. The people of the valley were clearly protected by the quality of their native foods.

Although few of the other traditional groups Price studied consumed dairy products (those who did were certain African tribes, including the Masai), raw, whole milk (both fresh and cultured), cheese, and butter were used in large amounts by the people of the Loetschental Valley. This milk, from healthy, well-exercised animals, was unpasteurized and unhomogenized. Such foods may play a major role in a health-building diet for people genetically able to utilize them well. For the people of the Loetschental, their milk products provided fat-soluble nutrients and minerals essential to maintaining optimal health.

Gaels on the Islands of the Outer Hebrides

The Isle of Lewis and the Isle of Harris, visited by Price after leaving Switzerland, are the chief of these islands off the northwest coast of Scotland. When Price and his wife visited them, they were isolated, and inaccessible much of the year because of constant rough seas. Most islanders lived traditionally, working at fishing, sheep-raising, and farming.

Fish was abundant, and many men went to sea daily. Cod, lobster, crab, oysters, and clams were readily available. Oat grain was the only cereal that grew well and was a staple. The islands were covered with peat, providing poor farmland and pasturage, and consequently people rarely kept dairy animals. Milk was practically unknown; so too were fruits.

Modern foods—white bread, jam, marmalade, canned vegetables, vegetable oil, sugar, syrup, chocolate, and coffee—were available for purchase in shipping ports. Together with some fish, these foods formed the diet of many people in the port towns. Their health was in stark contrast with that of the rest of the population. Children living on seafood, oats, and in summer, vegetables in primitive areas showed less than one tooth out of 100 with any decay. Tuberculosis, cancer, arthritis, and other degenerative diseases were unknown to them.

Children eating modern foods in the several shipping ports, on the other hand, showed an average incidence of 16.3 to more than 50 decayed teeth per 100 examined; even three-year-olds had decay. Tuberculosis was a great problem—some populations had been decimated by it. Wherever Price investigated, afflicted individuals had been eating modern foods. The authorities blamed tuberculosis on the fireplace smoke in the thatched-roof houses that for centuries had been the people's homes. Yet, former generations had been free of tuberculosis. Only the diet had changed.

Whole grains—rye in the Loetschental, oats in the Outer Hebrides—formed major parts of these traditional European diets. Grains were also important to the few African tribes Price studied. Everywhere else, fish, animals, and vegetables formed the bulk of traditional diets, and grains played little or no role.

Seafood was the other staple in the Outer Hebrides. Fish organs (especially the liver), fish eggs, the head, and the bones were all consumed. A dish considered especially important for children was made from the head and liver of codfish. Since there were no dairy foods, bones used in soups were important because of the calcium and other minerals they contained.

Fish, especially the liver, is a rich source of the vitamin D complex and other fat-soluble nutrients that were supplied primarily by butter, cheese, and milk in the Loetschental Valley. In every culture that Price found free of dental and degenerative disease, a rich source of these fat-soluble nutrients formed a substantial part of the diet—and it is precisely these nutrients that are strikingly deficient in the diet of most modern people.

NORTH AMERICA (1933)

Eskimos of Alaska and Northern Canada

A simple yet stirring story of primitive Eskimos tells of a time when food ran short during the long winter night north of the Arctic Circle, when for months there is no daylight. An Eskimo man takes to stormy seas in a kayak to hunt seal with a harpoon. In darkness, bitter cold, high winds, and rough seas, he searches the dark waters for food. A wave crashing over a kayak can snap even a strong man's back; as breakers approach, the kayaker rolls the vessel, submerging himself. The tight fit of sealskins between the upper edge of the kayak and his waist keeps water from entering. When the white water passes, he flips upright and continues the hunt, finally killing a seal and returning home with food for his family.

As impressive as Weston Price found the physical strength of primitive Eskimos in Alaska and northern Canada, even more impressive was their character—their courage, honesty, and openness, dedication to family and community, and ability to survive and thrive in the harsh northern environment. In village after village, among Eskimos living entirely on the native diet, Price found virtually no decayed teeth and no evidence of chronic disease. Among those partially subsisting on refined foods, decay and disease increased in direct proportion to the amount of refined food eaten.

The plight of the natives' modernized brethren was bleak. With no medical help to alleviate their suffering in the years immediately following the introduction of refined foods, many had been driven by the pain and misery of progressive tooth decay to take their own lives. In many small native settlements where the white man's food was available, some, however, refused it, subsisting entirely on the primitive diet. No evidence of decay or signs of chronic disease were found in them. Their fellow villagers, living the same life except for the fact that they consumed refined foods, had extensive decay, and some had tuberculosis. Among those who had eaten modern foods for several years, some also had arthritis.

In children born of parents who consumed refined foods, the majority had crowding and malocclusion of teeth because the dental arches were too narrow to accommodate the teeth properly. Several of Price's photographs contained in this chapter illustrate such changes. In contrast is the breadth of the dental arches and the perfect fit of the teeth shown in figures 1.1, 1.2, and 1.5; these Eskimos and other primitives exhibit nature's normal dental development, found wherever people subsisted entirely on native traditional foods.

This hereditary pattern, normally passed on from generation to generation in accordance with nature's laws, had been disrupted by the introduction of refined foods. Problems seen in the children of Price's patients in the United States were, for the first time, appearing in primitive cultures. "Intercepted heredity" was the term Price used for this: the hereditary pattern of perfect dental form, seen clearly in thousands of his photographs, had been intercepted by poor nutrition.

Observation reveals that most people today have crowded teeth; a small minority has the broad dental arches and perfectly fitting teeth that are normal in primitive cultures. And while most people today have the four wisdom teeth (the third molars) removed because of crowding, traditional people nearly always had room for all thirty-two teeth.

Traditional wisdom enabled successive generations to reproduce nature's perfect pattern. This wisdom in every culture prescribed specific kinds and quantities of foods known to ensure fertility, the birth of healthy babies, and the optimal development of growing children.

In terms of food consumed by the Eskimo cultures that Price visited, the diet, mostly fish and wild animals, was rich in animal fats. Salmon was important. Most primitive Eskimos had homes near deep water, making salmon relatively accessible from the sea. Much of it was dried and then smoked for winter use. When eaten, the fish was dipped in seal oil, rich in vitamin A and also used to preserve sorrel grass and flower blossoms.

Salmon eggs were dried raw and used in quantity; they constituted a source of great nutrition for small children after weaning. Rich in iodine, they were used by women of childbearing age to ensure fertility. The milt of male salmon were eaten by men for the same purpose; this too was eaten raw. Other foods in the Eskimo diet included caribou, especially the organs; kelp, gathered in season and stored for winter; the organs of large sea mammals; and certain layers of the skin of one whale species (analysis showed this was very high in vitamin C). Wild plants and berries were gathered in the summer and stored.

Indians of North America

Great areas of northern British Columbia and the Yukon Territory were still inhabited by Indians in the 1930s when Price visited these places. He went also to reservations in Canada, where Indians lived under more modernized conditions, consuming modern foods, and to Florida to study present-day Seminoles and the remains of pre-Columbian Indians.

Indians living in the Rocky Mountain range in the far north of Canada were unable to obtain any seafood, not even migrating salmon. Winter temperatures of seventy degrees below zero precluded the possibility of growing cereal grains or fruits or of keeping dairy animals. The diet of these Indians was thus almost entirely limited to wild animals.

One old Indian was asked through an interpreter why Indians did not get scurvy. He replied that scurvy was a white man's disease. Although it was not outside the realm of possibility that an Indian might contract scurvy, the Indians knew how to prevent it and white men did not. When asked why he did not tell white men how to prevent it, he replied that white men knew too much to ask the Indians anything. When asked how it *could* be prevented, the Indian replied that he must go to his chief for permission to divulge the secret. Upon returning—with permission—he explained that when an Indian kills a moose, he opens it up and finds a small ball in the fat above each kidney. He cuts these balls—the adrenal glands—into pieces that are immediately eaten, one by each person in the family.

We now know that the adrenal glands are among the richest sources of vitamin C in all animal or plant tissues. Cooking destroys vitamin C. The Indians' empirical knowledge and use of different organs and tissues of animals has certainly been verified by modern methods of analysis. Their wisdom preceded the discovery of vitamin C by thousands of years.

Such wisdom is again demonstrated in a story of a white man running out of supplies while crossing a high plateau in the far north country just before the fall freeze-up. A doctor of engineering and science, he was forced to march out of the wilderness when his prospecting plans went awry. While crossing the plateau, he went almost blind with a violent pain in his eyes that persisted for days. He nearly ran into a grizzly one day; an old Indian tracking the bear recognized the white man's plight.

The Indian led him to a nearby stream, and with a trap of stones, caught some trout. Throwing the fish on the bank, he told the prospector to eat the flesh of the head and the tissues behind the eyes. In a few hours the man's pain was largely gone. In a day his sight was returning, and in two, it was close to normal. He had been suffering from xerophthalmia, due to vitamin A deficiency.

The fatty tissue around the eyes is one of the richest sources of vitamin A in any animal's body.

For nine months of the year, the nutrition of these northern Indians was mostly wild game, chiefly moose and caribou. Emphasis was placed on eating organs, including the wall of parts of the digestive tract, which are rich in vitamin D. Some meat and organs were eaten raw; much muscle meat was fed to dogs. Bone marrow was consumed, especially by children. Plants were consumed in summer, and some bark and buds of trees in winter.

The thyroid glands of the male moose, greatly enlarged during the fall mating season, were eaten liberally by men and women in moose country near the Arctic Circle. The Indians said this caused a large percentage of children to be born in June, the best time to bring infants into the harsh northern environment. A known, direct relationship exists between thyroid gland activity and fertility.

The teeth of several primitive groups that Price examined showed no indication of decay. In these and other groups, a total of eighty-seven Indians living on the native diet were examined; only four teeth ever affected by decay were found. As well, there were almost no irregular teeth and no impacted third molars found. Inquiries were made about tuberculosis and arthritis; not a single case was seen or heard of among isolated groups.

However, many crippling cases of rheumatoid arthritis were seen at the point of contact with refined foods, and tuberculosis was taking a severe toll. Tooth decay was rampant, and crooked teeth with deformed dental arches were typical.

Josef Romig, a surgeon known then as the most beloved man in Alaska, was interviewed by Price at the government hospital in 1933. Dr. Romig had served primitive and modernized Eskimos and Indians for thirty-six years. He stated that cancer was unknown among truly primitive natives. He had never seen a case, though when the Eskimos and Indians began eating refined foods, it frequently occurred. Other acute medical problems requiring surgery, common among modernized Eskimos and Indians, were similarly rare among primitives.

Such experiences led Romig to begin sending modernized natives afflicted with tuberculosis back, when possible, to native conditions and a native diet. Though the disease was generally progressive and eventually fatal when patients remained on refined foods, he found that a great majority of them recovered when they reverted to a traditional diet.

During those years, a physician in Los Angeles with a keen interest in nutrition was using a strikingly similar diet in treating patients with tuberculosis and other chronic diseases. This physician, Francis M. Pottenger, Jr., would soon conduct and publish studies validating the use of a diet rich in high-quality animal-sourced foods, especially raw and lightly cooked organs. (Pottenger's investigations into the effects of cooking upon foods and his discoveries about the role of animal foods in healing chronic diseases will be presented in chapter 5.)

Price also interviewed the physician directing the hospital on Canada's largest Indian reservation in Brantford, Ontario. The doctor explained that during his twenty-eight years there, the services that the hospital offered had changed completely. He had had contact with three generations of Indian mothers. The grandmothers of the current generation had given birth without difficulty in wilderness homes, but current mothers often were in labor for days, and surgical interference was frequently necessary. As a result, the main function of the hospital had changed to address problems related to problems associated with maternity. All reservation Indians ate refined foods.

Seminole Indians in Florida were studied and comparisons were made with skeletal material from pre-Columbian Indians in museums. Some Seminoles still lived in relative isolation in the Everglades and in cypress swamps; others lived near communities consuming modern foods along the Tamiami Trail and near Miami.

Several hundred pre-Columbian skulls from burial mounds in southern Florida were examined; not one decayed tooth or a single dental-arch deformity resulting in crowded or crooked teeth was found. A comparison of the skulls' thickness with that of recent skulls showed the older skulls were much thicker, providing further evidence of superior physical development in the native culture. Pre-Columbian skeletons showed no evidence of arthritic joint involvement; many Indians eating modern foods had bony deformities derived from rheumatoid arthritis, along with tooth decay.

The original inhabitants of North America had great wisdom about utilizing foods native to the land. Most Indian cultures ate quantities of superior quality animals and seafood to maintain resistance to disease, great physical strength, and normal reproduction. As with the Eskimos, this often was accomplished on diets of mostly fish and wild animals, supplemented by plant foods.

Native Americans and other native cultures throughout the world had detailed information about using specific parts of animals and the unique importance of each part. Many sources also indicate a vast knowledge of the medicinal uses of herbs. The development of these cultures was not simply a matter of people randomly eating whatever was available. Rather, cultures passed on the accumulated wisdom of the group to the next generation. This wisdom was concerned with laws of nature that, when ignored, lead to sickness, death, and the degradation of succeeding generations.

We know not from where this wisdom came. We only know that it has disappeared from the consciousness of the vast majority of people alive today.

Western culture has mobilized the intelligence and resources to send men to the moon, make color televisions, and plumb the atom's depths. Yet, modern people have failed to recognize that the native people who were exterminated knew a great deal about maintaining the biological integrity of the human species. As millions of people continue down a path of disease and suffering, modern medicine obstinately refuses to recognize that the fundamental cause lies in the way most people eat. And the way a person eats is merely a reflection of the way he or she thinks and lives.

THE TROPICS

Melanesia, Polynesia, and Hawaii (1934)

The tropics were of interest to Price because he sought universal factors affecting people everywhere, regardless of climate, race, or environment. Melanesians (on New Caledonia and the Fiji Islands) and Polynesians (on the Hawaiian, Cook, Tongan, and Marquesas Islands, and the Tuamout group, including Tahiti) were visited. Arrangements had been made through government officials, leading everywhere to a cordial reception.

Detailed records on physical development, the condition of every tooth, the shape of the dental arches and face, and kinds of foods eaten were kept for each individual. Special or unusual physical characteristics were photographed. More isolated members of each tribe were compared with those living in the vicinity of the port or landing place of the island.

Government reports revealed exactly what was imported. Nearly always, 90 percent of the total value of imported goods consisted of white flour and sugar. This was true everywhere Price traveled.

The magnificence of the islanders of the South Seas—as reported by early European explorers—is legend. They were a strong, beautiful, and kindly people. The islands had been densely populated. But by the time Price arrived, these populations had been decimated—mostly by tuberculosis, but also by smallpox and measles.

He paints a distressing picture of the majority of the people remaining. Most used little of the seafood staples of their ancestral diets, and in addition to some vegetables and fruits, they ate foods made with white flour and sugar. Decay was found in more than one-third of the teeth examined. Many individuals suffered from tuberculosis, and dental-arch deformities were common in the youth.

Relatively isolated groups were found, though on many islands there were few such groups. The native diet was mostly shellfish and fish, eaten together with land plants, fruits, and sea vegetables, all selected according to a definite program. Much shellfish was eaten, often raw, as were many small fish. Underground ovens of hot stones were used for cooking. Taro root was dried and powdered, then mixed with water and fermented. The incidence of decay was about one tooth in every two hundred examined, and dental arches were uniformly broad, with no crowding of teeth.

Viti Levu, one of the Fiji Islands, is one of the larger islands in the Pacific. Price hoped to find natives in the interior living far enough from the sea to be dependent entirely on land foods. He could not. Everywhere in the interior, piles of seashells were found.

Food from the sea had always been considered essential, his guide told him. Even when at war with coastal tribes, arrangements existed whereby interior tribes sent special plant foods by courier to coastal tribes in exchange for seafood. The couriers were never harmed. Land animals, including pigs, an excellent source of vitamin D, and freshwater fish, supplemented what seafood inland tribes could get. No places were found where seafood was not eaten.

The same physical changes seen in natives eating modern foods in Switzerland, the Outer Hebrides, Alaska, northern Canada, and Florida were seen in the islanders of the South Seas who had abandoned traditional native diets. Similarly, tuberculosis and arthritis had become prevalent.

The isolated groups immune to these problems were largely eating animal-sourced diets, which provided large supplies of fat-soluble vitamins and other nutrients. The source in the South Seas was seafood.

Groups maintaining immunity to dental and chronic disease on diets consisting entirely of vegetable matter had been especially sought by Price but none were found. As his studies progressed, it emerged ever more clearly that healthy, free-ranging animal life of the land and sea provided humans everywhere with essential nutrients apparently unobtainable in adequate quantities from plants.

Many individuals have recovered from diseases on vegetarian diets. Most of these diets have included dairy foods and at least the consumption of occasional fish or poultry in their regimens. When well-balanced, such natural diets are far superior to the diets rich in white flour and sugar that most people consume today. Strictly vegetarian diets that exclude all animal foods (known as vegan diets) often initially result in better health and the alleviation of serious problems.

But the success of vegan diets is usually self-limiting. By avoiding all animal foods and animal fats, nutrients essential for the development of optimal strength, resistance to disease, and reproductive capacity are lacking. Individuals on strictly vegan diets may thrive for several weeks, months, or even years, but in the vast majority of cases, problems—including mental illness—eventually appear.

I recall my first philosophy teacher in naturopathic medical school. Crusty and old-fashioned, the doctor had practiced for many years. Surveying thirty-six rather thin and predominantly vegetarian students on the first day of class, he stated, "Most of you people look like you could use a good steak." Deciphering reality through the smokescreen of preconceptions is never easy. The idea that all natural foods build good health is a common preconception, but behind it lies reality: even when one eats mostly natural food, precisely which foods are emphasized determines the course of health and disease.

AFRICA (1935)

The magnificence of Africa has been partially captured in several films: vast rolling plains; primordial sunsets; thundering herds of wild animals; lilting, billowy clouds of long-necked snow-white birds; lions ripping and tearing at flesh before charging the camera. The Africa that Price visited was very beautiful but, like the other cultures he studied, its beauty had begun to vanish. But the land proved more permanent and less quickly damaged than the inhabitants, and even today much of its beauty remains.

Last to receive the sometimes dubious benefits of modern civilization, the African continent in 1935 contained scores of tribes living according to native ways. Price's travels in Africa covered more than six thousand miles. Thirty tribes were studied and more than twenty-five hundred photographs taken. Price's most indelible impression: the contrast between the rugged resistance of the natives to their harsh environment and the fragility of foreigners.

A racial difference this was not, for when the natives abandoned primitive foods for refined foods, they developed dental decay and became susceptible to infectious processes to which they were previously immune. These included malaria, dysentery, and tick-borne diseases such as sleeping sickness. The immunity experienced when eating native foods extended to chronic disease; an interview with the doctor in charge of a government hospital in Kenya revealed that in his several years of service among native people eating the native diet, he had seen no cases of appendicitis, gallbladder problems, cystitis, or duodenal ulcer.

In several tribes studied, no evidence of tooth decay was found, nor a single malformed dental arch. Several other tribes had nearly 100 percent immunity to decay, and in thirteen tribes no irregular teeth were found. Where some members had moved to cities and adopted modern foods, however, extensive decay *was* found. Children born of these individuals often showed narrowed dental arches with crowding of the teeth.

A wide range of diets was encountered, and differences between tribes were seen in physical stature and strength of typical individuals; stronger tribes dominated weaker neighbors. Among tribes studied were the following.

Nilotic Tribes, Including the Masai

Herders of cattle and goats, the people lived on milk, meat, blood from their steers, plants, nuts, and fruits. Blood was whipped in a gourd and the clot cooked. The liquid remaining, especially important in the nutrition of children, pregnant and lactating women, and warriors, was consumed raw.

These cattle people were superbly developed physically, brave, and mentally sharp. Every Nilotic tribe observed dominated its agricultural neighbors. This was not an undesirable trait or a sign of over aggression, for in the harsh African environment, as in all of nature, survival of the strong often was at the expense of the weak. The strength of the cattle people helped ensure their survival.

Protection of their animals from predators called for greater skill and bravery by the Masai than required of other African tribes. One or two men or boys often guarded entire herds with only spears. Price called the skill of Masai in killing a lion with only a spear "one of the most superb of human achievements." Scenes in films of lions in full charge—absolutely frightening images—give an indication of the courage involved in this practice.

Eighty-eight Masai were examined by Price; all were cavity-free.

The Kikuyu

These neighbors of the Masai were primarily agricultural, eating mostly sweet potatoes, corn, beans, bananas, millet, and insects. Smaller and much less rugged than the Masai, their teeth were quite good, but not up to the standard of cattleherding tribes; 5.5 percent of teeth examined showed cavities. Dental arches were generally well formed.

For six months prior to marriage, young Kikuyu women used a special diet including extra animal-sourced foods; these foods were also emphasized in pregnancy and lactation. Children were spaced at least three years apart and each pregnancy was preceded with special feeding. Such practices were typical of native cultures everywhere.

The Maragou

Strong and well-developed, these people ate quantities of fish, whole grains, sweet potatoes, and other plant foods. One tooth with a cavity was found in the nineteen individuals examined.

The Muhima

These cattle-raising people lived on meat, milk, blood, and wild plant foods. They were tall, strong, and dominant, defending their families and animals with spears. This was one of six tribes Price found that had no tooth decay.

Sudan Tribes, Including the Neurs

These herdsmen supplemented milk, blood, and meat with fish and shellfish from the Nile River. Among the Neurs, women were often more than six feet tall; men more than seven. No cavities were found in any people of this tribe.

They believed the seat of the soul was the liver and considered it their most important food. The growth of a person's character and body was said to depend upon feeding that soul by eating the livers of animals. In that sense, liver seems to have been considered a sacred food for this culture; a food with both physical and spiritual dimensions not found in other foods.

Other Agricultural People

The chief foods of other agricultural people were corn, beans, millet, sweet potatoes, bananas, and other grains. The people were smaller than herdsmen and tribes consuming large amounts of freshwater fish, and indeed, they had been dominated by such tribes.

Other groups that had a diet made up chiefly of whole grains were examined at ports and missions. The individuals were not eating as their ancestors had. Some kept a few animals and most consumed some milk and fish. Six to eight percent of the teeth of individuals in these groups had cavities.

Wherever natives had used large amounts of refined foods for some time, decay was rampant and tuberculosis prevalent; other chronic diseases appeared eventually. Dental arch abnormalities commonly appeared in the next generation.

Modernized natives were aware of a problem. Native boys at mission schools often asked why they were not as strong as boys growing up without contact with mission or government schools. As in other places that Price had visited, the contrast between traditional and modern natives was stark. These words of a mining prospector, spoken after twenty years among the native people of Uganda, echo the sentiments of many people who observed native cultures: "The heaven of my choice in which to spend all eternity would be to live in Uganda as the natives of Uganda lived before the coming of modern civilization." Perhaps he romanticized. Yet such reports were not uncommon, nor are they inconsistent with recent reports by contemporary anthropologists studying surviving hunter-gatherer cultures.

Tribes eating grain-based natural food diets had well formed dental arches and resistance to infectious diseases, but their physical development, resistance to dental decay, and strength was inferior to tribes eating more animal foods. The people strongest physically and often 100 percent resistant to dental disease were herdsmen-hunter-fishermen. In towns and ports where some groups ate a combination of refined and primitive foods, problems developed, but not to the extent occurring when native foods were abandoned entirely.

Native people everywhere discovered essentials of life and, following fundamental nutritional laws, lived in harmony with nature. Modern civilization has chosen to ignore these fundamental truths. The sophistication of our technical knowledge has bred an arrogance that precludes an appreciation of the so-called primitives' superior skill in interpreting cause and effect. The wisdom of native societies in understanding laws of nature and living in harmony with these laws is a treasure humanity must not lose if we ever wish to regain our lost strength and resistance to disease. And yet, each day that treasure slips further and further from our grasp as the few remaining native cultures are encroached upon by the expansion of civilization into their habitats.

Words like "primitives" and "savages" reveal our prejudices. Most writers have emphasized aspects of native cultures that reinforce these images. Representatives of a Western civilization exporting religion and refined food to the rest of the world refused to realize they gave little for what they took and were unable to see that nonwhite people had something to teach them. Immoral actions were accompanied by a lack of common sense; Westerners failed to learn from cultures that, through destructive ignorance and malicious exploitation, were being forever destroyed. The degradation of traditional moral values in modern societies is a matter of concern.

Herein we have concerned ourselves primarily with matters of a physical nature, however, references to the more spiritual and moral qualities of the native people Price met warrant some review. Dr. F. M. Ashley-Montagu, a world-renowned anthropologist and author of various popular and scholarly books, wrote in his article in

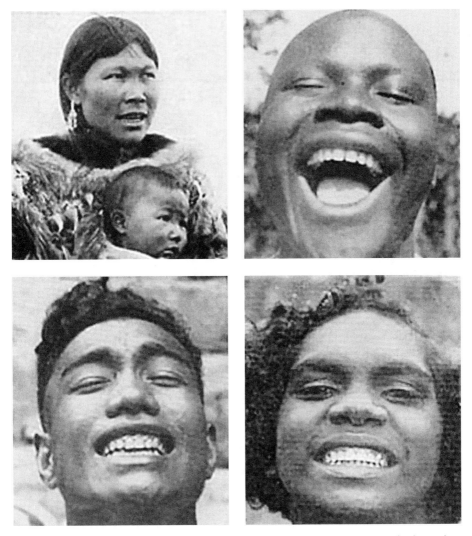

Figure 1.2. Further examples of the remarkable but quite natural physical development resulting wherever people ate according to the traditional wisdom of their culture.

Upper left: Eskimo woman and child

Upper right: African woman

Lower left: Samoan man

Lower right: Aborigine woman

the June 1940 issue of *Scientific Monthly*, "The SocioBiology of Man": "In spite of our advances, we spiritually and as human beings are not the equal of the average Aboriginal or Eskimo—we are very definitely their inferiors. We lisp noble ideals and noble sentiments—the Australians and the Eskimos practice them—they neither write books nor lecture about them." Decades later, the truth in this statement has become even more apparent.

Though currently many would prefer otherwise, nutrition is not a matter of opinion; nor are the ideals of truth, honesty, integrity, loyalty, and service that have been held in common in traditional societies the world over by thousands of generations. The price of modern society's decision to ignore natural laws governing these fundamental aspects of human life has resulted in the spiritual bankruptcy that threatens Western society today.

AUSTRALIA, THE TORRES STRAIT ISLANDS, AND NEW ZEALAND (1936)

Aborigines of Australia

Price wished to study many different cultures in order to witness as wide a range in their physical conditions as possible. More than one-half of Australia receives less than ten inches of rain per year. Poor soil and subsequent scanty plant and animal life in the interior regions made the physical condition and culture of Aborigines there all the more remarkable.

Their skill in tracking and trapping animals was renowned; they were said to see animals moving over a mile away. Their social organization too was quite remarkable. Aboriginal boys and girls were required to pass through a long and involved series of tests and trials (physical, mental, and moral) to enter adulthood. People knowing them well invariably stated that Aborigines never stole and were completely trustworthy.

They were a spiritual people who believed in an afterlife. The stars to them represented spirits of ancestors. Indeed, spirits of great character made up the constellations, and aboriginal youth learned their names. These were people who had conquered life's temptations and lived completely in the interest of serving others. Aborigine spirituality was built upon this principle.

In every isolated primitive group, Price saw physical excellence in all individuals. But the majority of Aborigines had been deprived of their homelands, placed on reservations, and enslaved as laborers. The contrast between them and those left alone was more extreme than any place Price had seen. Whites who enslaved Aborigines ate the same refined foods, and their physical degeneration was equally marked.

Aborigines from both interior and coastal districts were studied. Special effort was made to examine children aged ten to sixteen after their permanent teeth had come in. Only then could the developing shape of the adult dental arch and pattern of the adult face be determined, allowing a full assessment of the effects of the individual's nutrition.

A large number of skulls of Aborigines in museums at Sydney and Canberra were also examined. Aborigines living primitively all had broad, beautifully proportioned faces, with wide and well contoured dental arches. Museum skulls too were uniformly excellent.

Aborigines near the coast were larger than those of inland tribes, and skulls from near the coast were more massive. Coastal people ate quantities of fish, sea cow, a great variety of shellfish, sea plants, land plants, and fruits. Inland food was scarcer; people ate roots, stems, leaves, berries, seeds, large and small animals of every variety (including rodents, insects, beetles, and grubs), various animal life from the rivers, birds, birds' eggs—nearly everything moving or growing.

All of those examined in primitive groups from both coastal and inland places had excellent bodies, with almost no decay or abnormalities in the shape of the dental arch and face. Apparently this had been the case for thousands of years, for the primitive museum skulls were all perfect.

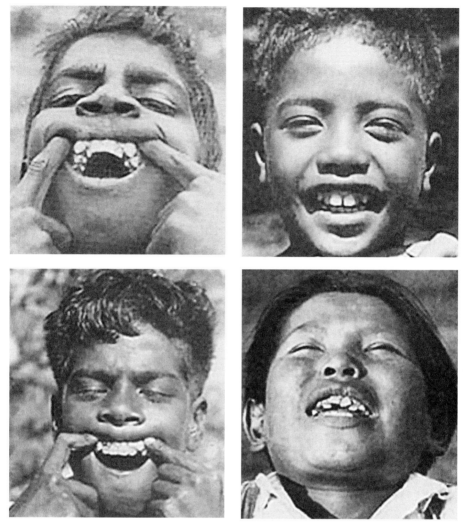

Figure 1.3. Typical changes occurring in the first generation born after the introduction of refined foods shows narrowing of the dental arches with subsequent crowding of teeth. These problems occurred in addition to the agonizing dental decay that both parents and children experienced.

Upper left: Aborigine boy

Upper right: Polynesian boy

Lower left: Torres Strait Islands boy

Lower right: Eskimo boy

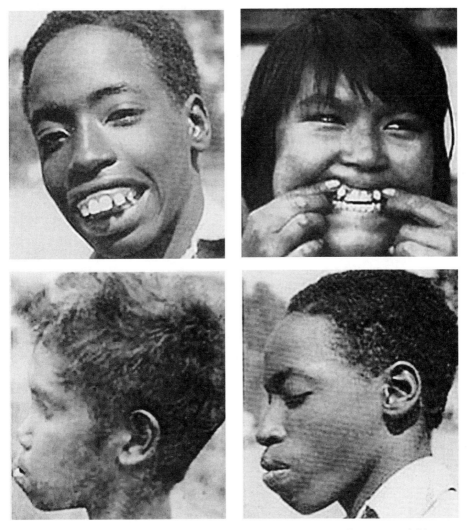

Figure 1.4. Further examples of degenerative changes typically seen in children born of parents eating refined foods.

> **Upper left:** African boy with extreme protrusion of the upper teeth and shortening of the lower jaw.
>
> **Upper right:** Eskimo girl with crowding of the upper dental arch, which has caused the bicuspids to protrude. This is often seen in cultures eating refined foods. Contrast this with the young people in figures 1.1, 1.2, and 1.5.
>
> **Lower left:** Aborigine boy. Changes in the shape of the face and dental arch have caused the lower jaw to be thrust forward. Price virtually never saw such changes in people eating native, natural food.
>
> **Lower right:** African boy with the same thrust of the chin found in a boy on the other side of the world. The cause is the same.

Those forced to eat refined foods showed, in the next generation, the same dental abnormalities present in white people. Tuberculosis and crippling arthritis became common, particularly among those with no access at all to native foods.

The story of the Aborigines is perhaps sadder than that of other native peoples decimated by contact with Western civilization because the Aborigines were so completely exploited. They are a reminder that the white man was not welcome in primitive lands; guns were his introduction and the arbiters ensuring his stay. Perhaps natives in some places welcomed Westerners at first, but had they seen everything that was to come, they almost certainly would have resisted initial contact more strongly.

The processes destroying traditional cultures were so insidious as to be perhaps unrecognizable in early stages. Who was to know that the white man's food would lead inevitably to sickness and death and that the biological integrity of thousands of generations would be disrupted? When conditions deteriorated, it was in most cases impossible to return to traditional ways.

Some native people exposed to Westernization chose to maintain traditional ways, however, entirely refusing to eat the white man's food. These people also maintained their strength, health, and integrity. Perhaps they served as models for any of their fellows seeking help.

Torres Strait Islanders

The Torres Strait is the body of water between northernmost Australia and southernmost New Guinea. Many small fertile islands supported populations of several hundred to a few thousand people when Weston Price visited this region. Government stores selling refined foods had in recent years been established on many of these islands. Before a local market economy took hold here, adults had reached maturity eating only native food; very few other factors in the environment had changed.

Surrounding waters were rich with fish and shellfish. Plant foods too were abundant and of such importance that Thursday Island, the location of the administrative center for the islands, was not originally inhabited because the soil was poor. The native diet consisted of a great deal of fish and shellfish of many kinds, tropical plants, seaweed, taro, bananas, papayas, and plums.

Natives living on native foods had practically no cavities. Most had broad, normal dental arches. They were a happy, peaceful, and contented people; there was almost no crime.

Thursday Island was the home of the majority of whites in the Torres Strait; imported foods had been available for several decades. Native people lived mainly on the rest of the islands and acutely resented the intrusion of modern ways, particularly refined foods. Government stores were seen as a danger, and on several occasions the issue had nearly provoked violence. Perhaps the people intuitively saw the threat posed by the "white man's foods."

The incidence of dental decay on a given island was directly proportional to how long a store had been present there. Children born after parents began using refined foods often developed abnormal dental arches, as did a large majority of white children on Thursday Island.

The government physician for the Torres Strait islanders stated that in his thirteen years with them, among the native population of four thousand he had never seen cancer. He had operated on several dozen malignancies among the white population of about three hundred. Among natives, any conditions requiring surgery were extremely rare.

The general health and resistance to disease of traditional cultures is demonstrated in interviews with the physicians who spent years with these people. Though Price focused primarily on dental health, his studies showed that a resistant individual developed neither dental disease nor other disease. He noted that people suffering from tuberculosis and rheumatoid arthritis nearly always had extensive dental decay. Physicians interviewed consistently stated that native people living on traditional diets remained nearly or entirely free of all disease. This was observed by early anthropologists, and confirmation has recently come in the form of several research articles, to be discussed later in this book.

New Zealand Maori

The reputation of the Maori among Western anthropologists has, since the first Europeans sailed to New Zealand, been that of the most physically well developed people in the world. An early study of two hundred and fifty Maori skulls revealed only one tooth per two thousand with a cavity, and nearly 100 percent had normally formed dental arches. This was superior to even the Eskimos.

According to Price, Maori have told a man at a telescope exactly when an eclipse of a satellite of Jupiter, supposedly invisible to the naked eye, was about to occur. Paintings in cave dwellings in other parts of the world reveal that some prehistoric people saw stars that we see only with telescopes.

Weston Price traveled eighteen hundred miles through twenty-five districts examining native Maori families and children in native schools that were in various stages of modernization; the cavities rate varied with the degree of change. In more isolated groups, 2 percent of the teeth had been attacked by decay, and in many districts 100 percent of the older generation had broad, normal dental arches. In modernized groups, from 40 to 100 percent of the younger people had abnormalities.

Tribal tradition placed much emphasis on shellfish, especially certain species, as was the case throughout the Pacific. Kelp (seaweed) and fern root were eaten in quantity. The Maori relied primarily upon the sea for nourishment.

SOUTH AMERICA

Ancient and Present-Day Peruvians (1937)

Long before Spaniards pillaged the Mayan and Aztec civilizations of Mexico and South America, cultures flourished in Peru, existing in the high plains country of the Andes Mountains and the arid desert region extending from the Pacific Ocean to the Andes. This desert, forty to one hundred miles in width, runs one thousand inhospitable miles

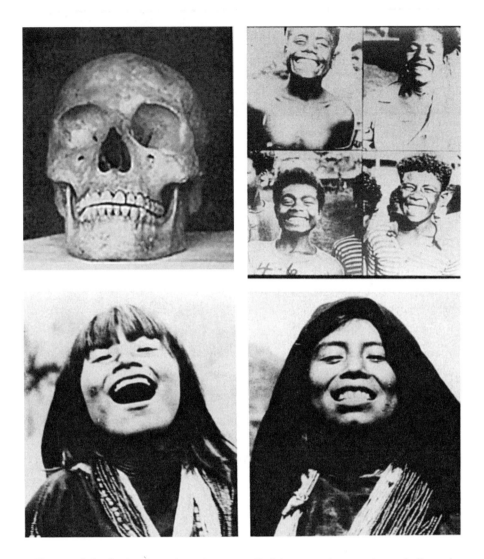

Figure 1.5. Archeological evidence studied in several countries—skulls and teeth from ancient cultures—showed in generation after generation that tribal patterns repeated themselves with no significant changes.

> **Upper left:** This ancient Indian skull was among the skeletal remains Price studied in North America, Australia, and Peru. In Peru, he examined 1,276 successive skulls without finding one with the narrowed dental arches of most modern people.

> **Upper right:** Melanesian boys. These four boys lived on four different islands and were not related. Each had nutrition adequate for the development of the physical pattern typical of Melanesian males; thus their similar appearance.

> **Lower left:** Peruvian jungle Indian girl

> **Lower right:** Peruvian jungle Indian woman

down the length of South America and is marked by vast sand dunes with scarcely a sign of greenery.

But throughout are found complex foundations of fortresses and extended residential areas from past civilizations. Great aqueducts brought water from the mountains, enabling people to grow quantities of corn, beans, squash, and other plants in river bottoms where alluvial soil from the Andes had collected for ages past. These foods, and the seafood consumed, nourished the cultures there.

Mummies of ancient inhabitants have been found in this desert region. Indeed, fifteen million mummies were estimated to be in the burial mounds found along the entire coast. Many articles were buried with these mummies, including jars containing food and items the dead person used in life. Nets and the tackle of fishermen were buried with many. The foundation of these cultures was ultimately the animal and marine life of the Pacific Ocean. Sweeping north from Antarctica, the Humboldt Current carries with it sources of food that support a vast population of fish and shellfish.

Thousands of mummified specimens, well preserved because of the dryness of the climate, existed in Peruvian museums. Skulls of 1,276 ancient people were studied by Price; not one significant deformity of the dental arches was found. Each showed normal broad arches capable of accommodating thirty-two teeth without crowding.

Villages were visited where descendants of one of these ancient cultures lived. Isolated on the north coast of Peru, they were fisherfolk who lived traditional lives and didn't consume modern food. Their physical development was excellent.

Cultural achievements of these ancient civilizations were considerable. Engineering feats remain unexplained. The great aqueducts of the coastal people, sophisticated and estimated to be capable of delivering sixty million cubic feet of water per day over distances of up to one hundred miles, were cut through boulders without hardened tools or blasting powder. Roads and suspension bridges built by the Incas crossed mountain divides fourteen to sixteen thousand feet above sea level, linking all parts of the empire to Machu Picchu, their mountain fortress. A superb engineering achievement, the walls were built of white granite lifted from quarries in a riverbank two thousand feet below.

The Tauhuanocan culture preceded the Incan and left magnificent monuments. One of the largest single stones ever moved and used in a building is found in one of their temples; it is thought to have been brought more than two hundred miles through mountainous country. Many structures from this culture are found in the Andean Plateau from Bolivia to Ecuador, all characterized by intricately fitted, many-sided large stones, some of them twenty feet long. The fit is such that most crevices do not allow for the passage of a knife point.

How were the stones cut and moved, and how were they and the white granite of Machu Picchu raised? No one knows.

The Incan society was a highly organized and perhaps successful socialistic state. Some sources report there was no hunger or crime, and that the ruling Incan carefully practiced laws his people were required to live by.

Foods in the high plateau country of the Incan and Tauhuanocan cultures were less diverse than those found at the coast. Plants and grains were consumed. These included potatoes, corn, several varieties of beans, and quinoa, a seed cereal. Llamas and alpacas were domesticated, and some wild game was available. A colony of guinea pigs was kept by each household for food; we now know they provided a rich source of vitamin D.

When Price visited, dried fish eggs and kelp were regularly obtained through commerce with the coast and were universally available in high-country markets; for centuries this had been so. The Indians said dried fish eggs were necessary to maintain fertility, and kelp was necessary to prevent the "big necks" whites often developed—the enlarged thyroid gland (goiter) that results when the body attempts to compensate for a deficiency of iodine.

Skulls from pre-Columbian burials in the mountains were studied.

All were free of dental decay, with broad dental arches and well-developed third molars.

Despite the severe climate of the mountains and the arid conditions of the coast, ancient Peruvians of both areas developed ways of eating and living that led to physical integrity and significant cultural achievements. The accumulated wisdom of their centuries of living in harmony with nature has been largely forgotten. Subsequently, people in these lands have developed diseases and structural, physical problems inherent to the use of refined foods.

Andes Mountain Indians

In high mountain plateaus of southern Peru and Bolivia, many descendants of the ancient Tauhuanocan and Incan cultures still lived according to their ancestors' methods. Market day was characterized by trade and socializing. On such days, Price had opportunities to examine several groups. Contact was arranged through local authorities.

The most isolated groups showed the lowest incidence of tooth decay and degenerative changes. No decayed teeth were found in one group of twenty-five; each individual had all teeth normal for his or her age.

Strength and endurance were characteristic of the Indians of the Andes Mountains who typically carried loads in excess of two hundred pounds all day long, day after day. In freezing weather they slept with ponchos about their heads; their legs and feet remained bare. Many lived at elevations of twelve thousand feet or more.

While native cultures in Switzerland and Georgian Russia used quantities of dairy products, Andes Indians achieved physical excellence without them, for dairy animals introduced to the Andean climate had never adapted to it. Llamas, wild birds, and guinea pigs were the animal foods consumed by inhabitants here.

Amazon Jungle Indians

The Amazon region of Peru begins in the eastern foothills of the Andes, where fertile soil, warm climate, and abundant rainfall generates fish-filled streams and forests rich with tropical vegetables, fruits, and wild animals. Price met and examined a group of thirty Amazon jungle Indians who lived in this area.

They were a proud, beautiful people with great strength. They exhibited no evidence of dental decay; each individual had perfect dental arches. Another tribe of the same ancestral stock was in contact with a mission and had reduced the use of native foods in favor of refined foods available through the mission. As a result, many members of this tribe had rampant tooth decay, and young children had dental-arch deformities. They were becoming civilized.

Decay and missing teeth were expected. But Weston Price's monumental study for the first time thoroughly and convincingly linked many other problems to inadequate nutrition. Among these problems were changes in the shape of the dental arches, head, and face; infertility, miscarriage, difficult labor, and birth defects; susceptibility to acute diseases; and prevalence of tuberculosis, arthritis, cancer, and other chronic diseases. Price also wrote of the relationship between inadequate nutrition and criminality and mental deficiency. His discovery of characteristic animal nutrients in the diets of all groups enjoying immunity from these problems further adds to the revolutionary impact of his findings.

CONCLUSIONS OF THE MEDICAL COMMUNITY PERTAINING TO DIET AND DISEASE

In response to controversy about the role of diet in degenerative diseases, a consensus emerged within the medical profession in the second half of the twentieth century that animal fats and foods rich in cholesterol were harmful. There is no truth to this assertion, which has been used to reach numerous faulty conclusions.

Analysis of the deterioration of the modern diet is complex. Beyond the decline in quality, traditional wisdom about the use of different organs and tissues of animals has been forgotten or ignored. Liver, for example, is seldom eaten today. But in all traditional cultures, liver is among the most important of foods.

The displacement of traditional foods by refined foods is the heart of the problem. Attempts to cite the single issue of animal fats and cholesterol as the chief problem and solution are misdirected and sidestep issues central to a reasonable approach to health and disease.

While Price was a pioneer, other scientists have studied traditional cultures and concluded that food is almost certainly responsible for the nearly complete protection that hunter-fisher-gatherers enjoy from dental and chronic disease. Recent publication of this work and research comparing oils and fats in fish and wild game with those in domestic animals will be reviewed shortly, after completing our travels with Weston Price.

3
PROTECTIVE CHARACTERISTICS OF PRIMAL NUTRITION

Dr. Weston Price's time in history was unique. The cultures he observed were still truly indigenous, with groups of people living entirely on the local foods. Photographic emulsion was commonly available for the first time, as was world travel. With one step in the old world and one step in the new, Price recorded his groundbreaking findings. A primary discovery was that the diets of native groups that were immune to dental and degenerative disease had several characteristics in common (these people hereafter will be referred to as "immune groups").

COMMON FEATURES OF NATIVE GROUPS STUDIED

Nearly all foods that were consumed by the native groups that Price studied were whole and unrefined. Many whole foods were concentrated, for example, butter and cheese in the Loetschental Valley of Switzerland, seal oil and other concentrated animal and fish-liver oils by Eskimos, lard by groups that utilized pigs and beef fat in the making of pemmican by Native Americans—all of which served to include more saturated fats in the diet!

The foods of each immune group had been used by the group for centuries or longer, were prepared in special ways, and were indigenous to the group's region. No imported foods were used. Customs dictated the importance of eating certain foods at specified times in life. Specific foods were known to prevent specific problems. Certain special foods believed to ensure the birth of normal, healthy offspring were particularly valued and were included in the preconception diet of both parents.

Most of the diets did not contain large amounts of fruit, which was used when available, but generally in limited quantities. Even where large quantities of fruit were available—for example bananas in the Amazon and in parts of Africa—fish and shellfish, animals, and vegetables were preferred.

Immune groups used none of the many foods commonly consumed today. The obvious ones include sugar, white flour, canned goods, and other supermarket standards. Less obvious are vegetable oils and fruit juices, both commonly used by health-conscious people. Nor were significant amounts of honey utilized by the immune groups, even though it often was the only sweetener available. Alcohol was consumed moderately if at all, in raw fermented beverages rich in enzymes and minerals. No vitamin pills were consumed.

Fish and shellfish were used in quantity by immune groups near the sea, supplemented by sea mammals, land animals, or both. Freshwater fish, animals, and sometimes milk and cheese were the most important protein foods for inland groups. Seaweed was consumed by every immune group living near the sea. Inland groups traded for it or, in the case of certain African tribes, special iodine-rich freshwater plants were used. In many groups, green vegetables and plants, gathered wild, were staples for all. Most cultures consumed at least some fruit. The organs of animals or fish or both were considered vital.

Given these common characteristics, we will now turn our discussion to specific fat-soluble nutrients, minerals, and raw-food proteins and enzymes. These biochemical and structural elements, abundant in primitive diets and lacking in modern ones, help to explain why the foods of traditional people largely protected them from disease.

FAT-SOLUBLE NUTRIENTS IN
FOODS OF ANIMAL ORIGIN

Foods rich in fat-soluble vitamins and fatty acids formed substantial parts of traditional diets. These foods fall into three categories:

1. Seafood, especially fatty fish such as salmon and herring.
2. Animal and fish organs, especially liver, brain, marrow, and intestines.
3. Dairy products from animals feeding on fresh green pasturage, particularly cheese and butter, which feature concentrated fat-soluble nutrients.

Vitamin D is richly supplied in these foods. Vitamin D is a complex of several vitamins. One, vitamin D_3, is produced in humans by the action of ultraviolet light on the skin. Vitamin D_3 helps regulate the absorption and utilization of calcium and other minerals. Other members of the vitamin D complex appear to play similar but complementary roles.

Sunlight does not appear to stimulate production of these other members of the D complex; they are supplied in the above-listed foods. This may be a reason that these foods proved to be essential in building immunity to dental and degenerative disease, for these other members of the D complex may play a role in maintaining health. Indeed, why would they be present in animals' bodies if each did not serve a function?

Weston Price found that when patients with active decay eliminated refined foods and ate sufficient protective foods, the decay process often ceased. This was the case in young people of the Loetschental Valley who experienced decay only while outside of the valley. The decay ceased without the need for the teeth to be filled with fillings—photographs in Price's book detail this. Present-day dentists occasionally observe cavities that have ceased to be active, by and large without realizing that this relates to specific dietary changes. The fat-soluble vitamins A, D, and K_2 are the keys to this. (Their interactions are complex, thus to articulate all of them in their entirety is beyond the scope of this book.)

Price's chemical analyses of dairy products from all over Europe and America showed the fat-soluble vitamin content was much higher in those dairy products that had been made from butterfat derived from animals fed fresh green pasturage. This fat-soluble vitamin content was highest when grass was growing most rapidly. Dairy products from animals *not* eating fresh grass did not contain significant amounts of fat-soluble vitamins. (As we will see in chapter 5, in Francis M. Pottenger, Jr.'s experiments, milk from cows fed fresh greens had significantly healthier effects on animals than milk from cows fed hay. This was due to an unidentified nutrient Price called activator X, now thought to be Vitamin K_2.)

Fish fats are rich in the omega-3 fatty acid, eicosapentaenoic acid (EPA). Wild grazing animals have small but significant amounts, yet domestic beef fattened on grains contains almost undetectable amounts. But all animal fats contain arachadonic acid, which is needed to balance EPA.

Desirable prostaglandins are formed from EPA; some are responsible for keeping arteries optimally dilated and platelets from clotting abnormally (platelets are small particles in the blood that aid in clotting). Other prostaglandins made from EPA seem to enhance the functioning of the immune system. Many other effects of EPA are currently being studied by medical researchers. Evidence indicates significant EPA consumption is one reason that Eskimos and other native people (consumers of large amounts of fish and wild game) rarely suffer from heart disease and other chronic and acute diseases. But again, balancing the level of EPA with a proper balance of arachadonic acid is critical, given that excess EPA can be harmful.

Analysis of wild African grazing animals found significant amounts of EPA, and we may assume milk from such animals contains EPA.

Analysis of domestic beef found almost no EPA; such animals are fattened on grains and fed little or no fresh grass the last few months of life, explaining the lack of EPA in their fat.

Seafood, organ meats, or raw dairy products of the proper quality are, in my experience, essential for full recovery from chronic disease and the maintenance of optimal health. Experiences of traditional cultures when these foods were displaced by refined foods indicate they are essential to also ensure normal development, birth, and growth of the unborn child and child. Considerations of the proportions and kinds of these foods best suited for individual tastes and needs will be discussed in later chapters.

MINERALS

Minerals originate and reside in the soil or the sea. In a forest, minerals leave the soil as vegetation and are returned by animal droppings, carcasses, and decaying vegetation.

Modern agricultural practices break that cycle. A few elements, without which the land would not produce crops, are replaced— nitrogen, potassium, and phosphorous. Others, however, including trace minerals, are not. Since life first emerged from the sea and gained a foothold on the barren masses of the primitive continents, a delicate balance of natural forces has worked in harmony to evolve its rich diversity. Chemical agriculture ignores that equilibrium.

These natural forces provided foods required for optimal health and strength. Modern commercially produced foods cannot. Evidence about the role of trace-mineral deficiencies in the development of disease has emerged in recent years. Such deficiencies may be directly traced to modern agricultural methods, which produce food for people along with the feed for animals that provide meat and dairy products. Modern agricultural practices simply do not return to the soil what is taken out. Refining processes further strip grains of minerals and other nutrients.

Price analyzed foods of immune groups for mineral and vitamin content. In every case, the foods supplied at least four times modern consumption levels for each nutrient tested. Calcium intake ranged up to seven times as much; phosphorous intake, from five to eight times as much. Magnesium intake for several groups was more than twenty times as much; iron and iodine intake was up to fifty times as much. Intake of both fat-soluble and water-soluble vitamins was in every case at least ten times the minimum daily requirement. Mineral supplements benefit many people; often health problems are accompanied by deficiencies of calcium and magnesium and of trace minerals. But excesses occur if overdoses are taken, and increased intakes of some minerals can cause deficiencies of others. Supplementary zinc, for example, can drive down body levels of copper.

Natural foods have been assembled in nature's laboratory over the course of evolution. The best way to get minerals is from foods; the full balance of accompanying nutrients is then supplied simultaneously. Special foods and supplements may be helpful in ensuring adequate intake or in correcting deficiencies.

Research and clinical experience indicate that a deficiency of minerals in modern diets contributes to health problems. The high incidence of osteoporosis among the elderly is an example; it is due in part to calcium deficiency. Liberal amounts of minerals in the foods of immune groups resulted from environments in which ecological balances were respectfully allowed to maintain and replenish themselves. Perhaps because humans took little, they were given a great deal.

We have since taken a great deal from forests, plains, and seas. Only a fraction of our wilderness and wildlife heritage remains. Unless we live with the land, rather than on it, and maintain it rather than rape it, whatever capacity the planet has left to supply traditional foods will be lost. The ability to resist disease, and much of the biological strength human beings have evolved over thousands of years, will be lost along with it.

RAW-FOOD PROTEINS AND
ENZYMES

Food-industry products are rarely raw foods—the industry has scant interest in researching the benefits of raw foods. Thus, the value of raw foods is little understood by either the public or food scientists. This pertains to enzymes, which are found in raw foods. Enzymes are catalysts made of protein that initiate and speed up the biochemical processes of life. The protein they are made of consists of chains of amino acids linked by chemical bonds. The body can make many of the amino acids it requires; the eight it cannot produce are called essential and must be consumed.

Textbooks of physiology and biochemistry state that dietary proteins are broken down in the small intestine into constituent amino acids that are absorbed into the bloodstream. (Enzymes in the body are also broken down or destroyed if the body's temperature exceeds approximately 107 to 108 degrees.) Scientists and medical students are taught that enzymes in foods have no nutritional value beyond that of their constituent amino acids. Since all proteins (and thus all enzymes) supposedly are broken down and reach the bloodstream as amino acids, standard teaching holds that enzymes in raw foods have no unique or special effects. The possibility that enzymes and other proteins in foods may be absorbed intact, or in large fragments having significant biological effects, has long been dismissed as the province of faddists seeing mystical properties in raw foods.

But evidence was published in the 1970s by W. A. Hemmings of the University College of North Wales and other researchers indicating that a significant portion of dietary protein is absorbed intact, in large fragments of many linked amino acids. Studies were done by feeding radioisotope-labeled animal protein to rats and measuring the radioactivity levels in different parts of the animal's body. The researchers found that about half of the ingested protein freely passed as intact protein and large identifiable fragments into the bloodstream. These proteins went to tissues throughout an animal's body and were broken down over a period of days or weeks. The researchers believe a similar process occurs in humans, indicating that different raw foods each have unique and potentially significant biological effects.

Such evidence supports the experience of healers who for thousands of years have stressed that raw foods are essential to the healing process and the maintenance of health.

As we will see in chapter 5, more than fifty years ago Francis Pottenger, Jr. proved that raw foods were required to maintain the health of cats. He applied elements of this knowledge to the care of his patients with tuberculosis and other chronic diseases, with excellent and well-documented results. Unfortunately, while his work was initially well received by the medical profession, in the ensuing years it has been largely ignored.

Every native culture Weston Price studied ate many foods raw; tradition often dictated which. The milk, cheese, and butter of Swiss villagers and African herdsmen were seldom heated. Organs in every traditional culture were often eaten raw or lightly cooked. Eskimos of Arctic regions, where no plants were available much of the year, ate some fish raw. This practice prevented scurvy; the vitamin C in meat and fish is destroyed by cooking. Much meat was eaten raw, lightly cooked, or smoked. Salmon eggs were important for coastal people; uncooked eggs were dried in fall for use in winter.

In the South Pacific, islanders and coastal Australian Aborigines ate much fish and shellfish raw. When shellfish were cooked, native people arranged them circularly about a small fire, with the animals' valve ends toward the flames. Just enough heat was used to open the valves, saving much work.

Dried raw seaweed was used by coastal people everywhere. Many vegetables and other plant foods were used raw, especially young greens. Fruits were nearly always eaten raw. Perhaps most importantly, fermented foods, an incredibly rich source of enzymes, were used universally.

PROTECTIVE NUTRIENTS AND
HIGH-QUALITY FOODS

When protective nutrients are lost from the diet, health problems are bound to ensue. Consuming enough of these nutrients is a step toward building strength and resistance to disease. Certain foods are more appropriate than others, depending on one's ancestry and tastes. The point in detailing traditional use of specific parts of animals, often raw, is not to suggest that one emulate this, though one might. Rather, the concern is finding adequate sources of nutrients that native wisdom teaches are important.

Raw and lightly cooked foods may be eaten in quantity if enjoyed; they should not be forced. A reasonable approach might utilize raw or lightly cooked egg yolks from free-range chickens (some of the B vitamin biotin is lost by binding with the protein avidin in raw eggs, and raw egg whites are difficult to digest and highly allergenic), raw milk, rare beef, and raw fish (sushi and sashimi). In some states, raw butter is available. In years past, millions of people safely used certified raw dairy products. The safety of raw beef, fish, and dairy products depends largely on the health of the source animals. In my opinion, the danger resulting from a lack of essential nutrients found in raw foods is far greater than that associated with eating the foods raw if they are derived from healthy animals.

If animal foods are used raw or lightly cooked, sources ideally should be similar in quality to animal foods of native cultures. More and more, such sources are now available.

Vegetables, especially salad greens such as lettuce and sprouts, are best raw, although cooked vegetables add variety and, in colder weather, warmth. Raw-food vegetarians may enjoy quite good health, particularly if the diet includes raw dairy products. The quantities of raw vegetables needed for caloric needs supply large amounts of enzymes. Those individuals eating no animal foods typically develop problems involving mineral metabolism, vitamin B_{12} deficiencies, and inadequate amounts of the fat-soluble vitamins A, D, and K_2. But until then many strict vegetarians may feel quite well. Such exclusively vegetarian diets may initially help people suffering from chronic diseases, but inevitably lead to serious problems if followed for any extended period of time.

Another consideration relates to the high quality of foods used in traditional native cultures. These animal and dairy foods were healthy and free of pesticide residues, antibiotics, and added hormones—as was seafood. Vegetables, grains, and fruits grew on living soils rich in elements natural to the soil and free of pesticides. Suffice it to say that health can be dramatically improved without eating organic foods, but optimal health requires them.

Foods of the highest quality are more expensive and may be difficult to find, however. Be that as it may, the financial rewards of consuming high-quality foods are considerable, especially if one succeeds in improving one's health to the point where visits to a physician are no longer a regular affair. This is a reasonable goal. Intangible rewards are even greater, for nothing equals the feeling of a smoothly functioning body.

In the next chapter we will look at the effect of diet on longevity by assessing the communities of different indigenous populations in three far-flung corners of the world.

4
THE LONG-LIVED PEOPLE OF VILCABAMBA, HUNZA, AND GEORGIAN RUSSIA

Reports of many people remaining vigorous into extreme old age are the stuff of popular legend, and Vilcabamba, Hunza, and Georgian Russia have generated their share. Isolated and remote when studied in the 1970s, Vilcabamba is a village in the Vilcabamba Valley in the Andes Mountains of southern Ecuador. Hunza too is remote and mountainous, an ancient kingdom near the borders of China and Afghanistan in the high valleys of the Himalayas in Pakistani-controlled Kashmir. Georgian Russia covers a much larger area, and it is mountainous as well. One of the three former Soviet republics of the Caucasus region, it has a population of some five million people.

VERIFYING AGES AND HEALTH STATUS

Many people in these three places have claimed to be well over 100 years old. Attempts to verify the stated ages involved several independent methods that were matched against each other. Documentation of dates of birth—such as church baptismal records—were considered the most reliable. Passports, old letters, and even the carved woodwork of some homes in which birth dates had been recorded all proved useful as well.

In the 1971 census, the village of Vilcabamba listed 9 individuals over the age of 100 in a population of 819. The number of other centenarians living on small farmsteads in surrounding mountains and hamlets is unknown. However, Ecuador is Catholic, and church baptismal records have been carefully made and preserved there for centuries. As we shall see, these church records were extremely helpful when validating the existence of centenarians in Vilcabamba. Many old people in Hunza claimed to be over 100, but there was no recording of births there, so ascertaining the veracity of this is more difficult.

In the 1970s, Georgia reported 1,844 centenarians, or 39 per 100,000 people; for some, birth records existed. In comparison, centenarians numbered 3 per 100,000 in America.

In Hunza and Georgian Russia, alleged experts on "life extension" have discredited all reports of great longevity there because a common practice in these places was for a man to take his father's or grandfather's name, and with it his age, to avoid compulsory military service. This may indeed have occurred, and some Hunzas and Georgians may well have exaggerated their ages to investigators. But these are not reasons to discredit *all* claims of great longevity among the men and women of these areas.

Several medical investigators took pains to verify the ages of oldsters in Georgia and Vilcabamba and have stated with reasonable certainty that a number of these people were more than 120 years old, and many others were well over 100. Soviet gerontologists report that Russia's oldest man died at the age of approximately 168.

In the studies undertaken in the 1970s, each oldster was questioned about his or her age at marriage, the time interval until children were born, and the present age of children. Memories of events of historical and local importance were recorded. Calculations of the person's age made from this data correlated well for 704 centenarians in Georgia whose ages were known from birth records; for 95 percent, the calculated age exactly matched the age on the birth record. For the rest, the error averaged 5 percent, and in no case was the error more than 10 years.

Verification was more difficult in Hunza because the absence of written records made it impossible to confirm exact ages. But as in Vilcabamba and Georgia, investigators agree that physical vigor in extreme old age, rather than the age itself, most impressed visitors. The old men and women lived in the mountains and were farmers, and often the men had been hunters or herdsmen (a few over 90 still were). Since early childhood, everyday life had involved much walking and other exercise, and these individuals continued to walk and work, usually until shortly before death.

THE WORK OF
DR. DAVID DAVIES IN VILCABAMBA

Dr. David Davies, then a gerontologist at University College in London, did a thorough job of documenting the ages of a number of centenarians in Vilcabamba. He made four trips to the Vilcabamba Valley and the surrounding mountains between 1971 and 1973. In *The Centenarians of the Andes* (1975), he describes these trips.

Davies spent a great deal of time in churches searching baptismal records. The priests would not let these books out of sight, thus the books never left the church premises. The earlier records were made of parchment with a skin covering; some dated back to 1655. Dry climate and care had preserved them in highly legible condition.

Baptismal records of people still living dated to 1847; one individual was 126 at the time of the investigation. Records were found for several others who were older than 120. Death certificates were found for four people who had lived to 150 and died in the 1920s and 1930s in the mountains near the Vilcabamba Valley. The records had been kept by Jesuits, who in those years controlled the export of Peruvian bark found in the area, at great profit. As a source of quinine, it was then the chief medicine for malarial fevers. Davies points out that the Jesuits certainly would not have wanted to attract visitors by creating a longevity myth, and one can think of no reason why they would have falsified the documents.

Civil registers were kept separately beginning around 1900 in state offices in the different villages; these too recorded births and deaths. In these registers, deaths of the old people, births of their children, and wedding dates were recorded. These dates of death matched those in the church records. Other dates were used to corroborate life-history methods of estimating age. These data were checked for correlation with the documentation and stated ages of individuals.

Children and grandchildren were also interviewed to further corroborate the ages of the centenarians, as were other oldsters of about the same age. Interviews were held separately to prevent possible prompting. Memories of the old people are described as remarkable, and the various methods consistently verified ages listed in baptismal records. Davies' reasonable conclusion: "We have been entirely satisfied that the ages of these centenarians are authentic."

He further reported these people were lucid, agile, and active in old age, and did not have cancer, heart disease, diabetes, high blood pressure, or other diseases afflicting people in modern cultures—diseases that were common in towns just fifty miles away. Even in the village of Vilcabamba and other villages in the valley, chronic disease had begun appearing with the introduction of refined foods. When centenarians who had moved down from the mountains to be near younger relatives were exposed to these foods, they were less healthy; in some, symptoms of diabetes appeared.

Centenarians had nearly always spent their lives on their small mountainside farms outside the villages. When remaining there, they eventually experienced a time when health declined and aging occurred rapidly. Typically, within a few months death came.

Davies discovered two problems in the health of Vilcabambans. First, mortality in infancy and early childhood was high. This he discovered in examining church baptismal records; 40 percent died of epidemics and viruses before the age of three. And second, the vast majority of older people, including most centenarians, lost most or all of their teeth at a fairly early age. The gums were firm; individuals could chew foods easily, but were without many teeth during their later years. This was in contrast with Georgians, whose teeth generally remained excellent into extreme old age. We'll return to these problems later.

THE WORK OF DR. ALEXANDER LEAF IN VILCABAMBA, HUNZA, AND GEORGIAN RUSSIA

An article that appeared in *National Geographic* in January 1973 entitled "Every Day Is a Gift When You Are Over 100," is an account of long-lived people by Dr. Alexander Leaf and John Launois. Dr. Leaf, a physician and teacher at Harvard University, spent parts of two years traveling in Vilcabamba, Hunza, and Georgian Russia. In the Abkhazia region of Georgian Russia, he interviewed a woman by the name of Khaf Lasuria who, he concluded, was more than 130 years old. She was the one who spoke the immortal words of the article's title: "Every Day Is a Gift When You Are Over 100."

She recalled events of her life for Leaf in great detail. She had retired from her work as a tea-leaf picker two years prior. After she had passed the age of 100, in the 1940s, she had held the record as the collective farm's fastest picker. Still independent, she took care of herself, regularly taking a bus alone to a distant village to visit relatives, keeping a garden, and caring for her chickens and pigs (which are rich in saturated fat).

She greeted the doctor with a toast of vodka; she drank a small glass of it each morning, and a glass of wine before lunch. Each household in Abkhazia had its own vineyard and made its own wine. The wine was dry and drunk fresh. It was a source of enzymes, minerals, and other nutrients, and many old people drank two or three glasses of it a day. On festive occasions, many Abkhazians drank considerable amounts of grape vodka (also homemade) and wine. But the older people often abstained from vodka and their wine glasses were smaller!

Rather amazingly, Khaf Lasuria smoked about a pack of cigarettes a day—and she inhaled! She began smoking in 1910. A small number of old people in these three regions smoked, but many reportedly did not inhale.

Leaf was surprised to find a handful of overweight centenarians in Georgia, but they too worked and walked vigorously in the mountains. Exercise is almost certainly one key to longevity.

OTHER GERONTOLOGICAL RESEARCH IN VILCABAMBA, HUNZA, AND GEORGIAN RUSSIA

A Russian gerontologist studied more than 15,000 people older than the age of 80 in Georgia and found that more than 70 percent of them walked regularly in the mountains and more than 60 percent of them still worked. Oldsters who failed to maintain useful roles tended to die sooner.

With modern investigative techniques, one Georgian cardiologist and gerontologist, Dr. David Kakiashvili, tested the hearts and lungs of many of the old. He found many had silent cardiovascular diseases that had never caused any symptoms. All had exercise-induced superior cardiopulmonary function, which he believed was protecting them. Dr. Miguel Salvador, a well-known and respected Ecuadoran cardiologist, extensively studied 338 elderly Vilcabambans and found only 1 with a weak heart.

In several studies (dating back to 1932) of the Abkhasians that were made by other Georgian gerontologists, only the slightest signs of heart conditions were ever found, these in some of the very old. No reported cases of cancer occurred in a nine-year study of 123 people who were more than 100 years old; the vast majority were also found to have good neurological and psychological stability. A study of the vision of another group over the age of 90 found that 40 percent of the men and 30 percent of the women were able to thread a needle without glasses; hearing was good in 40 percent of the group.

Further evidence of an absence of chronic diseases in Vilcabamba was provided by Dr. Jorge Santiana, a cancer specialist and an associate of Salvador. Santiana also visited Vilcabamba and examined many of its elderly. He found only one growth—benign.

Most old people in Georgia were married. The study of 15,000 Georgians older than 80 revealed that, with rare exceptions, only married people attained extreme age. Many couples had been married upward of seventy and eighty years. Among centenarians, 91 percent of the women had two or more children; 68 percent had four or more. Only 2.5 percent were childless. Among both men and women, a strong interest in sexual activity was considered normal into old age; an active sex life well into one's nineties was not unusual.

In contrast, Davies had found in Vilcabamba that most women older than 100 had never married. The life of married women there was considerably harder; they were overworked, treated as sexual objects, and exhausted by middle age. Of fifty married women interviewed, all but one over the age of 25 had between four and fourteen children, many more than the women in Georgia.

People of the cultures discussed above expected to live long lives; young people interviewed spoke of living to 100. Old people enjoyed high social status and were esteemed for their wisdom and experience. Multigeneration extended-family households were universal, and the word of the eldest family members was generally regarded as law. Even people well over 100 continued tending animals, gardening, caring for children, working in the fields on a limited basis, and performing domestic chores.

Common elements are present among long-lived people, but having a long and healthy life is an individual matter. In dietary matters as in other habits, each person—within the framework of what was available—set his or her own patterns. Individual diets undoubtedly had an influence on individual longevity.

Foods used in the three regions have much in common, but there is conflicting and somewhat confusing evidence. We'll now examine the diet of each place to provide a basis for contrasts, comparisons, and conclusions.

THE IMPACT OF DIET ON LONGEVITY

In Georgian Russia

Soviet gerontologists studied dietary habits of 1,000 people over the age of eighty, including more than 100 centenarians. These oldsters consumed plenty of animal products, including plenty of fatty pork and whole milk. They ate lots of vegetables as well, along with their meat, milk products, and eggs. The proportions were nearly identical to the average found in contemporary hunter-gatherer cultures and correspond with estimates of the diet of hunter-gatherer cultures existing at the beginning of the agricultural revolution.

The caloric intake of these Georgians was estimated at seventeen hundred to nineteen hundred calories per day. This is very low, especially considering their high level of physical activity. Soured raw milk, usually from goats, and raw-milk cheeses were consumed at nearly all of their meals. Eggs were commonly eaten as well. Most people kept chickens, goats, and often pigs and sheep. These animals were eaten regularly, always including the organ meats, and there were many meat courses on festive occasions. Protein intake was estimated to be between seventy to ninety grams per day.

Vegetable gardens were kept by most people. Fruits were common, but were not a large part of the diet. Grain staples included whole-grain bread baked in outdoor ovens and unflavored cornmeal-mush patties eaten with sauces spiced with hot red pepper. Homemade butter and homemade wine, as well as pork, were consumed daily, and many people enjoyed small amounts of homemade grape vodka.

In Vilcabamba and in Coastal Ecaudor

The village of Vilcabamba lies thirty miles southwest of Loja, a small town some five hundred mountainous miles south of Quito, the capital of Ecuador. *Vilca* means "sacred" and *bamba* means "valley" in the language of the Quechua Indians who once inhabited the area. Legend has it this valley was the original paradise of Adam and Eve; myths and romantic stories abound. Visitors say a very special atmosphere permeates the place.

The valley is nearly at the equator, and the altitude at the village is a little over five thousand feet. The temperature is steady year-round—usually about sixty-eight degrees at midday. Chief crops of the valley and adjacent mountain slopes are wheat, barley, yucca root, corn, and some grapes. Coffee and sugarcane are grown for export. A wide variety of green vegetables, legumes, celery, cauliflower, and cabbages are also grown.

Most of the elderly lived on small mountain farms and grew vegetables and raised animals. Soured milk products were consumed, though less so than in Georgia. By some reports, the Vilcabambans ate little animal protein—an average of twelve grams per day—according to an Ecuadoran medical team that studied the elderly there. But Davies details typical meals with centenarians that included raw or lightly boiled eggs, cottage cheese—high in fat, made fresh from cows' or goats' milk—and occasionally fresh meat. Many centenarian families had more meat because one member was a herdsman. Pigs were kept and pork was commonly eaten. Both eggs and cheese were commonly consumed as well, although less so than in Georgia because Vilcabamba was poor and its people could not keep as many animals as the Georgians.

Few English-speaking people had visited Vilcabamba when Davies wrote his book. Scant original information about their diet has been written; most accounts are repetitions of the few original reports, particularly that of the Ecuadoran medical team. Davies's book indicated that more eggs, milk products, and meat were eaten by old people than had been reported in several popular books by individuals who had never visited Vilcabamba.

Davies spent time in the mountains visiting centenarians, and he learned that they all kept chickens and dairy animals and often pigs. Davies tells of his stay with one centenarian family. At dawn, the old man hiked fifteen minutes up a steep mountainside to his fields, bringing back fresh corn while his wife gathered eggs around the house.

These foods would typically be lightly boiled and eaten with homemade brown bread, boiled beans, homemade raw cottage cheese, and perhaps yucca, wild potatoes, fruits, or green vegetables. Meat and organ meats were eaten if an animal had been killed recently.

Vilcabamban villagers, who were more accessible to other investigators, did not keep as many animals as the Vilcabambans who lived in the mountains.

The Ecuadoran medical team did not single out centenarians in their studies of the elderly; their data, based on a sampling of older people in the village, did not specifically reflect the average diet of centenarians.

The details of the diets of centenarians as a group and of individual centenarians might provide invaluable clues about longevity. A detailed examination of the food and lifestyles of individual centenarians (including analysis of fat-soluble nutrients and vitamin and mineral content) would add another dimension to our understanding of these people. Other considerations would include the quality of the soil and the health and diet of animals used for milk, meat, and eggs.

Many Vilcabambans had only limited amounts of animal foods; the amounts were not quite adequate for many of the people. More were available to Georgians, and fishermen centenarians certainly were richly supplied. The Vilcabambans suffered from loss of teeth, perhaps because their diets lacked adequate fat-soluble protective nutrients found only in animal-sourced foods. But foods available to them were of the highest quality and were sufficient both to protect them from most problems and to give many of them great longevity.

These issues are complex. While many claimed Vilcabambans lived so long because they consumed little food of animal origin, I believe that the evidence indicates they lived so long in spite of it. What they did consume was of the highest quality, and most likely provided high levels of fat-soluble vitamins.

Witness the Georgian centenarians. The very old eventually lost some teeth, but Davies and other investigators report that most had very good teeth. Mortality rates of infants and young children were low. The diet was rich in meat and dairy foods of the highest quality and also in fat-soluble nutrients, which were found in substantial quantities only in these foods and in fish. These nutrients are known to control mineral metabolism (thus the effect on dental health), benefit the immune system, and have a host of other profound beneficial effects. Like the Ecuadoran team's study, the study in Georgia of one thousand people over the age of eighty grouped all data and presented averages; no search was made for differences between diets of centenarians and those of the rest of the elderly.

The high mortality rates that Davies found among the young in Vilcabamba also may be explained in part by these same considerations; many simply did not have sufficient strength to resist disease. Apparently nutrition that is adequate in most ways for adults is not adequate for the very young or for pregnant women. Imagine a population living in a way conducive to good health and longevity, and eating optimal foods, but without quite enough of certain foods and associated nutrients. Some problems must appear somewhere—although the people as a whole may be healthy and many might live to be very old. Is it not logical and even expected that nature would find a way to limit the population and prevent further scarcity? Nature's way is to take the weakest of the young, both in human and in wildlife populations.

Birth control was practiced by virtually all native cultures that Weston Price studied. These cultures were conscious of the need to space children at least three years apart, and they accomplished this through customs and tribal laws. Further, to ensure healthy children, women ate special foods before and during pregnancy and while nursing. Young children ate special foods as well.

Any such customs regarding the spacing of children among Vilcabambans were lost as they became Roman Catholics after the arrival of the Spanish; the practice of any form of birth control was forbidden. Very large families, with no planned spacing of children, resulted, along with frequent deaths among infants and young children and reduced longevity among the women.

Among elderly Vilcabambans, even with the loss of teeth, their gums and jaws remained strong. The misery accompanying the decay and extensive loss of teeth that marked the introduction of refined foods in the cultures Price studied was conspicuously absent; teeth simply fell out in middle and later years. The people had the strength and resilience to adapt to this loss.

Vilcabambans ate more meat and milk products when they were available, for example, if one family member was a herdsman. Their consumption of animal foods was limited by scarcity rather than choice.

Several elements of Vilcabamban life are disconcerting, including the high death rate among the young and the dental problem. Davies also observed that the men often did not treat the women very well and tended to drink excessively quite frequently. Married women spoke of being unhappy with their lot in life, as did some very old women who had never married. Many people smoked (compared with only a few in Georgian Russia). The balance and happiness found in the people of Georgia was seldom seen among the Vilcabambans, except perhaps among the mountain farmers.

Two other men reportedly more than 125 years old both lived on the coast of Ecuador and had been fishermen, as was the case for the majority of that country's isolated individual centenarians. Davies did not investigate them because he believed that isolated, remarkable individuals might live to a great age simply because of their great stamina. His interest was in examining environments where large numbers of centenarians lived, looking for influences upon the aging process. But Davies writes that in his previous studies of surviving primitive cultures (he had led expeditions studying several primitive societies and had authored several books about his work) he often found individuals living to a great age near the sea.

This is a significant clue in understanding longevity because the quality of animal life of the sea is similar to that of the dairy products, eggs, and meat produced in the mountains of Vilcabamba, Georgian Russia, and Hunza. Protective nutrients richly supplied in fish, free-ranging animals, milk products, and eggs from such animals are common elements in diets of coastal and mountain centenarians throughout the world.

In Hunza

Hunza, in the Himalayas, was isolated when studied by Dr. Alexander Leaf in the 1970s. The nearest air travel was to Gilgit, Pakistan, and even then only in good weather, through a narrow mountain gorge. Several days' travel over difficult mountain roads was then required to reach Hunza. Permission to visit, granted by the Pakistani government and the ruler of Hunza, was difficult to obtain. Those who visited were unable to accurately document the ages of the elderly, for there was neither a written language nor birth records, and as a result, the reports of Western visitors are conflicting.

Sir Robert McCarrison, a British physician who worked in India for nearly thirty years, spent much of his time between 1904 and 1911 in Hunza. He later wrote in *Studies in Deficiency Diseases* that the people were "unsurpassed in perfection of physique and in freedom from disease in general. . . . The span of life is extraordinarily long. . . . I never saw a case of asthenic dyspepsia, of gastric or duodenal ulcer, or appendicitis, of mucous colitis, or cancer." The Hunzas and their diet inspired McCarrison's animal-feeding experiments.

John Clark's *Hunza, Lost Kingdom of the Himalayas*, was published in 1956 and detailed his twenty months in Hunza in 1950 and 1951. The holder of a doctorate in geology, Clark was a professor and research associate at Princeton University at the time of his book's publication. He had first spent time in the Far East as an army engineer during World War II, and subsequently returned on his own to see what he could do to help what he described as a small, poverty-stricken Asian country. He had training in anatomy, first aid, and public health, plus he had twenty years of field experience in first aid, obtained while working as a geologist in remote areas.

Clark's purpose in Hunza was both humanitarian and political; he wanted to teach the people technological expertise about farming, animal husbandry, and modern woodcrafting, which would enable them to raise their standard of living and turn away from possible Communist influences. While he did not formally survey the health and longevity of the people, he did record in detail his observations and experiences.

At the urging of the mir, the hereditary ruler of the country, Clark set up a medical dispensary upon his arrival. He describes the people as desperately poor, sometimes malnourished, and much in need of medical help for a variety of problems, including malaria, dysentery, worms, impetigo, goiter, dental decay, rickets, and tuberculosis. He saw many of these problems daily during his entire time in Hunza, often treating fifty to sixty people a day, using antibiotics, sulfa drugs, and antimalarials he had brought into the country. Eventually he was forced by the Pakistani government to leave; his plans for helping the Hunzas improve their way of life and escape poverty had been rejected.

The book *Hunza Land: The Fabulous Health and Youth Wonderland of the World,* by Renée Taylor, based on her travels in Hunza, was published in the early 1960s and was followed by a film, *Hunza: The Valley of Eternal Youth.* Taylor wrote several other books about Hunza, stating there was little or no sickness of any kind, no need for doctors, and that Hunza was "the land of just enough." She stayed at the Royal Palace and quotes the mir extensively. She wrote that many of the people were more than 100 years old and that virtually everyone was healthy and happy. No documentation was offered about the health status of any of the people.

Alexander Leaf wrote of Hunza that he had an impression of many extremely fit and vigorous old people moving about the very mountainous countryside. A picture of a man said to be the oldest in Hunza and claiming to be 110 is shown; Leaf regarded the age as approximate. Leaf apparently did little field work or interviewing in Hunza, and his only comment on the Hunzas' health and longevity was to report that the mir, from his personal knowledge of the states' history, verified the ages of many of the elderly.

The above accounts indicate that some people in Hunza likely enjoyed quantities of raw grass-fed dairy products, but that for many the diet may at times have been sparse in animal foods because few families could afford more than one or two animals. The country is in the high Himalayas, and villages and farms are largely built on steep valley hillsides; usable land is crowded. Clark wrote there was no winter pasture, and summer pasture was much overgrazed; the land would maintain few animals.

Chapatti was a mainstay of the diet. It is a flatbread made from wheat, barley, buckwheat, or millet flour freshly ground from whole grain—kneaded and baked over an open fire. Sprouted seeds were consumed, as were fresh vegetables; the people all farmed small plots of land. Apricots, mulberries, grapes, and walnuts were grown; the grapes were made into homemade wine. Apricot seeds were both eaten and made into an edible oil. When an animal was butchered, every possible edible portion was consumed. Clark wrote that this would typically be only twice a year; then meat would be eaten for a week or so.

Milk available was mostly from goats; milk and buttermilk was often used sour. Butter and cottage cheese were made. Those who cared for animals in high summer pastures likely ate much of these foods; most of the population had less.

Robert McCarrison's account of Hunza is an objective medical report by a physician who knew the country well. McCarrison was one of the fathers of modern nutritional science; a list of his experiments, research papers, and the honors he received during his career would fill pages. His character, creative intelligence, and ability to record objectively the situation in turn-of-the-century Hunza cannot be questioned.

Reports since then are both scarce and conflicting. John Clark's previously mentioned book, *Hunza, Lost Kingdom of the Himalayas,* is a well written and carefully constructed account of his nearly two years of living among the people of Hunza. The illnesses he reported were acute infectious processes and deficiency states, rather than chronic diseases. Prevailing problems may well have reflected deficiencies of adequate nutrients from animal sources, compounded in some cases by inadequate total caloric intake. The Hunzakuts went through a period each spring, just before fresh foods began growing, when very little food was available.

The legend of Hunza was strong before John Clark's time in the kingdom. He writes in his preface: "I wish also to express my regrets to those travelers whose impressions have been contradicted by my experience. On my first trip through Hunza, I acquired almost all the misconceptions they did: The Healthy Hunzas, The Democratic Court, The Land Where There Are No Poor, and the rest—and only long-continued living in Hunza revealed the actual situations. I take no pleasure in either debunking or confirming a statement, but it has been necessary clearly to state the truth as I experienced it."

There is no reason to doubt Clark. Taylor's and other later accounts were written by some of the few Westerners who were allowed into the country; their visits were brief. As guests of the mir who stayed at his palace, they may have seen no more than the ruler wished. A film was made, this too perhaps influenced by official decisions about content. The creation of a myth may have been considered desirable. The myth has been further perpetuated by popularizers of vegetarian and largely vegetarian diets.

Early and reliable reports such as McCarrison's established Hunza as a rather special and healthy place; hence it was that much easier to later create and perpetuate a popular legend. But if McCarrison's account of Hunza from 1904 through 1911 and Clark's account of Hunza in 1950 and 1951 are both accurate, we are left to account for why things changed.

This is difficult. The capacity of the land may have been overextended; by the time of Clark's tenure in Hunza every square inch was in use. But in a land that prospered for more than two thousand years, why did problems develop in less than fifty? It seems likely that some refined foods had been introduced. For whatever reasons, John Clark's book makes clear that by 1950, a small but significant percentage of the people of Hunza suffered from problems directly caused by inadequate nutrition; he reports treating more than five thousand people during his time in the country.

CONCLUSIONS ABOUT LONG-LIVED PEOPLE

Conflicting reports generate controversy, but we are left with reasonable proof that people in Vilcabamba and Georgian Russia lived to be very much older than most authorities state is possible, and that they did so with great vigor. This may have been the case in Hunza as well. An extremely active, emotionally rewarding life and a special kind of natural diet featuring foods from grass-fed animals appear to be the influences most responsible.

Georgians have demonstrated the most resistance to health problems, whereas Vilcabambans and Hunzas suffered from problems uncommon in Georgian Russia. The Georgians alone obtained sufficient amounts of protective nutrients, especially fats that were richly supplied by their grass-fed meat and dairy foods.

IMPACTS OF THE TRADITIONAL AMERICAN DIET ON LIFE EXPECTANCY

Foods that rural preindustrial America relied upon were similar to those consumed by the residents of Georgian Russia. One hundred twenty-five years ago, half of Americans lived on farms. They made bread from whole grains; grew vegetables and stored and preserved the surplus; raised beef cattle on grass without chemicals and hormones; kept chickens, pigs, and dairy animals at pasture; fished in creeks and rivers; and hunted for wild game. Many people living near the coast fished daily; others combined elements of farming and fishing life. People spent their days outdoors, working. They walked a lot.

Their milk and cheeses were raw and high in fat, their gardens free of pesticides, their grains whole, their animals healthy, free of hormones, and eating their natural diets. The diet of American farm people included lots of butter, cream, and lard. This was roughly the diet of Georgian Russians and of traditional people everywhere who cultivated plants and kept animals for food.

These people were largely free of the diseases of civilization—hypertension, heart disease, arthritis, colitis, obesity, diabetes, cancer, and stroke—to name the more common. Well into the twentieth century in America, these diseases had nowhere near the prevalence they have today.

The average age of death in America in 1900 was forty-five to fifty years of age. But one-third of all babies died in infancy or early childhood, keeping the average down. Sanitation in cities was poor, and the nutrition of people in cities did not begin to compare to that of people who lived on farms. Antibiotics and advances in public health, combined with resultant improvements in sanitation, have drastically reduced death among the young. Average life expectancy is thus up to seventy-five years, but the average forty-year-old today can expect to live only four years longer than the average forty-year-old could expect to live in 1900. Health and quality of life for the elderly have declined; the very prevalence of chronic disease implies extended suffering that in the past occurred on a much more limited scale.

One hundred years ago, many deaths at very young ages caused the average life expectancy to be only forty-five to fifty years, despite the fact that many people lived to be sixty, seventy, eighty, and older. A somewhat larger percentage of people today live to those ages; the claim is made that this is why there is a rising incidence of chronic disease. But the moderate increase in the percentage of people living longer today has been nowhere nearly enough to account for the increases of several hundred percent that have occurred in the incidence of each of the diseases mentioned above. Each now afflicts many people before they reach fifty or even forty. While unusual or even rare among the population as a whole 100 years ago, most of these diseases were then nearly or literally unheard of at age forty or fifty.

Protective nutrients are found in the native diets Weston Price studied, in the raw-food diets of Pottenger's experiments and clinical work (detailed in the next chapter), in ancestral and contemporary hunter-gatherer diets, and in the diets of long-lived people. When present, these nutrients exert extremely beneficial effects; their relative deficiency in modern diets may well prove to be the ultimate cause of the growing epidemic of modern degenerative diseases.

In the next chapter we will examine the nutrients that are found in raw foods, and detail the work of Dr. Francis Pottenger, Jr., who studied the effects of raw food in cats.

5
THE BENEFITS OF RAW FOOD AS DETERMINED BY DR. FRANCIS POTTENGER, JR.

Archaeological evidence indicates humans used fire at least four hundred thousand years ago; splintered and charred bones of large mammals that Peking man hunted littered his caves. These early humans probably used fire to help get at the marrow, and they may have roasted some meat.

Cooked food is more quickly chewed than raw and thus the change from an entirely raw to a partially cooked diet freed some time formerly spent eating. The time was now spent cooking. Cooking has always been both social and practical, combined with elements of ceremony, habit, convenience, and pleasure.

A home heated by wood gathers people near a fire for hours in cold months. In caves and later primitive shelters, cooking and sharing meals around the warmth of fire was an everyday routine; it has been so in all native cultures since. And yet in every native culture examined, anthropologists find that customs dictate certain foods be eaten raw. Reasons given by the people invariably relate to preventing disease, ensuring fertility, and promoting optimal growth in children.

THE WORK OF DR. FRANCIS POTTENGER, JR.

Francis M. Pottenger, Jr. was a physician and researcher whose work demonstrated that raw foods contain unique nutrients vital to human beings. Part of his research included a now-classic series of controlled experiments that involved more than nine hundred cats for more than ten years. He also kept detailed records of his thousands of human patients for more than thirty years. He discovered correlations between the cat experiments, the discoveries of his contemporary Weston Price, and his clinical work treating people with chronic and acute diseases.

The son of the physician who founded the once-famous Pottenger Sanatorium for the treatment of tuberculosis in Monrovia, California, Pottenger completed his residency at Los Angeles County Hospital in 1930 and became a full-time assistant at the sanatorium. From 1932 to 1942, he also conducted what became known as the "Pottenger's Cats" study.

In 1940, he founded the Francis M. Pottenger, Jr. Hospital at Monrovia. Until closing in 1960, the hospital specialized in treating nontubercular diseases of the respiratory system, especially asthma. Pottenger maintained his private practice until his death in 1967.

A regular and prolific contributor to the medical and scientific literature, Pottenger served as president of several professional organizations, including the Los Angeles County Medical Association, the American Academy of Applied Nutrition, and the American Therapeutic Society. He was a member of a long list of other professional organizations.

Pottenger's Cats and Raw Foods: The Ten-Year Study

Extracts from adrenal glands of cows and steers were part of treatment that patients received at the tuberculosis sanatorium, which manufactured the extracts from fresh glands shipped from Denver and Los Angeles. No laboratory assays capable of determining hormone content of biological extracts existed in the 1930s. To determine potency, cats that had had their adrenal glands removed were kept alive with extract; the amount required to maintain animals adequately determined the level of that batch's potency.

Despite careful surgical techniques and a diet of raw milk, cod-liver oil, and meat scraps from the sanatorium kitchen, many cats died after the surgery to remove their adrenal glands. There was no obvious explanation, but the cats showed signs of nutritional deficiencies. Many had problems reproducing, and many kittens born in the laboratory pens had skeletal malformations and internal malfunctions.

Pottenger had a keen interest in nutrition; a high-protein and fat natural-food diet was an important part of treatment at the sanatorium. Liver, tripe, brains, sweetbreads, and heart were fed to patients; scraps, all cooked, were fed to cats. When the cat population grew because Pottenger's neighbors donated so many, he began securing raw meat scraps for some cats.

These cats were, before long, in plainly better health than cats consuming cooked meat. Their postoperative mortality markedly decreased, they reproduced more easily, and their kittens were healthier.

This inspired Pottenger to embark on a series of controlled experiments. Because pathological problems in cats eating cooked meats were similar to those in his patients, he believed a controlled-feeding experiment with animals would isolate variables of importance in human nutrition as well.

The experiments met the most rigorous scientific standards of his day. Pottenger's outstanding credentials earned him the support of prominent physicians. Alvin G. Foord, M.D., professor of pathology at the University of Southern California and pathologist at the Huntington Memorial Hospital in Pasadena, co-supervised with Pottenger all pathological and chemical findings of the study.

The technology of science has grown more sophisticated since Pottenger's study, as the search for causes of disease has moved to the intracellular level. But because of the strength of his insights, Pottenger's inquiries and observations provide demonstrations about fundamentals of nutrition and disease.

Two areas of inquiry in particular address questions modern science has largely ignored. First, what is the nutritive value of heat-labile elements—nutrients destroyed by heat and available only in raw and undercooked foods? Second, what determines the difference in nutritional value between one animal and another, one egg and another, one glass of milk and another? Pottenger's ten-year study answers these questions through an inquiry into the difference between raw and cooked meat, raw milk and pasteurized milk, and fresh greens versus dry greens. We will examine these areas of study in further detail next.

Raw Meat versus Cooked Meat

Effects of a raw-meat diet fed to one group of cats versus those of a cooked-meat diet fed another were measured in the initial experiment, begun in 1932. The raw-meat diet consisted of raw meat, including bones and organs such as liver, heart, brains, kidneys, and pancreas; raw milk; and cod-liver oil. The cooked-meat diet was exactly the same except for the fact that the meats were cooked. In both diets, raw milk was "market-grade"—milk available commercially. A high-grade raw milk from cows kept at pasture or fed fresh-cut greens was later used in select experiments.

Cats were kept in large outdoor pens, and successive generations were followed. The raw-meat group reproduced easily, and as each generation developed there was, for each sex, striking uniformity in size and skeletal development. A broad face with wide dental arches and no crowding of teeth was the rule. Fur was uniform, with good sheen and little shedding. Inflammation and diseases of the gums were rare.

These animals were resistant to infections, fleas, and other parasites. They were friendly, even tempered, and well coordinated—when dropped from up to six feet or thrown, they always landed on all four feet. Miscarriages were rare, and litters averaged five kittens. Cause of death was generally old age, or occasionally fighting among males. Autopsies invariably revealed normal internal organs.

The cooked-meat group showed many contrasts to the raw-meat group, contrasts that grew with successive generations. Litter mates varied greatly in size and skeletal structure, particularly in dental and facial pattern. Often by the third generation bones had become so soft as to be actually rubbery. Vision problems, infections of internal organs and bones, arthritis, heart problems, underactivity of the thyroid gland, inflammation of the joints and nervous system, skin lesions, allergies, intestinal parasites and vermin, and a host of other pathologies were common. Coordination was poor—when tossed a short distance, the cats had trouble landing on all four feet. Pneumonia and lung abscesses were the most usual causes of death in adults; pneumonia and diarrhea were the usual causes in kittens.

At autopsy, analysis of the bones of cooked-meat animals determined calcium and phosphorous content for second- and third-generation kittens to be one-third to one-half that of raw-meat kittens. A marked difference between the two groups was also found in the average calcium to phosphorous ratio (2.08 to 1 for raw-meat kittens versus 2.63 to 1 for cooked-meat kittens).

Many cooked-meat kittens exhibited behavioral changes; females were irritable and aggressive, while males were often docile and unaggressive with little interest in females but keen interest in other males (an interest never seen in males fed the raw-meat diet). Abnormal sexual activities also were seen between females in the cooked-meat group. At autopsy, females often showed small ovaries with a congested uterus; males frequently showed testes that had failed to develop the ability to produce sperm.

Cats born outside the Pottenger Sanatorium, donated to the study and placed on the cooked-meat diet, were called first-generation deficient cats. Kittens born of them and fed the cooked-meat diet were called second-generation deficient cats. Kittens born of second-generation deficient cats and fed the cooked-meat diet were called third-generation deficient cats.

The miscarriage rate among first-generation deficient females was about 25 percent, among second-generation deficient females, about 70 percent. Many cats died in labor; deliveries were difficult; many kittens were born dead or too frail to nurse. The kittens born of cooked-meat mothers weighed an average of nineteen grams less than those of raw-meat mothers.

No fourth-generation deficient kittens were ever born in the ten years of the study. Third-generation deficient kittens always died before reaching six months of age, terminating the strain.

Raw Milk versus Pasteurized Milk

Four groups of cats were used in this part of the study. For one-third of the diet, all of them received raw meat, which included organs and cod-liver oil. The other two-thirds were either raw milk, pasteurized milk, evaporated milk, or sweetened condensed milk. The rawmilk, raw-meat diet produced many generations of healthy cats, while the various heat-processed milk and raw-meat diets produced successively sicker cats unable to reproduce by the third generation. The inclusion of one-third raw meat in the cooked-milk diets did not prevent severe problems.

The most degeneration occurred in cats fed sweetened condensed milk; they became extremely irritable and nervous and developed heavy fat deposits and marked skeletal deformities. Cats fed evaporated milk were nearly as damaged. Those fed pasteurized milk showed lesser damage, similar to that seen in the animals of the prior experiment that ate cooked meat—that is, skeletal changes, decreased reproductive capacity, and infectious and degenerative diseases (problems that were among those seen in the sweetened condensed-milk and evaporated-milk groups).

In a variation of this experiment, the effects of raw milk from cows fed fresh greens versus those of raw milk from cows fed dry feed were compared. Cats fed cooked meat and raw milk from fresh-feed cows did significantly better than cats fed cooked meat and raw milk from dry-feed cows. The latter produced deficient kittens and had difficulty nursing. Deficiencies were much less marked for animals fed cooked meat and also fed raw milk from fresh-feed cows.

The fresh greens apparently contained critically important nutrients that were lost when the greens were dried.

Fresh Greens versus Dried Greens

Guinea pigs were used to compare the effects of fresh greens versus dried greens directly. A group of these animals was fed grains, cod-liver oil, and field-dried alfalfa. Deficiency symptoms appeared—loss of hair, diarrhea, pneumonia, paralysis, and high infant mortality. Fresh-cut greens were then introduced (grass cut after sundown, sacked, and delivered before sunrise). The animals gained weight, infant deaths decreased, loss of hair decreased, and no new cases of paralysis developed.

Some guinea pigs that had developed severe symptoms initially and had not fully recovered were then allowed to feed on grass and weeds growing outside their pens. Within a few weeks, all diarrhea and loss of hair stopped, and their hair was soft, shiny, and velvety; the animals appeared even healthier than those kept inside the pens on fresh-cut greens. Seeking an explanation, Pottenger discovered that the temperature inside sacks of cut grass used for feed was from five to thirty degrees warmer than the outside air. The grass had become somewhat cooked in the sacks, and heat-labile nutrients apparently had been altered. The health of the animals suffered as a result.

THE WORK OF DR. ROBERT MCCARRISON

Pottenger was not the first to maintain experimental animals for extended periods on natural food. From 1902 until 1935, Robert McCarrison, a British physician in the Indian Medical Service and founder of the Nutrition Research Laboratories at Coonoor, India, studied goiter and other health problems of the Indian people. He did extensive experiments with large populations of laboratory animals and in 1933 published a report containing statistics about several studies.

In conjunction with those studies, McCarrison kept a control colony of about one thousand white rats for more than three years. The animals were killed and autopsied when they were two years old. In more than fifteen hundred autopsies, no sign of disease was ever found. In the three years, there was no illness, no death from natural causes, and no infantile mortality. The animals were fed whole-wheat-flour cakes of unleavened bread lightly smeared with raw butter, sprouts, raw carrots, cabbage, raw milk, raw meat, and bones once a week. All foods were fresh; the animals lived in large, airy, clean rooms, and were exposed to the sun daily.

PARALLELS BETWEEN POTTENGER'S AND PRICE'S WORK

While the experiments of McCarrison and Pottenger show the value of raw foods in keeping animals remarkably healthy, one might wonder about relevance to human needs. Cats are carnivores, humans omnivores, and while the animals' natural diet is raw, humans have cooked some foods for hundreds of thousands of years. But humans, cats, and guinea pigs are all mammals. And while the human diet is omnivorous, foods of animal origin (some customarily eaten raw) have always formed a substantial and essential part of it.

Problems in cats eating cooked foods provided parallels with the human populations Weston Price studied; the cats developed the same diseases as humans eating refined foods. The deficient generation of cats developed the same dental malformations that children of people eating modernized foods developed, including narrowing of dental arches with attendant crowding of teeth, underbites and overbites, and protruding and crooked teeth. The shape of the cat's skull and even the entire skeleton became abnormal in severe cases, with concomitant marked behavioral changes.

Price observed these same physical and behavioral changes in both native and modern cultures eating refined foods. These changes accompanied the adoption by a culture of refined foods. In native cultures eating entirely according to traditional wisdom resulted in strength of character and relative freedom from the moral problems of modern cultures. In modern cultures, studies of populations of prisons, reformatories, and homes for the mentally delayed revealed that a large majority of individuals residing there (often approaching 100 percent) had marked abnormalities of the dental arch, often with accompanying changes in the shape of the skull.

This was not coincidence; thinking is a biological process, and abnormal changes in the shape of the skull from one generation to the next can contribute to changes in brain functions and thus in behavior. The behavioral changes in deficient cats were due to changes in nutrition. This was the only variable in Pottenger's carefully controlled experiments. As with physical degenerative changes, parallels with human populations cannot help but suggest themselves, although the specific nature of the relationship is beyond the scope of this discussion.

Human beings do not have the same nutritional requirements as cats, but whatever else each needs, there is strong empirical evidence that both need a significant amount of certain high-quality raw foods to reproduce and function efficiently.

THE NEED FOR A UNIFIED BIOLOGICAL THEORY

Beginning with Albert Einstein, theoretical physicists have sought a single encompassing theory uniting the theories of relativity, electromagnetism, and gravity. Although details of such a theory may remain elusive, many believe an encompassing explanation for the physical phenomena of the universe will indeed be found.

Such a theory, however, will not explain the biology of the degenerative physical and mental changes that have accompanied the abandonment of humanity's traditional primal foods and the adoption of the refined foods of modern industrial society. To explain our modern predicament—and guide us out of it—we need a unified biological theory, based on an understanding of humanity's roots; one that attempts to work in harmony with forces inexorably shaping us. Physics seeks an understanding of physical forces affecting the universe; human health requires an understanding of biological forces in foods that affect human destiny.

THE BENEFITS OF RAW FOODS

Enhanced Calcium Metabolism

Pottenger maintained inpatient facilities and an outpatient practice for more than thirty years, giving him an opportunity to study the effects of his nutritional programs on many patients. He observed problems with calcium metabolism in a majority. Poor development of the teeth is the first and most obvious sign. Later, arthritis appears; nearly all older people in America today show symptoms of it.

Other problems commonly connected with faulty calcium metabolism include back problems and other skeletal disorders. These include spondylitis; gallstones and kidney stones; atherosclerosis, often leading to coronary heart attacks; hardening of the arteries of the brain, often leading to strokes; cataracts; and bursitis. Deposition of calcium in abnormal places is their common denominator.

Though many people develop these problems eating diets deficient in calcium, so too do others consuming diets rich in calcium. A diet rich in calcium (including calcium supplements and vitamin supplements to aid in the assimilation of calcium) does not prevent or reverse these problems unless the diet contains adequate amounts of fresh raw foods.

Pottenger found clues about calcium problems in X-ray studies documenting changes in the skeletal system of his patients (the dangers of X-rays were little understood in his time). One study compared skeletal structures and bone age (the development of the growth center of bones in relation to the standard for a child of that age) in 150 children drinking four different types of milk—breast milk, raw-certified milk, pasteurized milk, and canned milk.

The only group with consistently excellent development of the bones and skeleton and with normal bone age was the group drinking raw-certified milk. Nearly all of the children drinking pasteurized milk or canned milk developed either very fine small bones, disturbances in the calcification of bones, or marked weaknesses in joints and ligaments. Bone age in a majority of these children was below normal.

Among children fed breast milk, development of bones was dependent on the diet and state of health of the mother. Children of mothers using high-quality foods, including raw-certified milk and raw greens, had well-developed bones displaying normal bone age. Children of mothers using diets including the cooked milks had bones with delayed development of growth centers and poor calcification, and weak joints. Breast milk is superior to raw-certified milk only if the diet of the mother is of proper quality.

Chronic Disease Deterrent

Dr. Josef Romig told Weston Price that modernized Eskimos and Indians with tuberculosis usually recovered when returned to their native villages and native diets. Native Eskimo and northern Indian diets were similar to the diet Pottenger successfully used for patients with tuberculosis and other diseases. Liberal amounts of liver, heart, pancreas, kidney, brain, tripe, meat, fish and shellfish, fertile eggs, and raw milk were used; organs were emphasized.

Much of this diet, including the organs, was served raw, in a variety of recipes. Much of the food, including the meat, was ecologically produced. Food was cooked as lightly as was palatable for the patient. Raw vegetable salads with sprouts were served twice daily. Breads made from sprouted whole grains were baked at low temperatures, minimizing the destruction of nutrients. Bone meal and marrow were also prepared at low temperatures. Small quantities of fruit and sesame seeds were consumed, and the use of vegetable oils was minimized. This type of diet, carefully individualized for each patient and usually including some fish and shellfish, is integral to the approach to chronic disease that I have used successfully for many years.

RAW FOODS AND THE DIGESTIVE SYSTEM

The digestive system adapts well to raw foods introduced at a rate appropriate for the individual. An acute inflammation in the digestive tract—gastritis, ulcers, colitis, certain types of diarrhea, for example—may be easily irritated by raw vegetables or fruits, which should in such cases be slowly introduced only when the acute problem has resolved and healing has begun.

But for most people, becoming accustomed to more raw foods in the diet involves mental more than physical obstacles. While cooking or fermentation does indeed make many foods more digestible, the healthy human digestive system is fully capable of digesting a wide variety of foods raw. Many foods may be more easily chewed when cooked, but for the fully functioning human digestive tract, many foods are most easily digested when they are eaten raw or lightly cooked. This is particularly true of most animal foods, salad greens, and fruits. But many people really cannot digest raw vegetables and some of these vegetables—kale, spinach, cabbage, potatoes—should not be eaten raw.

Colloidal cellulose and pectins in plants can withstand greater temperatures than can proteins; this is why cooking has a less pronounced effect on the digestibility of most plants than on that of animal-sourced foods. In fact, uncooked pectins and certain other fiber can be harmful, and cooking makes many vegetables more digestible. While cats indeed thrive on an all-raw diet, humans do best on a modern primal diet that includes a balance of cooked and raw foods.

In the ten-year cat study, the cats that had cooked foods were consistently found at autopsy to have much longer intestines than the cats that had been fed raw food. Intestines of the former had many distensions and a general lack of tone; the length was often up to twice that of the raw-food cats. The argument has been made that the length of the human digestive tract demonstrates that humans are best suited for a vegetarian diet; remains of the digestion of animal flesh may putrefy when stagnant in the rather long human intestines. I believe that the eating of overrefined and overcooked foods contributes to that length; problems that are due to flesh being in the intestines for an extended length of time are partly due to intestines that are too long. The low fiber content of refined foods further contributes to this problem.

SAFETY, PERSONAL TASTE AND CONVENTIONS

Evolution, anthropology, animal experiments, and clinical experience aside, the usefulness of information about raw foods justifiably hinges on questions of safety, personal taste, and convention. This pertains more to animal-sourced foods than to plant-sourced foods. In either case, however, and as mentioned earlier, the amount of raw or slightly cooked food in the diet should be increased rather slowly, allowing the body to adapt gradually. The mind also requires time to grow used to new and changing ways. Occasionally, individuals highly motivated by a desire to recover from serious health problems or to prevent them succeed in making these changes more rapidly.

Safety

In terms of animal-sourced food, there are two other primary considerations about the safety of its consumption raw or lightly cooked: the health of the source animal and the health of the individual eating the food. Both healthy animals and healthy people are highly resistant to disease. And by definition, healthy animals do not carry disease.

Be this as it may, most animals are raised today in a manner that raises questions about their health and desirability as food for human beings. Consider a steak ordered rare—in many restaurants served nearly raw in the middle. That meat has passed through an inspection system of sorts. The steer was fed hormones, antibiotics, and grains containing residues of a variety of chemical poisons; varying amounts of each are in the meat, be it well-done or raw. Government inspection supposedly guarantees that the meat contains no harmful organisms; it is accepted as safe. But mistakes, oversights, and occasionally corruption occur in the inspection system.

Meat and organs from pasture-fed, naturally raised cattle must also be inspected. Such meat is more desirable than the usual commercial varieties. Though available in many areas now, meat of this quality in much of the country is still hard to find.

It has been reported that brucellosis, or undulant fever, may be contracted by eating the meat or drinking the raw milk of infected animals, but this is debatable. Although modern commercial meat and dairy animals rarely contract this disease, their health is often poor as a result of overcrowded quarters, a lack of fresh grass and exercise, overuse of chemicals in their management, and perhaps due to a diet comprised of GMO corn and soy. These animals are best kept at least partly at pasture and in uncrowded conditions. With exercise and proper feeding, they produce milk and meat that is healthy and safe.

Occurrence of brucellosis in cows was correlated with trace-mineral deficiencies in Pottenger's article "Brucella Infections" (*The Merck Report*, July 1949). Minerals present in tissues of healthy cows were found on spectrographic analysis to be missing in tissues of cows with brucella infections. Cows fed the trace minerals manganese, cobalt, copper, and iodine were immune to brucellosis when exposed to the disease in other animals.

In subsequent work with more than eighteen hundred patients with brucellosis, Pottenger found that supplements of these minerals (together with his dietary program) consistently resulted in significant improvements in blood picture, visible symptoms, and the patient's sense of well-being. The previous diet of nearly every patient indicated a state of malnutrition long before symptoms of brucellosis first came to attention. This underscores the susceptibility of weakened individuals to infection from contaminated foods.

The corollary of increased susceptibility of weakened individuals to the spread of disease from animals is that healthy individuals are resistant to such spread. This is why primitive Africans were resistant to organisms causing so much disease among whites in Africa, and it is why traditional people everywhere ate animal life without fear of infection. The animals were by and large healthy, but the first line of defense was the superior resistance of the people consuming them. That this resistance was in part the result of eating the animal life—much of it lightly cooked, some of it raw—completed the circle of cause and effect.

Most Caucasian Americans are descendants of people from western, northern, and central Europe and Russia; a smaller number are of southern European and Middle Eastern origin. Foods have been cooked in northern regions since early explorations by prehistoric hunters. In southern Europe, the Middle East, and African regions where ancestors of African-Americans originated, cooking played a smaller but still significant role in the traditional preparation of food. Every culture Weston Price visited used at least some cooked foods. To eat an entirely raw-food diet is to ignore this heritage.

Personal Taste and Conventions

Socially, the consumption of an all-raw diet may put an individual on the fringe; eating is a social event, and the strictly raw-food person may find his or her diet quite limiting in this respect. One can, however, eat in a somewhat unconventional manner—if done with flair—and still be accepted by one's friends. Indeed, some interesting conversations may result.

In terms of social convention, very rare meat is socially acceptable, and so too is certain raw flesh—carpaccio, steak tartare, oysters, and clams. (This obviously has nothing to do with safety. Taste as well as convention is served by cooking; a charcoal-grilled very rare steak has considerably more flavor than raw meat.) The consumption of raw fish has been accepted in America, though sushi here is deep-frozen for at least fourteen days. Most sushi is derived from ocean-going fish, and while most oceangoing fish do not harbor organisms that are harmful to humans, some do. Deep-freezing kills any such harmful organisms.

Most other fish may be lightly cooked to the point of flaking apart, which is undercooked by most standards—many individuals prefer it cooked a bit more. Restaurants generally overcook fish; by ordering it "a bit undercooked," one may avoid having it served overcooked.

In any event, for the unconventional eater, compromise is required in social situations as well as with one's own taste buds. Raw and lightly cooked foods simply cannot be forced. As with all food, it must be enjoyed if lasting habits are to develop. While one may strive to try new things, let the first consideration be the selection and preparation of natural foods that are enjoyed. Upon this base may be built a long life-time of refinements.

6
THE UNIQUE
NUTRIENTS OF
SEAFOOD

Dr. Weston Price, in his studies of native peoples, found that they consumed much seafood (both scalefish and shellfish) wherever available; indeed, fishing cultures were among the most physically well developed and disease resistant found. Let's explore why this may have been so. This discussion includes the results of several studies that have been done to determine the benefits of seafood.

EFFECTS OF THE
NUTRIENTS IN SEAFOOD

Much recent medical research has focused on the physiological effects of fish consumption and on the fatty acids in fish oils. Essential fatty acids have collectively been referred to as Vitamin F. Fatty acids consist of chains of carbon atoms bonded to hydrogen. "Unsaturated" means that some of the chemical bonds in the carbon chain are unstable; oxygen may form bonds with the carbon atoms adjacent to these unstable bonds and cause rancidity. A highly unsaturated oil can stay liquid at cold temperatures, while saturated fatty acids such as those found in butter or meat are solid at room temperature.

Eicosapentaenoic acid (EPA) is found in high concentrations in certain fish. As mentioned earlier in the book, EPA is a long-chain, highly unsaturated fatty acid that can be used in metabolism to make some important prostaglandins, as can several other fatty acids, including gamma-linolenic and arachidonic acids. Prostaglandins are hormone-like substances exerting control over events throughout the body, for example, the production and release of chemicals by blood platelets and cells lining the walls of blood vessels. These chemicals control the tendency of the platelets to form a clot. They thus influence the chances of a thrombus (clot) forming, lodging in the coronary arteries, and causing a coronary thrombosis (heart attack).

Linoleic and alpha-linolenic acids are essential fatty acids; the body cannot make them and they must be supplied in the diet. Though experimental animals freely convert alpha-linolenic acid to EPA, some researchers believe that EPA should also be considered essential for humans. This is due to the fact that we have, at most, a limited ability to make EPA, and it has unique and beneficial effects.

Many prostaglandins made from either EPA, dihomo-gamma linolenic acid (DGLA) (linoleic acid is a precursor of DGLA), or arachidonic acid affect the same bodily functions, though in different ways. For many functions, the body can utilize prostaglandins made from any of the three. All produce critical prostaglandins. What seems to be required for optimal function is properly balanced production of prostaglandins made in the body, on the one hand, from arachidonic acid, and on the other, from DGLA and EPA. Prostaglandins made from arachidonic acid are called the series 2 prostaglandins; those made from linoleic acid and DGLA are called the series 1 prostaglandins; and those made from EPA the series 3 prostaglandins. Figure 6.1 details the metabolic pathways of the fatty-acid precursors of these three series of prostaglandins. EPA is concentrated in the fat of marine (saltwater) fish and shellfish, especially the cold-water varieties. Concentrations of a closely related fatty acid, docosahexaenoic acid (DHA), occur in the same sources. DHA is also concentrated in the brain and in retinal cells of the eyes of mammals, including humans; the significance of this will be demonstrated in experiments discussed later.

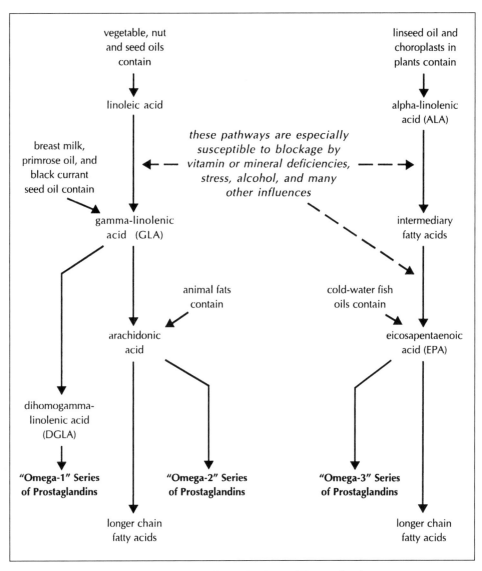

Figure 6.1. Foods, Fatty Acids, and Prostaglandins

Chloroplasts—the green cells in plants—contain small amounts of alpha-linolenic acid, which mammals can convert to EPA. While grazing animals convert alpha-linolenic acid to EPA, the extent to which the human body can do so is not clear. One research team in the Clinical Chemistry Department of Aalborg Hospital in Denmark gave a volunteer one tablespoon of cod-liver oil three times a day for one week (far more than what should be consumed on a regular basis). Cod-liver oil is about 10 percent EPA. A tenfold increase in the EPA content of the blood fats occurred within the week. Linseed oil was given to the same person two months later, in the same dose; after one week the individual showed only insignificant increases in EPA.

The human body nevertheless may well make the conversion of alpha-linolenic acid to EPA under certain circumstances, the EPA then being utilized for synthesis of prostaglandins. All of the prostaglandin pathways are inhibited by many influences, including deficiencies of magnesium, zinc, iron, vitamin B_6, or other nutrients; excessive alcohol consumption; cortisone-like drugs; increased adrenaline associated with stress; aging; and especially the presence in the body of unnatural fatty acids such as those found in margarine and hydrogenated vegetable oils.

In converting alpha-linolenic acid to EPA, the proportion of different kinds of fatty acids in the diet has a major influence. Had the individual been on a diet very low in arachidonic and linoleic acids—unlikely, since they predominate in most modern foods—he may have formed measurably more EPA from the linseed oil.

Balance is critical. Sources of linoleic acid include most vegetable, nut, and seed oils. Sources of EPA, DHA, and alpha-linolenic acid include fish and shellfish and green vegetables, including lettuce and other salad greens. Arachidonic acid is richly supplied in meat and dairy foods.

A STUDY OF FISH CONSUMPTION AND HEART DISEASE

In an article entitled "The Inverse Relation Between Fish Consumption and Twenty-Year Mortality from Coronary Heart Disease," which appeared in the *New England Journal of Medicine* in 1985, a team of Dutch researchers detailed the results of a twenty-year study of

852 middle-aged men in the town of Zutphen, the Netherlands.

Men free of known heart disease were selected in 1960. Dietary histories were obtained from the participants and their wives, with special attention being paid to fish consumption. Twenty percent of the men ate no fish in 1960. Among the rest, the intake varied from a fraction of an ounce to 11 ounces per day. The average for all the men was 0.75 of an ounce per day.

The research team followed these men for twenty years; 78 of them died of coronary heart disease. Statistical analysis was done on all data. The conclusion: an "inverse dose-response relation" existed between the amount of fish a man ate and his chances of dying of coronary heart disease. The more fish consumed, the less risk of heart attack; this relationship held true from trace amounts up to the maximal intake.

The results of the men who were eating an average of at least 1 ounce of fish per day were compared with those eating no fish; their death rate from coronaries was more than 50 percent lower. Statistical analysis proved these results independent of all other factors for coronary heart disease; fish consumption was a protective factor, independent of all variables. The influence of EPA on clotting tendencies is one possible reason for these results, but another that has emerged in recent years is the beneficial effects of the vitamin D that is richly supplied in fish.

The men were divided into groups by the amount of fish consumed. Those with the highest intake averaged 2.5 ounces of fish per day. Two-thirds of it was lean (cod and plaice) and one-third fatty (herring and mackerel), providing about 0.4 grams of EPA per day, mostly from the fatty fish. However, the consumption of lean fish also proved to protect against heart disease, and the more consumed, the greater the protection. Nutrients in addition to EPA seem to be involved.

While more fish gave greater protection, the men averaging only 1 ounce a day of any fish—one or two modest portions a week—had less than half the death rate from heart disease than those eating no fish. The conclusion is that regular inclusion of some seafood in the diet seems prudent. Traditional Greenland Eskimos, shown in several studies to have an extremely low incidence of coronary heart disease when living on their native diet, eat upward of 14 ounces of fatty fish per day.

A STUDY OF FISH OILS
AND HIGH BLOOD FATS

An article by B. Phillipson et al., entitled "Reduction of Plasma Lipids, Lipoproteins, and Apoproteins by Dietary Fish Oils in Patients with Hypertriglyceridemia," appeared in the same issue of the *New England Journal of Medicine* as the Dutch study on fish consumption. Hypertriglyceridemia refers to the presence of excessively high triglycerides in the blood. Triglycerides are normal fats found in the blood; they are a type of plasma lipid. Excessive amounts have been correlated with the overconsumption of carbohydrates, especially refined carbohydrates. Heart disease and circulatory disorders are related to high triglyceride levels.

In this study, twenty patients were placed on three successive controlled diets differing only in the kind of fat included. The first diet was low in fat and contained no fish oil. The second contained fish oil (in fish and in supplements) amounting to 20 to 30 percent of the daily calories. The third substituted an equal amount of polyunsaturated vegetable oils for the fish oil of the second diet.

In every patient, blood triglyceride levels fell while on the diet rich in fish oils. In four weeks triglycerides fell an average of 64 percent for the patients with moderate elevation of triglycerides, and they fell an average of 79 percent for the patients with severe elevation. The new levels were, on the average, less than one-third of the old. Cholesterol levels fell 27 percent for the moderate group and 45 percent for the severe group. It is important to note that while triglyceride levels are significant, cholesterol levels are a phony issue and in fact are not related to heart disease. Numerous studies have demonstrated that the incidence of coronary artery disease is not connected to blood cholesterol levels and that the use of cholesterol-lowering drugs does not result in increased survival. Also note that virtually all of the diets Weston Price studied were rich in cholesterol, and the people had no heart disease.

The reductions were from the levels measured while the patients were on the low-fat diet prior to the diet rich in fish oil. Many then still had milky looking blood plasma, a characteristic of fatty blood. Within days on the diet rich in fish oil, this disappeared.

When the patients were taken off the fish-rich diet and placed on the diet rich in polyunsaturated vegetable oils, they experienced alarming developments. Among those who had moderately elevated blood fats prior to being on the diet rich in fish oil, levels of triglycerides rose considerably, but remained below previous levels. Vegetable oils are known to reduce triglycerides; they proved less effective than fish oils.

The vegetable oils caused more striking effects in the patients who had severely elevated blood fats prior to being on the diet rich in fish oil. These people had experienced large reductions in triglycerides and cholesterol while on the diet rich in fish oil. Within three to four days on the diet rich in vegetable oils, all had increases in triglyceride levels. After ten to fourteen days, levels had on the average tripled. Because abdominal pain and liver tenderness was developing in many of these patients, and because of the severely elevated blood fats, the vegetable-oil-rich diet was discontinued at that point. The plan had been to continue it for four weeks, the same length of time the diet rich in fish oil was used.

A return to the diet rich in fish oil was followed by the disappearance of the abdominal pain and liver tenderness. The triglycerides dropped to the previous levels, and eventually became even lower as the diet was continued.

These dramatic results demonstrate the danger of believing advertisements implying alleged health benefits of polyunsaturated vegetable oils. Because early studies determined that in most individuals these oils caused reductions in some blood fats, the public was led to believe large quantities were beneficial. More recent studies have shown that these oils do not reduce the blood fats thought to do the most harm when elevated, that is, the very-low-density lipoproteins (VLDL) and associated triglycerides. These fractions of the blood fats are most affected by fish oils.

Polyunsaturated vegetable oils are suspected of being cancer-causing agents and of speeding up biochemical processes involved in aging. Some of the fatty acids that vegetable oils supply in large quantities are essential nutrients, but the diet rich in fish oil supplied adequate amounts without the inclusion of vegetable oils. Limiting dietary polyunsaturated vegetable oils aids the body's ability to convert the alpha-linolenic acid in plant chloroplasts to EPA, and thus increases production of more favorable prostaglandins. Olive oil contains about one-tenth the polyunsaturated fatty-acids found in most vegetable oils; I recommend moderate use of 100 percent extra-virgin olive oil.

The diet rich in fish oil in the study just described supplied from 20 to 30 grams of EPA per day (nearly twice that of even Eskimo diets, and far too much for proper fatty-acid balance); 2 ounces of fatty fish such as mackerel or salmon supply about 1 gram of EPA. Both the twenty-year study and the fish-oil study point toward great benefits from seafood consumption. This is not to be taken as a recommendation to take fish-oil supplements. However, I do recommend a modest amount of cod-liver oil, up to one-half teaspoon a day, to supply vitamins A and D, along with small amounts of EPA and DHA. This should be consumed in the context of a diet rich in saturated fat. Take cod-liver oil in small quantities, for overdosing is possible.

A STUDY OF
FISHERMEN AND FARMERS IN JAPAN

Further insight into the amount of seafood one might eat for optimal protection against coronary heart disease, as well as other disorders involving abnormal clotting of the blood, is provided in a study by a group of Japanese researchers (Aizan Hirai et al.) in the British medical journal *Lancet* in 1980. The main source of dietary protein in Japan is fish, and the Japanese have a low incidence of heart disease. (It is important to note, however, that many groups we have discussed ate little or no fish and had scant evidence of heart disease.) Believing EPA might be a major reason for the low incidence of heart disease, the researchers carried out platelet aggregation studies to look for differences between the people of a fishing village and those of a farming village.

In the fishing village, the average daily intake of fish among the people was 9 ounces per person, supplying 2.5 grams of EPA. In the farming village, the average was 3 ounces, supplying 0.9 grams of EPA. In the fishing village, the people had significantly higher blood levels of EPA.

In the platelet aggregation studies, the platelets of the people in the fishing village showed significantly less tendency to adhere and form a clot. Consistent with EPA's role as a precursor of prostaglandins that cause decreased platelet aggregation, the tendency of platelets to clot is directly related to the level of EPA in the blood.

The difference in platelet aggregation between the fishermen and the farmers was apparently due to the greater fish consumption and subsequently higher blood levels of EPA of the fishermen. The farmers ate as much fish as the group of men who were the biggest fish eaters in the twenty-year Netherlands study—an average of 3 ounces a day. The fishermen ate three times as much, approaching the consumption of Greenland Eskimos.

While the Netherlands group (eating an average of 3 ounces of fish daily) had more than 50 percent less coronary heart disease than those eating no fish, they were not immune; some had heart attacks. Decreased platelet aggregation among fishermen eating 9 ounces of fish a day, compared with farmers eating 3 ounces a day, suggests that optimal levels of fish intake may be closer to 9 ounces per day than to 3.

A STUDY OF A MACKEREL DIET
ON BLOOD PLATELETS

As described in an article in *Lancet* in 1980 (Siess et al.), mackerel nearly exclusively constituted the diet of seven volunteers studied by West German researchers; the daily intake was from 18 to 29 ounces. Blood studies were conducted, with particular attention being paid to platelets.

A platelet is formed when certain bone-marrow blood cells called megakaryocytes fragment. Each platelet has a membrane surrounding it, and this membrane is a storehouse for fats. The researchers found that the composition of these fats, while the subjects were on the mackerel diet, became similar to the composition of fats in mackerel; within a few days of beginning the diet, the volunteers' membranes became rich in EPA.

The tendency of the blood to clot thus changes when eating large amounts of foods rich in EPA; changes occur in the structure of the cells responsible for clotting. Recall the old saying: "You are what you eat."

Concern has been expressed that EPA-rich diets may cause problems related to an inability of the blood to clot, and Eskimos on their native diets in fact have longer bleeding times than most Americans. But their blood does clot well and their wounds heal well. An EPA-deficient diet may shorten bleeding time. Bear in mind, though, that EPA may be overdone.

THE ROLE OF FISH OILS IN
VISION AND INTELLECTUAL FUNCTION

In a 1985 article in *Transactions of the Association of American Physicians*, researchers stated that sharpness of vision and brain development are related to blood levels of EPA and DHA. These fatty-acids are essential for good vision. DHA is a normal constituent of the cells of the retina, and the amount present is dependent upon the amount in the diet. Animal tests at Oregon Health Sciences University in Portland indicated that deficiencies reduced the ability of retinal cells to be stimulated, with consequent reduction in sharpness of vision.

In other studies at the Oregon Regional Primate Center, the development of vision during gestation and early life was impaired when female monkeys were fed a diet deficient in EPA, DHA, and linolenic acid for two months prior to and during their pregnancies. The infant monkeys were then fed the deficient diet; when twelve weeks old, their vision was only half the strength of monkeys fed a normal diet. The cells of the retina and brains of animals with deficient vision were analyzed; the fat content showed very low levels of EPA and DHA, explaining the loss of sharp vision.

The ability of Maori to see the moons of Jupiter with the naked eye was apparently related to the rich supply of EPA, DHA, alpha-linolenic acid, and other fatty acids supplied in their foods (they certainly did not take any fish-oil supplements!).

EPA and DHA, especially DHA, are also found in high concentrations in the cerebral cortex of the normal human brain. Deficiencies may impair the functioning of the brain—learning, reasoning, and overall intellectual powers. Rats fed a diet deficient in these fatty acids were unable to learn to run a maze as well as rats fed a control diet.

The wisdom of primitive diets is demonstrated by this research; every traditional culture Weston Price studied emphasized foods rich in vitamins A, D, and K_2. Seafood, organs, and in some cultures dairy products from pasture-fed animals were particularly emphasized for mothers to be (prior to and during pregnancy, and later during lactation) and young children. Recent research has indicated the human brain acquires about half its fat composition before birth, and most of the rest during the first year after. Native people did everything that research now indicates people should do to ensure the optimal development of the next generation.

THE RESEARCH OF DR. WESTON PRICE AS IT PERTAINS TO VITAMINS A, D, AND K_2

Dr. Price measured vitamins A and D in dairy products, as well as his unknown activator X. Dr. Price presented evidence in *Nutrition and Physical Degeneration* that this fat-soluble activator X played an essential role in immunity and the utilization of minerals. He measured the amount of it in dairy products, and found the substance in the milk fat of only those cows that ate rapidly growing green grass. X-Factor butter oil is extracted, without heat, from the dairy fat of cows that eat 100 percent rapidly growing pasture.

Price determined that the activator X (now known to be vitamin K_2) was critical for the normal growth and maintenance of bones and teeth. We now know also that it is responsible for calcium deposition throughout the body and is of critical importance in maintaining the integrity of the circulatory system and thus the health of the heart.

The wide facial structures and freedom from cavities seen in Price's photographs of native people are examples of typical physical development in people consuming optimal amounts of natural vitamins A, D, and K_2 in the proper balance as proffered by the foods they typically ate. Modern diets are sadly lacking in these vitamins, which may be derived from the dairy products of grass-fed animals, especially butter and cream, as well as from seafood and grass-fed meats and organs.

Cod-liver oil is an excellent supplemental source of vitamins A, D, and K_2; it may be used to complement dietary sources. Natural, unadulterated cod-liver oil contains substantial amounts of vitamins A and D in their natural ration of ten to one. Cod-liver oil boosts immunity, enhances and maintains brain function, regulates blood pressure, eases pain and inflammation, and helps alleviate depression. It really is something of an elixir.

Bone broth made from the bones of grass-fed animals is a great way to include natural vitamins A, D, and K_2 in the diet. To learn more about the wonderful health benefits of broth, see *Nourishing Broth* by Sally Fallon Morell and Kaayla Daniel. The book includes a detailed account of how broth also supplies collagen, another nutrient missing in the modern diet and crucial in maintaining truly vibrant health and recovering from disease.

PART 2

DIET AND DISEASE

Planning for Health and Recovery

Now that we have a fundamental understanding of the value of traditional, natural foods in the diet, in the second part of *Primal Nutrition* we will provide an overview of other important areas and questions to address in our search for good health. Specifically, we will review the role of the primary physician as it fits into our overall picture of a more holistically based regimen.

We will also review some well-known diets, each of which has proved helpful to many individuals. Some of these diets stress the importance of raw foods, and some make no mention of the issue. All are successful to varying degrees, however, we will see that the most successful have a deep understanding of the value of raw-food nutrients. After a review and analysis of these diets, we will then segue into a synthesis that will incorporate our several sources of knowledge of native foods into a plan you may use to begin creating your own best primal diet, suited to your own unique circumstances. Ideally that diet will evolve as your health evolves.

The last chapter in this second part of the book will review specific medical conditions, and discuss how the diet may impact these conditions in a positive, healing manner.

7
GUIDANCE ON THE PATH TO GOOD HEALTH

Though food is the dominant subject of this book, it is a book about health, and this chapter is one of guidance as it pertains to that. This guidance falls into two areas: important considerations when selecting and working with a primary physician, and important considerations about popular diets today. In both cases, I offer advice about what to look for and incorporate into a new health regimen, and what to avoid. As we undertake our search for improved health and well-being, challenging but realistic goals may be established once one understands what may realistically be expected. An understanding of one's health goals and a sound relationship with a physician who is sympathetic is key. Also germane is to understand how and why popular diets that purport to be beneficial may actually need to be avoided in our search for health.

CRITERIA FOR SELECTING A PHYSICIAN

To progress toward better health, one must make decisions. Reasonable decisions are based on information, and the most basic information required for decisions about health concerns is a solid answer to the question: Where do I stand now?

An individual with a problem that has not been examined should see a physician. A detailed knowledge of one's current condition provides both a baseline for measuring improvement and a means of deciding how seriously the business of improving health should be taken. Even when under a physician's care, one may continue to ask questions that the physician may not ask. Done thoroughly, a self-assessment complements a professional medical assessment. At times the latter may not define or diagnose the problem; an individual may nevertheless realize something is wrong and seek other opinions or take appropriate nutritional measures independently.

Self-assessment questions may relate to growing older without fear. One might ask, "Is my body feeling as if it will carry me through for the duration without becoming diseased?" We all grow old, and when the biological clock inside has run its course, we die.

This does not frighten us. But disease does, and rightly so. Old age and death are as natural as life. Disease is not.

A gentle suggestion: In taking stock of your own personal health situation, ask questions that will help you to learn to live in health. Success in your endeavor may bring genuine happiness and peace of mind.

A physician may help in the search for improved health. Although most doctors think more in terms of disease than in terms of health, a working relationship with a caring and competent doctor who is respectful of individual needs and goals enables one to understand medical conditions and make reasonable decisions about courses of treatment.

A physician's first duty is to use his or her medical expertise to gather information in order to best assess the patient's status. This is the purpose of a thorough medical history and physical examination, and of laboratory tests and any special diagnostic procedures.

The physician's next duty is to explain his or her findings clearly and simply. If a doctor understands the broad spectrum of conditions that may exist between robust good health and overt disease, and recognizes the numerous subclinical problems people eating modern diets develop, there will be much to talk about. A doctor with this knowledge may help one prevent early symptoms from developing into major problems.

Most physicians find conditions satisfactory if no problems that are treatable with drugs or surgery are present. But when such conditions are discovered, the individual style, personality, and character of the physician greatly influence subsequent events.

Almost every doctor realizes that whatever the condition, choices about methods of treatment exist. But because most also believe strongly in some particular method, each tends to recommend that particular method to patients. While this is understandable (often the physician has little knowledge of alternate ways of dealing with the problem), the *most* competent physicians are aware and knowledgeable about methods outside of their own area of expertise. When telling a patient of a medical problem, such a physician is willing and able to explain the existing options. If the physician's own particular approach is the one most suited for the individual and the problem, this will become apparent. The patient is always free to make his or her own informed choice.

This issue is complex even before bringing in the matter of treating disease through nutrition. Surgery and drug therapy are commonly a matter of one physician's opinion over another's; hospital studies have shown that patients receiving certain drugs or surgical procedures statistically fared no better—or fared worse—than those with similar conditions receiving no treatment. Often there is considerable debate between physicians over whether a given condition in general, or a given patient in particular, should be treated surgically, pharmaceutically, or not at all (nutrition, alas, is seldom considered).

Most conditions commonly treated with drugs or surgery are indeed treatable through nutrition, and this complicates matters further. Many physicians do not accept this, however, or accept it only on the most limited basis. Without the knowledge and experience to treat medical problems in this manner, most physicians cannot offer the alternative—treatment through proper nutrition—to their patients.

The realization that you may know more about these matters than your physician can be a matter of life and death. To your doctor's evaluation of the situation, you must add your own. For some people, the recommended course of drug or surgical treatment is the most appropriate course to follow. For others with the discipline, knowledge, tenacity, and courage to steer their own course, there are times when it is not.

This is not a recommendation that anyone embark on a course of self-treatment for a serious medical problem; the help of a competent and understanding physician may be immeasurably important. But there are times when a recommended drug or surgical treatment is not in the best interest of an individual patient. The discerning patient must be prepared to recognize when this is the case.

Seek out a physician who understands all of this. Local chapters of the Weston A. Price Foundation can help you find a holistic physician in your area (westonaprice.org). Usually doctors who take the time to know their patients as individuals are responsive to these issues. Long ago and far away, most of us had a family doctor, a general practitioner with whom we grew up. This doctor knew us well, knew our families, histories, and idiosyncrasies. In this age of the specialist, too often a medical problem is seen as an isolated issue in a single part of the body, rather than as a signal that the body will break down further if one does not change one's ways. In years past we were more willing to listen, and general practitioners and naturopathic physicians were willing to give us these frank appraisals we needed to hear. Perhaps their time has come again.

THE SIGNIFICANCE OF THE MEDICAL HISTORY AND THE PHYSICAL EXAM

The body is an integrated whole, and the symptoms we suffer relate to one another and to how we live. For the physician, the medical history begins a process similar to putting together a jigsaw puzzle, whether the patient has come to her for preventive care, has been previously diagnosed elsewhere, or is ill with undiagnosed symptoms and signs. (Symptoms are subjective feelings, while signs are objective and physically detectable or measurable.) All of these cases may be equally challenging, because the proper questions elicit responses revealing patterns in the puzzle that soon give shape to a picture remarkably unique for each individual.

And yet, patterns of problems are seen in much the same form in many people. Which pattern dominates at a given time in life is determined by an interplay of one's genetic background, ways of reacting to stress, and individual dietary and exercise habits. We call these patterns diseases, symptom complexes, diagnoses, or illnesses. These labels are useful when used to organize information; they help relate problems to one another and ultimately to causes and solutions. But a physician should not forget that the names are but labels, and whatever the label, each individual's set of medical problems is unique.

Information gained from the medical history helps shape the physical exam. While circumstances necessarily dictate the thoroughness of the initial exam, a physician must know an individual's physical condition well if a solid and cooperative relationship is to be established. A competent physician observes, measures, and intuitively senses hundreds of bits of information in a fifteen-minute examination. The meaning of symptoms discovered in the history may be explored, clarified, and amplified. The possible need for special laboratory tests or further diagnostic procedures may be investigated and determined. Out of this process comes a sense of the individual's overall condition.

The medical history and physical exam thus generate a record of where an individual stands medically; laboratory tests and special diagnostic procedures clarify and enlarge upon that record. (Please note: appendix 3 contains a discussion of some common laboratory tests.) A description of symptoms with their history, physical findings, emotional state, pertinent family history, dietary history, exercise habits, and current medications—this information is all relevant, and may be used to begin creating an appropriate plan reflective of the individual's needs and goals.

THE IMPORTANCE OF SETTING GOALS

Set goals. Achievements come with goals and a realistic means to reach them. Determine the specifics and plan timetables; one must then take these goals seriously.

Be realistic, but take on challenges. Health goals may involve foods, feelings, plans for self or family, and/or the elimination of troubling conditions—but whatever the goals are, know that they are possible. Unlike any other aspect of life, one has complete freedom about what one eats from this moment until one's death. Health is one result of wisely exercising that freedom; others include greater self-control and freedom in other areas of life.

Learn to welcome change—including the changing of goals. Defeat leads to destruction only when nothing is learned. Learn, and change. Learning to eat as one knows is best takes time, and the modern world does not make this easy. Achieving health is a genuine challenge.

The enemy is apathy. We sometimes ask, what is it all for? We love family and friends; yet in some moments we wonder, why bother? What is it for, then—the food, the exercise, the caring, the search for health?

The belief that some mysterious powers live in each of us may overcome apathy. What Native Americans call the Great Spirit gives me life, energy to do for myself, and to do for others. I've been granted the gift of life—the strength to run fast and free on a mountain ridge, to walk peacefully on a quiet beach, to feel confident of my body, indeed, to understand that "the most supreme instrument in life is a perfect body," as Havelock Ellis wrote about indigenous people. My goals of health and independence intertwine, and the resulting feeling—one of physical and psychological strength—may become a sustaining force. The foundation, though, is love, as well as the sense that we are all brothers and sisters, equal in the eyes of creation. Love is fundamental to life.

That which is for oneself and that which is for the people we love are sometimes inseparable. When we eat living, natural food, we act in harmony with forces at the very core of our being. We attempt to attune ourselves to the collective human spirit, and I believe we bring ourselves closer to each other and to the Great Spirit. Living naturally in good health helps us to replace feelings of apathy with feelings of strength and love—which even in apathetic moments we may choose to make a part of our goals.

Overcoming apathy, then, is a good goal to strive for!

Next we will review several popular diets to determine whether or not they may be useful for us in our search for health moving forward.

A REVIEW OF SEVERAL WELL-KNOWN DIETS

Scores of dietary regimens have become popular today. Many contain elements and principles that are useful in understanding the effects of food on health. These include the Pritikin Diet, two high-protein weight-loss diets (the Atkins Diet and the Scarsdale Diet), the Gerson Diet, raw-food diets (which may incorporate fasting), and the macrobiotic diet of Michio Kushi.

Each contains elements of traditional diets. All recommend mostly fresh, unrefined foods. Each has helped many people but yet has drawbacks; a common one is restrictiveness. Inflexibility is another; individual problems occurring in response to certain foods may be difficult to adjust. A lack of flexibility is often a problem even as one's health improves, for a diet should change as an individual changes. A program initially bringing marked improvement often later fails to maintain health.

It must also be noted that although these dietary regimens have been of great value to many individuals, none incorporates fully the principles behind traditional human diets—principles necessary for designing nutritional programs in accord with our deepest physiological and psychological needs. But an integration of strengths from each of these diets, into knowledge of traditional human foods, yields a better understanding of the relationship between food and human health.

The Pritikin Diet

Nathan Pritikin established an inpatient diet and exercise rehabilitation center in Santa Barbara, California, in 1976. His program grew popular; one of his books, *The Pritikin Program for Diet and Exercise*, has sold more than two million copies.

The diet severely restricts all fats, vegetable and animal alike, especially cholesterol (though technically not a fat, cholesterol is often classed with fats). Fresh raw and cooked vegetables and whole grains are emphasized; animal protein is restricted to four ounces daily. The Pritkin regimen also includes an exercise program of extensive walking, and later on, jogging.

The fatty-fish and fish-oil diets described earlier in this book are successful in lowering abnormally high triglycerides. Differences between fats in fish and those found in commercial animals (and subsequent effects on metabolism) are not recognized in the Pritikin Diet, nor are differences between food derived from healthy animals (seafood and pasture-fed farm animals) and food derived from conventionally raised animals.

As previously discussed, in the early 1980s I worked in a large medical practice in New York. My colleagues and I employed the Pritikin Diet to treat individuals with heart and circulatory problems. Larger amounts of high-quality animal foods, especially fish, shellfish, and liver, enabled people on the diet to follow the routine more consistently and yielded greater improvements than seen in individuals following the standard Pritikin regimen.

Pritikin had some success—people switching from the standard American processed food diet to just about any kind of natural food regimen often see improvements. But his claim that his diet was "the world's healthiest diet . . . the most significant breakthrough in man's age-old quest for rejuvenation," and that "for centuries the hardiest, most long-lived peoples in the world have thrived on these foods" is not true. He followed his diet for more than twenty-five years, apparently reversing the course of his heart disease and controlling the leukemia that eventually led to his hospitalization and subsequent death. Pritikin committed suicide.

For centuries, the hardiest, most long-lived peoples in the world have indeed thrived on fresh vegetables and in a few cultures, properly prepared whole grains—among other foods. But healthy cultures everywhere, cultures in which cancer, heart disease, and other degenerative diseases were unknown or extremely rare, used substantial portions of high-quality, grass-fed animal-sourced foods. Primal foods.

Pritikin's work is significant and important, demonstrating the power of a program that emphasizes giving up unhealthy habits and adopting a more natural lifestyle. But selective use of circumstantial evidence is misleading, and Pritikin did not discuss many other health problems that occurred in individuals following his one-size-fits-all program. Evidence from the disciplines of anthropology, human evolution, and recent medical research is ignored. Frequent references are made to the African Bantu people, who are said to eat a low-animal-protein, low-fat, high-fiber diet and enjoy resistance to diseases of the cardiovascular and digestive systems. Yet no mention is made of their significant consumption of insects (high in fat) and their fermentation of grains and tubers. No reference is made to other traditional cultures that eat large amounts of animal protein and fat and enjoy similar resistance. Many different natural-food diets produce good health relative to that seen in modernized cultures. But only when all of the principles Weston Price discovered are in place can truly optimal health be obtained.

The same program that may help initially often does not maintain an individual's health over time. Changes to reduce or eliminate sugar, refined flour, alcohol, smoking, the consumption of commercial dairy products and food products derived from confinement animals, coupled with changes to increase one's level of exercise and intake of natural food, may bring improvement and feelings of well-being, often for some time. But fatigue, depression, digestive disorders, and even cancer and other chronic diseases follow in the long run when traditional wisdom about the importance of incorporating food products derived from grass-fed animal fats is ignored.

Building lasting health and resistance to degenerative processes is complex, and there is danger in oversimplification. Only a truly primal traditional diet incorporating the principles that Dr. Price discovered can lead to lasting health. The magnitude of what has been fragmented and mostly lost—the wisdom of our ancestors—is such that only by being open to learning from all available sources can one hope to put the pieces back together. Pritikin contributed to our understanding, and we thank him for that, but he also demonstrated the folly of being overly sure that one has all the answers.

High-Protein Weight-Loss Diets

Several weight-loss diets that emphasize protein foods have also become popular in recent years. Two of the most well known appeared in books that were bestsellers: *Dr. Atkins' Diet Revolution* and *The Complete Scarsdale Medical Diet.*

The Atkins Diet eliminates nearly all carbohydrates in early stages, forcing the burning of fats for energy and producing ketones, by-products of fat metabolism that the body can partially use for energy instead of glucose. Ketones are not completely burned when metabolized and are subsequently excreted; this may aid in weight loss. Their presence suppresses hunger; individuals eating mostly protein and fats (meats, eggs, fish, dairy products, fatty sauces) as the diet suggests, experience little hunger and yet may lose a great deal of weight. Salads and some fruits are also allowed on the Atkins Diet.

The Scarsdale Diet also causes ketosis (the presence of ketones on the breath and in the urine) and thus operates on much the same principle, although in this diet, an average of 35 percent of calories are derived from carbohydrates. Weight loss results from low caloric and low fat intake; the strict part of the diet (suggested for use no more than two weeks at a time) averages one thousand calories a day, 20 percent from fats. The use of lean meat, fish, skim milk, and low-fat cheeses restricts fat and calories. This low-fat regimen is actually very dangerous because too much protein and not enough fat is consumed; the diet lacks critical fat-soluble activators.

Elimination of refined carbohydrates (sugar, white flour, and most alcohol) and restriction of even whole foods containing many carbohydrates (whole grains, foods made from whole grains, and fruits) may cause the dieter to eat more foods of animal origin and more vegetables. Most people with weight problems have eaten diets high in refined carbohydrates, so such changes are beneficial.

But the quality of the animal foods used is an important issue. The Atkins Diet in particular stresses the use of fatty foods; the book presents evidence that refined carbohydrates rather than animal fats are the villains of the American diet. There is truth in this, but as we have seen, fats derived from modern commercial animals and milk products are very different in quality from those derived from animals living under natural conditions. In particular, they lack adequate quantities of the fat-soluble activators I have made reference to above (vitamins A, D, and K_2).

These diets may achieve goals of weight loss and decrease the risk for diseases associated with being overweight. This is no small accomplishment for the overweight person who has found it impossible to remain on other weight-loss regimens. But the individual wishing to optimize his or her health must adapt a diet built on primal wisdom.

The Gerson Diet

Max Gerson was a physician who began practice in the mid-1920s in Bielefeld, Germany. He studied under Professor Ottfried Foerster, a renowned neurosurgeon of the day. Gerson's specialty was diseases of the nervous system.

Because Gerson cured his own migraines with a natural-food diet, he began treating his migraine patients similarly; they did well also. One such patient reported that his skin tuberculosis or lupus (*cutaneous lupus erythematosus*) cleared up as well. Gerson found this hard to believe, for lupus was supposedly incurable. Laboratory reports and slides proved the lesions were indeed healing, and Gerson began treating other lupus patients. They too recovered.

Because Gerson was a specialist in nerve diseases, the medical community claimed he could not treat skin diseases and attempted to revoke his license. The case went to court, and the judge asked the physicians charging Gerson if they cured lupus. They replied that lupus was incurable. The judge responded, "Well, then, why don't you let this doctor do it?" and dismissed the case. Gerson went home, removed his shingle on which were the words "Internal and Nervous Diseases," and put another one up in its stead: "General Practitioner."

He began treating tuberculosis, meningitis, and other diseases with his natural-food diet. The wife of Albert Schweitzer, in very serious condition with tuberculosis, in 1928 went to Gerson. She recovered fully under his care. Years later, her husband, at the age of seventy-five, recovered from diabetes under Gerson's care; he lived to be ninety. On the cover of Gerson's book we find Schweitzer's words: "I see in Dr. Max Gerson one of the most eminent geniuses in medical history."

In 1929 Gerson began treating cancer, often with favorable results. His dietary regimen then consisted initially of fresh vegetables and fruits (many raw) and freshly prepared juices. During the course of treatment, buttermilk, pot cheese, yogurt, and egg yolks, all raw, were added. A mineral supplement was used, as were frequent enemas.

As he developed his therapy in Germany and then in America after escaping and emigrating here in the late 1930s, other health-enhancing elements were added to the diet. They included fresh green-leaf juice, fresh raw calf's-liver juice, injections of raw liver extract, iodine, desiccated thyroid gland, potassium supplements, and coffee enemas. The details of this therapy and theory are presented in his book, *A Cancer Therapy, Results of Fifty Cases,* published in 1958. Gerson died in 1959.

His book presents proof, with complete medical records, X-rays, and diagnoses of terminal cancer by accepted, established medical authorities, that a significant number of Gerson's patients (previously diagnosed as terminal) recovered from cancer. All fifty of the cases reported were alive and free of all signs of cancer at the time of the book's publication. Most had initially become Gerson's patients in the 1940s and early 1950s.

For more than twenty years, Gerson submitted reports of his work to medical journals. The medical establishment steadfastly blocked publication of it, even attempting unsuccessfully for years to revoke his license for practicing "unorthodox medicine." The cancer orthodoxy has long maligned Gerson's work as unproven and dangerous, grouping it with that of others who have dared suggest better ways of treating cancer patients—ways that do not involve surgery, radiation, and chemotherapy.

An account of Gerson's story is told by journalist S. J. Haught in a book first published in 1962 and entitled *Has Dr. Max Gerson a True Cancer Cure?* (reprinted in 1983 as *Cancer? Think Curable—The Gerson Therapy*). Haught's original intention was to expose Gerson as a fraud; his story was to be called *The Unveiling of a Quack*. He was converted to Gerson's side by the evidence.

In the years since Gerson's death, many people have applied his therapy. His daughter Charlotte established a clinic in Mexico and attempted to incorporate recent developments in natural therapy, while dropping critical elements such as the raw liver juice and other animal foods.

In Gerson's time, chemotherapy for cancer patients was in its infancy, and most people seeking his help had not been exposed to toxic chemotherapeutic agents. Because these agents depress the immune system, poison the liver, and leave the body weakened, he found that after chemotherapy people did not respond well to his dietary regimen. Today, most cancer patients seeking nutritional therapy have already had chemotherapy, although many seek to improve their nutrition while on chemotherapy.

Also enhancing Gerson's results was the superior food widely available in his day. More people had been raised on fresh, high-quality foods superior to those generally available today, and this may have enhanced their ability to recover from cancer. The foods readily available for use in his therapy were similarly superior.

The most intangible element in any therapy is the influence of the physician on the patient. Gerson's therapy is difficult both psychologically and physically, requiring a strict dietary regimen, months of hard work, and attention to detail. An inspirational and even charismatic physician-healer can make an immense difference in the patient's outcome, simply by virtue of his ability to inspire the patient and the family to follow his program with care. By all accounts, Gerson was such a man.

Several aspects of the Gerson Diet are of special interest in light of our knowledge of traditional diets. Fresh raw calf's-liver juice and fresh raw green-leaf juice are the central foods; both supply nutrients richly provided in primal diets.

Gerson wrote that liver juice is the most powerful weapon we have against cancer. (For most patients, drinking raw juice was more tolerable than eating raw liver.) The high vitamin A content of the juice is, in the opinion of many experts, the key to the success Gerson had. The therapy calls for three preparations daily, each made from eight ounces of liver. The juice concentrates essential nutrients, especially vitamin A. Gerson used a special press, the Norwalk juicer, to extract the juice from the liver. He stressed that liver utilized must be fresh, raw, and taken from animals raised without the use of hormones, antibiotics, or pesticides. Such liver is difficult to find fresh today.

Injections of crude liver extract and vitamin B_{12} were also part of the therapy. Gerson noted that leukemias in particular required greater doses of liver juice, liver extract, and vitamin B_{12}.

Research by Dr. Albert Szent-Gyorgyi gives an indication of the importance of nutrients found in liver for successful cancer therapy. Szent-Gyorgyi received the Nobel Prize for medicine and physiology in 1937 for his isolation and identification of vitamin C. He also discovered the function of bioflavonoids, and his work on contractile proteins is a foundation of muscle biochemistry and physiology. He reported in

1972 that his experiments had demonstrated that the growth of inoculated cancer in mice was strongly inhibited by extracts of liver. Other researchers have reported similar findings.

Fresh raw green-leaf juice is the other dietary mainstay of Gerson's therapy. As with liver, the use of juice allows the patient to take in far more nutrients than possible with solid foods alone.

Salads, lightly cooked vegetables, fruit and fruit juices, and some whole-grain foods were used, as well as buttermilk, raw cottage cheese and yogurt, and egg yolks. Other foods of animal origin Gerson considered essential were thyroid and pancreas. Thyroid tablets were used to stimulate metabolism, for Gerson had found that nearly every cancer patient had an underactive thyroid gland. Pancreas tablets taken with meals aided digestion. Iodine and iodide were given liberally.

Consistencies in the work of Gerson, Weston Price, and Francis Pottenger, Jr. are evident. Cancer remains the most difficult clinical problem that patient and physician must face. The Gerson therapy is no panacea, but many physicians and other healers today successfully use parts of Gerson's regimen given that many elements of the Gerson therapy are of benefit in treating cancer and other chronic diseases. An understanding of Gerson's work provides an essential piece of the puzzle that must be solved in order to effectively treat and prevent these diseases.

Raw-Food Diets and Fasting

Raw-Food Diets

Some diets advocate the exclusive use of raw foods. The program known as natural hygiene was described in books by Herbert Shelton, who for many years maintained a health spa in San Antonio, Texas. The natural-hygiene diet is strictly vegetarian—no animal foods are included (this is known as a vegan diet). Sprouts, fruits, and raw vegetable juices are emphasized. The regimen is frequently combined with therapeutic fasting as an approach to treating chronic diseases. While Shelton promoted an exclusively vegan diet, he was known to eat animal foods. I've noted over the years that this is common in longtime advocates of a strict vegan diet.

A strength of this program is that raw vegetables (especially sprouts and greens) and their juices are for many people very beneficial foods. An exclusively raw diet eliminates harmful foods, and individuals partaking of them often experience improvements and may even apparently recover from serious chronic diseases.

Improvement or recovery may be tenuous, however. Deficiency symptoms typically appear sooner or later, and there is usually difficulty staying on the strict regimen. Tremendous cravings often occur—the body knows something is lacking. The gaunt, hollow appearance of individuals who have followed a vegan raw-food diet over long periods of time speaks to a need for missing nutrients.

One case of mine was a four-year-old girl whose mother had been a strict raw-food vegan since the sixth month of her pregnancy with the child. This child had never consumed any food of animal origin, eating only raw vegetables, sprouts, nuts, seeds, and fruits. Markedly undersized for her age and with tiny bones, the pains she experienced in her legs suggested rickets. She was chronically tired, with little energy for playing or learning.

I suspected deficiencies of essential fatty acids, fat-soluble activators vitamins A, D, and K_2, calcium, vitamin B_{12}, and protein. I persuaded her mother to include grass-fed raw milk and eggs in the child's diet, though she would not include cod-liver oil or fish. Within a month, the child had gained weight and had more energy, and the pains in her legs had disappeared. Within a few months her fatigue was gone and, although still small, she had grown considerably.

Her case is typical of children who have been on vegan raw-food diets for extended periods of time. While the mother had not encountered major problems of her own, the diet lacked nutrients required for the growth and optimal development of her child.

Fasting

Many people who advocate a raw-food diet recommend periods of fasting, sometimes for a week or two or even more. In my opinion, a brief fast is optional. The elimination of harmful foods allows the body a rest, and extended periods of fasting may achieve good results. Although a fast helps cleanse the body, nutrients must nevertheless soon be provided. Individuals not undernourished, however, may fast for several or more days with considerable benefit and no great discomfort. A consistent recovery from chronic disease, with much less discomfort to the patient, may be achieved when proper foods are introduced.

Most chronically ill patients need not necessarily fast to recover their health. The individual experiencing an acute gastrointestinal problem is an exception. When recent internal bleeding has occurred, fasting under a physician's supervision until the bleeding has stopped may be the best course. This may take up to a few days. The proper foods, carefully prepared, may then be introduced, including broth, soups, and cooked vegetables.

A brief fast is almost without exception the best natural way to deal with acute illness or recovery from surgery. The acutely ill have no appetite; food is taken only at the urging of family members or out of boredom and habit. A sick child, like a sick animal, will not touch food. The natural response to the onset of illness is loss of appetite. When no food is taken, the body can most efficiently marshal its energy to fight illness, rather than being forced to channel energy into digestive processes. Stored reserves are more than adequate for energy. Recovery from colds, flus, and other acute illnesses is most rapid when a fast is initiated at the first sign. Rest is in order, and feeding usually should not begin until the temperature is normal and a strong appetite has returned.

Fasting is but one way to treat acute illness and is at times best combined with other methods. Antibiotics are overused, but they may be lifesaving in certain acute problems. Herbal medicines are of benefit in most situations. When in doubt, seek a competent physician.

The Macrobiotic Diet of George Ohsawa and Michio Kushi

By the early 1900s, refined foods were being widely used in many Japanese cities.

Yukikazu Sakurazawa, born in Japan in 1893, became ill eating these foods. He recovered by eating brown rice, miso soup made with fish broth, vegetables, fish, and other traditional Japanese foods.

While living in Paris in the 1920s, he adopted the pen name, George Ohsawa, and called his teachings "macrobiotics." The word *macro* is Greek for "long" or "great;" the word *bio* is Greek for "life." The term *macrobiotics* was used by Hippocrates to describe healthy, long-lived people. Other classical writers also used the term, which came to mean living and eating in a simple and natural manner.

For forty years, Yukikazu Sakurazawa's pupil Michio Kushi was the leader of the worldwide macrobiotics movement. The author of books on the subject, he did a great deal to popularize the use of whole and natural food.

Macrobiotics as taught by Kushi and his followers is a way of life, emphasizing a need to live in harmony with nature and one's fellow man. The core is the macrobiotic diet, somewhat individualized for each person according to age, gender, climate, geography, activity level, and personal needs. A principle of the diet is that whole grains should be the major portion of everyone's diet. Claims are made that the macrobiotic diet has been followed by ordinary people throughout history, that early humans and their forebears skewed more toward being herbivores than omnivores, and that whole grains were the principal food in all previous civilizations and cancer-free societies.

The standard macrobiotic diet consists of cooked whole grains (about 50 to 60 percent of daily food by volume); fresh vegetables, mostly cooked (25 to 30 percent of daily food); soup, featuring sea vegetables, and fermented soy products (5 to 10 percent of daily food); beans (5 to 10 percent of daily food); and small amounts of fruit, fish, and desserts prepared with natural sweeteners. Vegetables and fruits used should be those indigenous to the region where one lives. Tropical varieties are avoided, as are all dairy products, eggs, and meat.

In the Far East, population growth in geographical areas with limited resources necessitates the consumption of more grains and less food of animal origin. But traditional cultures have always utilized more animal foods than the tiny percentage that a macrobiotic diet advocates. The notion that whole grains formed the basis of the diet of all cancer-free societies is entirely contrary to information from scores of anthropologists, nutritionists, and medical researchers who have investigated this subject since the turn of the twentieth century. Both whole grains and animal-sourced foods of the proper quality have proved capable of forming an important part of the diet of cancer-free societies.

Macrobiotics as taught by Kushi and others can be a helpful regimen for a time. Individuals have recovered from chronic diseases on macrobiotic diets. One well-known case is that of Anthony Sattilaro, a physician who recovered from advanced bone cancer on a macrobiotic regimen, as detailed in his book, *Recalled by Life*.

Case Histories of Patients Following a Macrobiotic Diet

But a macrobiotic diet also has limitations. In one case, a fifty-seven-year-old man came to me with a recent diagnosis of lung cancer, a spot the size of a quarter on his lung. He did not want conventional therapy and began a metabolic program integrating elements of the Gerson therapy with other approaches I have studied and developed. The tumor remained stable for nearly a year, to the surprise of his family doctor, who continued to monitor his condition. This was an oat-cell carcinoma, a type of rapidly growing lung cancer with a poor prognosis—few patients live more than a few months after diagnosis.

Growing impatient with the rigors of his therapy and the tumor's continued presence, my patient learned about macrobiotics. After consulting with a macrobiotic nutritional counselor, he stopped his therapy and began a strict macrobiotic regimen. At that point, X-rays showed his tumor stable and still the size of a quarter. He reasoned that if macrobiotics failed, he would quickly return to the program I had designed for him.

His condition deteriorated within weeks, his lungs filling with fluid; he required hospitalization. His tumor had begun growing rapidly and a few days later he died.

Another case of mine was that of a twenty-three-year-old woman who had eaten the macrobiotic way for several years. She had a gradual onset of marked and occasionally severe abdominal and pelvic pain over the course of forty-eight hours. She consulted both a macrobiotic nutritional counselor and a medical doctor. The former modified her diet somewhat. Her symptoms became worse, and her medical doctor recommended hospitalization if she did not improve shortly.

I suspected appendicitis, but physical findings and symptoms were more suggestive of an ovarian cyst. She had continued eating, though she had no appetite. I immediately instituted fasting, enemas, and herbal medicines; unless she improved by morning, or at any sign of her condition's worsening, she was to be hospitalized.

Her symptoms had improved by morning. They had largely disappeared within seventy-two hours of instituting the fast, and she began eating small amounts of food, using considerably more raw vegetables and fish than called for in the standard macrobiotic diet. No further problems requiring treatment occurred.

Small children eating macrobiotic diets with their parents sometimes exhibit failure to thrive (being underweight, lethargic, and exhibiting slow growth) due to deficiencies of fat-soluble vitamins (especially vitamin D), vitamin B_{12}, essential fatty acids, calcium, and perhaps other nutrients. These children and their parents, who are often fatigued and sickly, suffer from a lack of raw food and animal-sourced nutrients; dietary adjustments invariably have led to marked improvement within weeks.

Some individuals do well for a time following a macrobiotic diet, while others do poorly. The amount of fish included in the diet has an influence—most people need more. In his recovery from bone cancer, Anthony Sattilaro regularly consumed modest amounts of fish. Vegetarian macrobiotic regimens including little or no fish most often lead to problems. I suggest adding fish broth made with fish heads, which are rich in vitamin A. Careful use of recommended amounts of beans, sea vegetables, and other special foods are required for balance in the macrobiotic diet.

A craving for sweets is common among people eating a macrobiotic type of diet. Naturally sweetened desserts are regularly consumed, and followers often report eating additional sweets. In contrast, loss of a taste for sweets is often a side effect of a whole-food diet that includes substantial portions of animal-sourced food.

The Spiritual Underpinnings of the Macrobiotic Diet

An expressed concern of the macrobiotic movement is world peace, a fine sentiment used to lure people into an ultimately dangerous diet. Whole grains as the staple food for mankind is seen as an important means of promoting this end, for more people may then be fed and more equal distribution of wealth achieved. Food plays a role in personality; this relates to the observation that people eating a grain-based diet may exhibit more passive and less aggressive tendencies than those eating a diet based on the consumption of animal food. Ironically, the macrobiotic and other vegetarian or near-vegetarian diets often make people angry, due to a vitamin B_{12} deficiency. Hitler comes to mind.

Food certainly does play a pronounced role in shaping biological and cultural evolution. Government and industry leaders determining national policies seem unaware of this, as are most people. Macrobiotic leaders, however, are aware that the acceptance of a macrobiotic diet by large segments of the Western world's population would have sociological as well as physiological effects. Perhaps it would be a step toward one world government—but what kind of world, and at what cost? The quantity versus the quality of life is at issue.

In the nuclear age, survival of the human species as we know it depends on controlling aggressive tendencies; the same aggressive traits that carried us through the evolutionary process now threaten to destroy us. But loss of our biological strength has resulted in an epidemic of disease, physical and mental abnormalities, and lost reproductive capacity that has caused far more suffering than any war yet fought. This suffering is directly due to changes in diet. The macrobiotic goal of reduced aggressive tendencies is laudable, but if we are to regain our biological strength and have both quantity and quality of life, we must maintain access to traditional animal-sourced foods, while largely eliminating the refined foods that have assumed so prominent a role in the modern diet.

Changes taking place in the American diet have been mirrored by changes in national health. The interrelationships are obvious when one considers the implications of our study of our evolutionary ancestors, primitive cultures existing in the earlier part of this century, contemporary hunter-gatherers and long-lived people, and current medical research on nutrition. Each of the diets considered in this chapter in some way utilizes beneficial aspects of traditional foods.

The next logical step—the creation and implementation of one's own diet for optimal health—is a complex process that may appear deceptively simple. We begin that process in the next chapter with a consideration of the elements of change, balance, and proportions in relation to food.

8
CREATING A PRIMAL DIET FOR HEALTH AND LONGEVITY

This chapter is meant to be an aid to selecting foods for a modern primal diet, one that is suited to individual tastes, personality, and genetic background. These are guidelines for experimenting with diet. By studying reactions to various foods, one may create an optimal nutritional program. When medical problems are present or suspected, see a competent physician, preferably one familiar with the concepts presented in this book.

Effects of specific foods upon different conditions will be discussed in the next chapter. Particularly if any of these or other serious conditions exist, the services of a knowledgeable and understanding physician may be invaluable.

PHYSICAL SYMPTOMS OF NUTRITIONAL IMBALANCE

The body's needs constantly change, and an optimal diet is dynamic. To maintain balance, a sense of which foods are most needed now is required. Foods eaten at the last meal, and in the last day or two, strongly affect this. But there are longer cycles during which a need to emphasize certain foods may be experienced. Some cycles relate to seasonal availability of foods; others are internal and may last for a few days, months, or even years.

Several signals may be monitored as a guide in food selections. Difficult bowel movements with hard stools and straining may signal a need for better hydration and more fats and salt, raw vegetable salads, fermented vegetables, or cooked vegetables. Exercise—daily walks, jogging, running, resistance training, or vigorous exercise like tennis that is actually fun—aids regularity by stimulating both the intestines themselves and the consumption of more food. (Please see appendix 4 for more information on ways to enjoy exercise.) One reason traditional people took in large quantities of vitamins, minerals, and other nutrients was that they led active lives, which included the playing of games. This required more food, which meant more nutrients.

Appearance of excessive mucous in the respiratory system—sinus or nasal congestion, postnasal drip, or early symptoms of a cold—is often a sign the body is reacting poorly to dairy products. Raw-milk products may cause these symptoms, too, when they are from grain-fed animals.

The skin is an organ of elimination and often is the first part of the body to reveal a nutritional imbalance. Abnormal redness of the skin—pimples, rashes, small blemishes—may result from eating sugar and sweets. Honey and other sweeteners, fruit juices, dried fruits, and even excessive amounts of fresh fruit may cause redness. The person eating no concentrated sweets for a time may have the quickest reaction when sweets are eaten—the body is well-balanced and immediately eliminates excesses.

Certain fruits may cause marked intestinal gas. Dried fruits, nuts, seeds, beans, and certain combinations of foods also often cause flatus, depending upon the amount eaten. Improperly prepared grains may similarly cause distress. Excessive gas, stomach or intestinal, is a sign the foods eaten have been improperly digested. When one eats correct proportions of properly prepared foods, digestion is smooth as silk.

BASIC FOOD GROUPS

I divide all foods into the following six groups, which inform us about what I call the Primal Principle:

1. **Grass-fed animal foods and fats.** This group includes wild fish, shellfish, and fish eggs; grass-fed meat, organs, bones, fat, and broth; pastured fowl and eggs; raw milk, yogurt, kefir, cheese, butter, lard, and ghee.

2. **Salad greens, raw and cooked green and other vegetables, fermented vegetables, sprouts, fruits, and sea vegetables.** These include lettuces and other leafy greens palatable raw in salads, parsley, celery, and sprouts. Cooked green vegetables include kale, broccoli, green beans, brussel sprouts, and others. Additional vegetables include carrots and cauliflower, both healthy and palatable whether raw or cooked. A wide variety of fruits eaten in moderation are both tasty and healthful. Sea vegetables include dulse, kelp, nori, and others. Fermented vegetables are wonderful traditional foods as well.

3. **Properly prepared whole grains and foods made from whole grains, nuts, seeds, and beans.** The key to a healthy use of these foods is proper preparation (typically involving soaking) and moderation. These foods may be part of a healthy diet, but they are not for all people at all times.

4. **Healthy oils and vinegars, spices and seasonings, and alcoholic and other fermented beverages.** One hundred percent extra-virgin olive oil and cold-pressed coconut oil are essential in daily food preparation. Other healthy and beneficial oils to use in moderation include macadamia nut, avocado, sunflower, sesame, and pumpkin oils. Raw apple cider vinegar and balsamic vinegar may be used in salad dressings. Sea salt—I prefer Celtic salt—may be used to taste. Freshly ground black pepper and other spices enhance the flavor of many foods. Wine is a

traditional drink that enhances appetite and the flavor of food and is enjoyed the world over in its own right. Beer too may be enjoyable and generally presents no problems, though beer is grain-based and those avoiding grains may wish to avoid it. But handcrafted unpasteurized microbrew beers are a healthy complement to kombucha and other fermented beverages when used in moderation. There is an old question: "Do you eat to live, or live to eat?" The items in this fourth group quite simply help make the answer to that question a resounding "Both!"

5. **Special foods, vitamins, minerals, and food supplements.** This group will have its own chapter later in the book. Suffice it to say for now that when carefully selected for individual needs, these items may complement even the best primal diets to aid recovery from health problems, build optimal health, and enhance longevity. Examples relevant for most people include carefully crafted cod-liver oil, krill oil, organ and gland supplements, iodine supplements, and nutrient formulas that help protect vision and memory as we inevitably age. Other people may benefit from supplements that help to correct dietary deficiencies or deal with environmental stresses.

6. **Everything else (refined and manufactured foods, particularly sugar and white flour).** Foods not included in the above five groups are not natural foods and are, for the most part, best avoided. The degree to which one can tolerate their occasional use depends on the state of health of the individual. Recovery from most medical problems is greatly enhanced when "everything else" is studiously avoided. Sugar in particular is highly addictive and indeed poison for many people when even the smallest amounts lead to overconsumption, a common occurrence.

THE PRIMAL PRINCIPLES

1. *Foods in groups 1 and 2 are the most primal, fundamental, basic foods, essential for prevention, healing, and recovery from disease.* That is the most important sentence in this book. Most of your diet should consist of foods in groups 1 and 2.
2. Use the foods in groups 3 and 4 in moderation.
3. Take advantage of modern wisdom about primal diets and health to help correct medical problems and achieve optimal health by utilizing the items in group 5.
4. Avoid the foods in group 6 like the plague.

CONSIDERATIONS OF PROPORTION, FLEXIBILITY, AND HABITUATION

The proportions of different foods most appropriate for each person vary from individual to individual, depending on one's genes, state of health, stage of life, tastes and inclinations, and health goals. Those ideal proportions will change as you go through life. I believe that by following the framework outlined in this chapter, you will find your way to utilizing the best proportions of the food you ingest. It helps to have an experienced guide, a mentor if you will. He or she might even be a physician. The word *doctor* is, after all, the Latin word for "teacher."

The critical fat-soluble vitamins A, D, and K_2, essential for immunity and mineral metabolism, are found together only in certain seafood (especially fish eggs, fish liver, fish-liver oils, fish heads, and shellfish), in meat and dairy fats from grass-fed animals (especially the organs), and eggs. These are the foods that Weston Price found richly supplied in the diets of immune groups. For raw-food nutrients, raw milk, butter, fresh raw greens and sprouts should be emphasized, especially if little raw meat and fish is consumed.

An example of a balanced regimen would be one-third animal food (fish and shellfish, meat and broth, organs, eggs, raw milk, kefir, yogurt, butter, and cheese); one-third raw salad greens and sprouts; and one-third mostly other vegetables and fruits, with some foods from groups 3 and 4. Cooked vegetable consumption increases in winter as raw vegetable consumption decreases. In late spring, summer, and early fall more fruit is consumed; consumption of grains may at such times decrease and even approach zero. Raw vegetable consumption too goes up in summer, when animal foods are usually eaten more infrequently. Again, these proportions may vary widely according to individual needs at different times and stages of life—but the principles apply to all of us throughout life.

I have spent weeks on the coast of Washington eating only salad and salmon—more than two pounds of the latter a day, cooked lightly with lots of butter. During my vegetarian days, late one Kansas summer, I ate little but muskmelons and watermelons for two weeks. Cross-country drives in younger times were spent eating brown rice, raw greens, and canned sardines for days at a time. The earth provides a wide variety of foods that will sustain us, at least for a while, though I certainly am not recommending any such regimens.

I've also fasted for up to seven days on springwater, though most uncomfortably. Literature about fasting describes how after a day or two, hunger disappears, and as cleansing proceeds, one does not experience hunger pangs until fat reserves are depleted and true hunger returns. Alas, by the third day, I experienced what felt like the excruciating pangs of advanced starvation. Seven days was eternity; the fast ended. That was many years ago; brief fasts of one or two days have since provided sufficient cleansing. (Fasting may cleanse, but it does not heal. Eating the right foods does.)

These are examples of variance; obviously none exemplifies a balanced diet. Balance in diet is best achieved by seeing one's body and one's health in the long term, while sensing how your needs may vary from day to day. Flexibility is essential. When principles are understood, nutrition may be approached in a creative way. People often complain they become tired of simple foods eaten daily and yearn for the variety of refined and prepared foods. But once one acquires a taste for whole and natural food (and it *is* an acquisition for those of us who grew up on refined foods), they never are boring or tiring when the primal principles embodied in our six food groups are carefully followed.

Experiences of Arctic explorer Vilhjalmur Stefansson illustrate this point. Despite adherence to medical advice of the early 1900s about the prevention of scurvy, expeditions of early Arctic and Antarctic explorers suffered severely from the disease. Stefansson's expeditions were a notable exception. Rather than carrying fruits and vegetables, lime juice, and other provisions of a "balanced diet," he and his men lived much as Arctic Eskimos did, eating nothing but seal and some polar bear meat for months, much of it raw and the rest lightly cooked. Eighty percent of the diet was fat. They got no scurvy. The little vitamin C in raw meat and fish, normally destroyed in cooking, provided adequate protection from the disease.

Stefansson found his men always became accustomed to the all-meat diet and eventually enjoyed it. The first week was difficult; some men ate little or nothing. Gradually they ate more until soon they were eating heartily, though with many complaints. Stefansson guessed that if sometime during the first three months they had suddenly been rescued from the seal meat and given a diet of varied foods, most would have sworn never to taste seal again. If it had been three or four months, a man may or may not have been willing to go back to seal again. But if the period had been six months or more, Stefansson claimed, none would have been unwilling to go back to the all-meat diet. (Please see appendix 1 for more on Stefansson and the all-meat diet.)

This is consistent with the experience of many people I have introduced to simple natural-food diets. There may be considerable discomfort initially, followed by a period of grudging acquiescence. But if the individual stays with the diet for three to six months, he or she usually will never go back to refined foods. I have found that the key to success is that the diet contains adequate fats, as occurs when the primal principles are carefully followed.

NUTRITION DURING PREGNANCY

A remarkable discovery of Weston Price's was that in cultures where little or no dental decay was found, physical abnormalities of any kind were almost nonexistent in children. Wisdom about special foods and spacing the birth of children by at least three years are the two factors most responsible for this.

This traditional wisdom about spacing childbirth is sound. Many psychologists believe that such spacing is also ideal for the emotional development of older siblings forced to compete at too early an age for the time and attention of the parents when siblings are born too soon after their own birth.

For at least six months before conception, the optimal nutritional program described earlier in this chapter should be followed. Most women particularly should place an emphasis on the foods in group 1. Iodine-rich sea vegetables such as dulse or kelp enhance fertility in women and an optimal development of the fetus. Their use as well by the prospective father before conception should ensure maximum viability of sperm and minimize chances of birth defects. During pregnancy (and lactation), a rich source of calcium such as raw milk or other quality dairy foods is important, particularly during the last trimester. Careful selection of special foods and food supplements in group 5 enhances fertility and helps ensure a healthy pregnancy. The diet itself should include foods such as organ meats, butter, egg yolks, fish eggs, raw milk, and cod-liver oil.

For more details, see the outstanding pregnancy diet section of the website of the Weston A. Price Foundation (www.westonaprice.org). Sally Fallon Morell's book *Nourishing Traditions* is also a wonderful resource on pregnancy and motherhood, as is Weston Price's work, and diets that follow the principles he discovered.

During pregnancy, exercise such as gardening, walking (or doubles tennis for a woman accustomed to it) continued on a regular, daily basis enables a fair volume of food to be eaten without exorbitant weight gain. Such volume and lots of animal fats should ensure freedom from the constipation that troubles many pregnancies. Avoidance of sugar and consumption of only the smallest amounts of alcohol and white flour—empty calories—further promotes the consumption of adequate animal foods and vegetables.

Price's evidence that such a program produces maximally healthy and well-developed babies is overwhelming. Women following such a program of diet and exercise have, in my experience, invariably had healthy pregnancies, births, and babies.

Many of the same foods emphasized immediately prior to conception and during pregnancy and lactation are especially important when treating disease through the utilization of food. These and other considerations important in treating specific conditions are discussed in the next chapter, as we continue to define how each individual may best select foods most suited to them.

9
DIETARY CONSIDERATIONS FOR SPECIFIC CONDITIONS

This chapter is about specific conditions, but a specific diet for each condition will not be described. Different people with the same diagnosed condition have different nutritional requirements; sometimes these differences are marked. Detailed recommendations may be made only after individual assessment. Tastes and emotional states should never be overlooked, for the finest plan is of no help if not followed. With this in mind, we'll discuss considerations pertaining to the following conditions.

COLDS, FLU, MONONUCLEOSIS

Colds and Flu

Colds and flu disappear most rapidly when a fast is started at the first sign of symptoms. Everyone has individual characteristic signs marking the onset of colds and flu—for some, fatigue and a headachy feeling or perhaps a loss of appetite, for others, a vague but growing soreness in the throat. The latter is often the first sign in those with no tonsils, which as a part of the immune system, protect the throat from bacterial and viral invasion; their loss leaves one more susceptible to sore throats.

Symptoms typically grow worse over the course of a day or two, as the illness becomes established. If a fast is instituted at the first sign, minor symptoms will usually begin to abate within twenty-four hours. The cold or flu can then often be avoided by eating very carefully for the next few days.

The human body is remarkable; when allowed, corrective action comes naturally. The acutely ill feel no hunger because food consumption during acute illness interferes with natural responses. But hunger may be strong when the earliest symptoms appear, for the illness is not yet established. Awareness and discipline aid greatly; too often we eat out of habit or boredom, or because of the expectations of others. The temptation to eat before we have fully recovered may be strong, but doing so often brings back the symptoms and blocks recovery.

After the fasting stage, the wisest diet is one that is comprised, simply, of non-starchy vegetables with lots of butter, broth, fish, chicken, or meat. The classic Jewish mother doles out chicken soup; this wisdom originated when the chicken was fed and raised in the barnyard. A soup made of beef, chicken, or fish stock, and greens, carrots, onions, and garlic is excellent. When a virulent bug takes hold and can't be shaken off in a day or two, this diet is the next best thing to fasting.

People often express disbelief about the effectiveness of a short fast. One patient called late one Thursday afternoon with flu symptoms. Her weekend travel plans were threatened; she felt ill and was feverish (101.5 degrees). She hoped to feel well enough to travel the next afternoon. A fast was recommended, consisting only of water, herbal tea, vitamin C, and cod-liver oil. "Nothing else," I told her. "Just rest. Don't eat tonight or tomorrow. No food, no juices. Take a warm-water enema, body temperature, with a quart or so of water, once tonight and again in the morning. By noon tomorrow, the fever should break, and if your temperature is normal by late tomorrow afternoon and you feel up to it, take your trip. Don't eat tomorrow night either. Begin eating Saturday—but only vegetables, some soup, and fish, chicken, or meat. Do not overexert yourself. If symptoms reappear, fast again."

Despite her doubts, she followed my directions. By morning, her temperature was close to normal; by evening she felt well enough to travel. She had aborted a bout with a cold or the flu. Natural, food-sourced vitamin C is useful, two or three hundred milligrams daily.

Recently, Michael Schachter, M.D., reported to me that in the acute stages of flu, patients greatly benefit from taking 50,000 IU of vitamin D and 100,000 IU of vitamin A for three to five days.

Mononucleosis

Mononucleosis is an infectious viral disease marked by fatigue, high fever, sore throat, and swollen lymph glands. The diagnosis is made from characteristics of the blood cells seen microscopically. While people in their teens and twenties are usually the most susceptible to it, middle-aged people with mono may go undiagnosed for months if the possibility is not considered when symptoms are present.

Conventional medicine has no treatment for mono; since it is viral, antibiotics are ineffective, though they may be given if a concurrent bacterial infection is suspected. While effective against some bacterial infections, antibiotics may further weaken the patient and place an added strain on an already overburdened liver. The usual course is several weeks of bed rest followed by several more of gradual recovery.

Recovery from mononucleosis with carefully supervised natural treatment may be dramatic. Even when the disease is well established, an initial thirty-six- to forty-eight-hour fast usually brings the fever under 100 degrees and reverses the course of any concurrent bacterial infection. By then the patient typically feels better and has some appetite; if so, some food may be taken.

With continued rest and careful eating only when the appetite is strong, patients are up and around and feeling fairly well, though still weakened, within a few days. Ninety-percent recovery within one to two weeks and full recovery within two to four weeks has been the rule.

Mono is not life threatening, but it can drag on for months and be most debilitating. Although unusual, some individuals suffer relapses, which may actually be flare-ups of a low-grade but continuing presence of the disease. Although no causal link has been established, patients with a history of recurrent mononucleosis have later developed Hodgkin's disease, a type of cancer of the lymph system. The chronically weakened immune system leaves an individual susceptible to the development of cancer. A healthy immune system eliminates the small number of cancer cells we all constantly develop spontaneously.

ACUTE ILLNESSES IN INFANTS

In most cases, no food should be given to infants or babies showing signs of acute illness until the temperature returns to normal; usually this takes from twelve to twenty-four hours. Even an infant may be safely fasted for a day or two if sufficient water is given. An acutely ill infant has no desire for food. Short tepid baths (water at seventy-five to eighty degrees for a few minutes) and small amounts of aspirin if the temperature is over 105 degrees usually lowers the fever in infants to under 105 degrees. If the problem seems serious or is accompanied by continuing diarrhea, if there is doubt about its nature, if the fever stays over 105 degrees, or if it persists longer than twenty-four hours despite these measures, the infant should immediately be seen by a physician.

The breast-fed baby is profoundly affected by the diet of the mother; if the baby is ill, the mother's diet is almost invariably to blame. The above described dietary measures usually quickly eliminate illness in the baby.

Acute illness is a warning sign of more serious things to come, and it may for the most part be avoided by a healthy lifestyle and diet. The simple and straightforward measures discussed effectively deal with most occasional, acute problems that do arise, in a safe and nontoxic way.

ALLERGIES

Allergies too are early warning signs that foods are creating imbalances. The worst offenders are often conventionally produced milk and cheese; removing them from the diet eliminates many allergies.

In young children, allergies most often manifest as coughs, colds, and recurrent middle-ear infections, all of which usually clear up when refined carbohydrates and conventionally produced milk and cheese are removed from the diet. An example is the case of a six-year-old boy whose marked hearing loss due to recurrent middle-ear infections was causing him difficulties in school. Surgical implantation of drainage tubes was planned, but his parents decided to try natural treatment first.

Acute infections in both ears cleared within a week; within three weeks the boy's parents and his teacher noted a clear improvement in his hearing. Subsequent audio testing showed his hearing returning gradually to normal over the next six months, and surgery was avoided. This little boy was a marvelous patient; within a week on the diet we planned together, he grew to love its foods. He once explained how he hadn't eaten any cake at a birthday party the day before because he was happy to be hearing better, and that was more important than cake. Eventually, he was able to have cake on occasion without any problems.

Despite having been corrupted by sugar, children's tastes often change rapidly; they tend to embrace good food when that's all there is to eat. Firm guidance is needed; they may refuse to eat in an attempt to pressure parents into giving them what they want. The alternative of good food or no food typically ends hunger strikes within a day or so.

Allergy tests are popular because of confusion about what constitutes a proper diet; they attempt to provide a sophisticated solution for a simple but subtle problem. Yet the proper diet for an individual may be determined without these tests.

Many people test positive for pollens and other environmental factors. Conventional allergy treatments are designed to neutralize the effects of these allergens (substances triggering the allergic response), and many people get relief. But adverse reactions to trees, grasses, flowers, dust, dogs, and cats are not normal and indicate that the immune system is unbalanced and failing to function properly. The cause of the imbalance is almost always poor food selection. Offending foods often cause no overt response when eaten. Rather, chronic symptoms such as postnasal drip, congestion, itchy eyes, fatigue, or others are continually present, masking responses occurring when the food is eaten.

The individual then at times has a gross and obvious allergic response to pollens and other environmental factors. The response is real and is directly stimulated by the environmental factors, but it has developed because foods disturbing immune function have been regularly eaten. Refined carbohydrates—sugar and white flour products—and conventional dairy foods are usually the worst offenders. Raw milk from grass-fed animals is very helpful for allergies, as are bone broths and natural vitamin C. The elimination of caffeine from the diet is also helpful.

When traditional diets are followed, allergy problems clear up. Trees, flowers, and cats are not supposed to make people sick; when they do something is wrong. Pottenger noted the development of allergies, and even of allergic bronchitis, in cats fed diets of cooked and refined foods. The naturally fed animals suffered no such aberrations. Unlike cats, people do not require an all-raw diet. But for human beings, allergies are caused by the modern diet.

CHRONIC FATIGUE AND THYROID PROBLEMS

Chronic fatigue is a very common complaint. Some people feel tired throughout life and accept fatigue as normal. Others feel tired for up to several months prior to the diagnosis of a chronic disease. If, however, the results of laboratory tests and a physical exam are normal, little attempt is usually made to treat fatigue. While it may be a sign of a serious but undetected problem, it is often considered a vague complaint that people must live with.

Chronic fatigue is a classic symptom of low thyroid function, or hypothyroidism. The thyroid gland is not an entity unto itself, and its effects on metabolism are best considered as one part of the overall picture. Low thyroid function is common, especially in middle-aged and older people. Laboratory tests for thyroid function often are normal in people exhibiting low thyroid function as well as some of the symptoms of hypothyroidism, which besides fatigue may include dry skin and hair, a tendency to gain weight easily, constipation, and sensitivity to cold weather. Seldom are all of these symptoms present; low thyroid function affects people differently.

The one common characteristic is a low basal body temperature as indicated by the underarm temperature upon first awakening in the morning (best taken at the same time daily before moving about or arising from bed). The most definitive readings in women are taken during the first three days of the menstrual cycle.

The physician first describing this test, Broda Barnes, initially trained as a physiologist, studying thyroid function in animals. He associated low thyroid function in people with the development of chronic diseases and other conditions, including migraines, emotional and behavioral disorders, infectious diseases, skin problems, menstrual and fertility problems, hypertension, heart disease, arthritis, diabetes, cancer, and premature aging. Presence of symptoms associated with low thyroid function and a consistent basal temperature below 97.8 led him to treat with thyroid tissue. In his thirty-five-year career, he treated thousands of patients this way, using the basal body temperature test as one means of monitoring progress. He suggests 97.8 to 98.2 degrees to be a normal range. In my experience, the lower end of the temperature range Barnes used is a bit high; the range of normal should be from 97.2 to 98.2. An individual in the 97.2 to 97.7 range may or may not have low thyroid function; many symptomless people fall in this range, but so do many people with overt symptoms. Those with basal temperatures below 97.2 nearly always show symptoms; people with chronic diseases usually are in this range.

Hormones produced in the thyroid gland control the metabolic rate of every cell in the body. The thyroid thus affects pathological conditions as they arise and develop, and low thyroid function contributes to a developing chronic problem. Many clinicians have noted this relationship. Medical literature since early in the twentieth century reveals many reports of beneficial effects of thyroid medication on a host of chronic conditions. Max Gerson noted that his cancer patients almost invariably suffered from grossly low thyroid function, and he included substantial amounts of thyroid tissue in his therapy.

Barnes kept records that revealed his patients taking thyroid had markedly lower incidences of chronic diseases, especially heart disease and cancer, than statistically expected. This is consistent with the experience of many physicians who find most patients with chronic diseases show some symptoms of low thyroid function and a low basal body temperature. Fat-soluble vitamins A and D are in short supply in most modern diets but are a must for a healthy thyroid.

When prescribing thyroid, endocrinologists and internists usually call for a synthetic hormone rather than natural, animal thyroid tissue. This allows a standardized dosage not possible with precision when using the natural product because tissue from different animals varies slightly in potency. But people on synthetic thyroid may show conflicting symptoms of underactive and overactive thyroid function, and low basal temperatures. Several in my experience have had recurrent heart irregularities—irregular rhythms and palpitations—while on synthetic thyroid. Such irregularities have not been noted in individuals on carefully regulated amounts of natural thyroid.

As chronic conditions improve, symptoms of low thyroid function improve also, and basal temperature rises. Proper diet and adequate iodine intake are essential for healthy thyroid function, as was elegantly demonstrated by Robert McCarrison. He showed that the weight of the thyroid gland as a percentage of total body weight in white rats varied significantly when a natural-food diet rich in raw milk, vegetables, whole-grain flour, and meat was changed to one of refined foods. Classic symptoms of hypothyroidism appeared when the animals were fed refined foods.

The first signs of improvement for many individuals with low thyroid function who are making dietary changes are increased energy with less fatigue and more frequent bowel movements. Improved glandular function, particularly of the thyroid gland, likely provides the stimulus for these changes.

ARTHRITIS AND BACK PROBLEMS

Most people over the age of fifty (and many much younger) suffer at least some early symptoms of arthritis. With added years, the problem usually becomes worse. The bent posture, stiff hands, and slow gait of most elderly Americans is in stark contrast with the energy, activity, and strength noted among the very old in Georgian Russia, Vilcabamba, and Hunza.

No adequate explanation for the development of arthritis has been put forth by conventional medicine. Deposits of calcium are found in affected joints, and involvement of an imbalance in calcium metabolism is accepted. These deposits occur early in osteoarthritis, the common arthritis of aging. In rheumatoid arthritis, they appear considerably later.

What causes these deposits of calcium in the arthritic process? Calcium serves a host of functions, and the absorption and utilization of dietary calcium is complex. Bones are a storehouse for calcium, and normal blood levels of calcium are maintained by an interplay of dietary calcium and calcium released from and taken into the bones.

Abnormal calcium deposits in the joints are due in part to disturbances in calcium metabolism caused by poor diet and subsequent lack of vitamin K_2. The MK4 type of vitamin K_2, rather than the MK7, is the most beneficial. Published studies of its use in osteoporosis indicate that the ideal dose may be 15 mg three times daily. When dietary calcium is inadequate, the bones steadily lose calcium to maintain adequate levels in the blood. This leads both to osteoporosis (defined as an abnormal loss of calcium from the bones) and to abnormal deposits of calcium; often osteoarthritis and osteoporosis are present simultaneously, and clinicians often have difficulty distinguishing between them.

A loss of calcium from the bones often leads to the spontaneous fractures of osteoporosis, especially of the hips in the elderly. Bones have become so weak in these cases that the break occurs under normal stresses of daily living. The loss of bone calcium leading to this takes place over many years. Studies show radiologists are not unanimous in interpreting an X-ray as showing osteoporosis until at least 30 percent of the calcium in the bone has been lost. This means lesser losses are often not detected; we may assume many middle-aged and older people have an undetected loss of calcium from the bones. This bone loss of calcium leads to the above problems involving calcium deposits.

People eating traditional diets consumed four to eight times the calcium and far greater multiples of vitamin K_2 than official standards recommend today. Food rich in calcium should be consumed, especially by people with calcium-related problems. But arthritis also develops in people receiving adequate dietary calcium. Eating refined carbohydrates, particularly sugar, causes disturbances in blood levels of calcium and phosphorous. Such disturbances are a major factor in the development of arthritis. Sweets of any kind aggravate symptoms of arthritis in most patients. Significant improvements in symptoms often lead to a "treat," a few cookies or similar sweets, soon followed by the reappearance of pain and other symptoms. This is no coincidence.

Commercial dairy products also may aggravate arthritis. Pasteurization changes the way calcium is arranged in milk and disturbs its normal utilization. Often young and early-middle-aged adults with back problems have been large drinkers of commercial milk. Calcium metabolism problems are seldom encountered in raw-milk drinkers. The evidence of Pottenger's cats is revealing; those fed pasteurized milk developed inferior skeletal structures and eventually mild arthritis, while those fed sweetened condensed milk developed gross skeletal abnormalities and debilitating arthritis. Those fed only raw foods including raw milk maintained perfect health.

The chronic bad back of a young adult often is an early stage of the osteoarthritis of an older individual. Dental decay in children and young adults and periodontal disease in middle-aged and older adults all indicate disturbances in calcium metabolism. These problems respond well to primal diets rich in fat-soluble vitamins A, D, and K_2.

These nutrients control mineral metabolism and have profound effects. As we have learned, cod-liver oil, grass-fed butter, egg yolks, liver, and cheese are excellent sources. If individuals chronically lack adequate dietary calcium, then cod-liver oil along with special foods rich in calcium, or calcium hydroxyapatite supplements, may have a rapidly beneficial effect within days, especially upon chronic back problems. Elimination of commercial dairy products and refined carbohydrates and inclusion of raw vegetables in the diet enhances results, as does the inclusion of grass-fed raw milk.

Excess fruit, particularly citrus fruits and fruit juices, usually aggravate arthritis. Night-shade vegetables—tomatoes, potatoes, green peppers, and eggplant—also usually aggravate the symptoms. A problem with nightshades is a sign of vitamin K_2 deficiency. My own decades-long allergic reactions to tomatoes largely disappeared when I began taking vitamin K_2 supplements (particularly the MK4 type) and eating more grass-fed animal sourced foods. Removal of most fruit, fruit juices, and nightshade vegetables from the diet may be an important part of a program for those serious about reversing an arthritic condition through careful nutrition. Later, moderate amounts may be better tolerated.

Arthritis is often accepted as a part of growing old, perhaps until the pain becomes great. But pain is a great motivator, and people with osteoarthritis are often very successful patients. Literally every patient of mine who has seriously attempted to follow the principles of nutrition outlined above has experienced significant relief from arthritis.

The degree of improvement correlates with the care taken with the diet. Many people find they can control arthritis by eating with some degree of care while continuing to eat some refined foods; arthritis is more easily controlled than other chronic diseases. Others following recommendations fully have experienced a complete reversal and no longer have symptoms. A return to refined foods sooner or later results in a relapse of symptoms. This seems true of all chronic diseases.

Fresh raw-vegetable salads may be important in arthritis, if well tolerated and enjoyed; they are rich in live enzymes and in calcium and other minerals. Juice made from raw greens and carrots may also be helpful. But collagen-rich broth made from the bones and tissues of grass-fed animals is perhaps the most powerful food in reversing arthritis and should be consumed in quantity daily. Fermented vegetables are an excellent source of enzymes and beneficial bacteria. Raw egg yolks blended into eggnog with grass-fed raw milk are excellent as well, as are various sprouts used in salads. Fresh or frozen wild seafood may form a significant portion of the diet; cook it with lots of butter derived from grass-fed animals.

Rheumatoid Arthritis

Rheumatoid arthritis differs from osteoarthritis in that the immune system malfunctions and produces antibodies that attack tissues of the body, particularly in the joints. Similar autoimmune problems occur in other tissues in lupus.

These problems respond to careful and thorough nutrition. Rheumatoid arthritis is less common than osteoarthritis and often more difficult to treat. Patients are usually younger than those with osteoarthritis; the disease typically occurs in middle-aged and younger adults, and occasionally in children.

Extreme sensitivity to certain foods is usual, and in particular sugar and gluten are problems. Fruits may not be tolerated. Commercial, conventional dairy foods usually cause marked reactions; dairy foods from grass-fed animals, best raw, are usually helpful.

One of my patients was a three-year-old girl first seen in 1981 one week after a diagnosis of rheumatoid arthritis. The joints of her wrists, fingers, and ankles were swollen, red, and painful, despite the use of aspirin. Her blood test was positive for rheumatoid arthritis. Offered steroid drugs, her parents elected to see me and try nutritional therapy.

The swelling, pain, and redness in her joints were gone within a week of beginning the careful diet I planned for her, and she no longer needed aspirin. She remained free of symptoms except for one period of several days when she had some joint pain. Her mother explained that the family had been careless with her diet for a few days prior. When she was returned to her usual diet, her symptoms again disappeared.

Unfortunately, rheumatoid arthritis may be much more difficult to treat when well established for many years. For some reason, many adults with this problem have found it difficult to follow a diet to the extent necessary for dramatic relief—more so than people with most other diseases. They have often expressed a feeling of being deprived when giving up sugary, refined foods, and some refuse to follow a careful diet and would simply rather suffer the symptoms of the disease.

Even with careful compliance, progress may be slow. Much depends on the degree of destruction in the joints; the longer the disease has been established, the more difficult treatment is. Extensive use of steroids such as cortisone, common in those long with the disease, makes recovery more difficult. Nevertheless, many middle-aged and older rheumatoid patients find they may largely control their symptoms with attention to diet. Mild improvement in symptoms or even simply preventing the problem from becoming worse may be all some people desire; many choose to eat with some care in exchange for partial relief. My rheumatoid patients who have made concerted and extended efforts to follow primal nutritional programs have made good to excellent progress.

Results with the other autoimmune diseases have been similar; individuals who carefully follow the details of dietary recommendations have had marked improvements. Many have found all their symptoms disappear and been pronounced cured by their medical doctors, who have often claimed "spontaneous remission" and expressed astonishment at the idea that diet could have anything to do with it. This attitude has changed somewhat more recently, however. Today more doctors now speak words to the effect of, "Well, whatever you're doing, keep doing it." I await the day when, as one or two have done over the years, more will contact me and ask me for details about their patients' recoveries.

HEART AND CIRCULATORY DISORDERS

For people with cardiac and circulatory disorders, one of the most important foods is fatty cold-water species of fish such as wild salmon.

Raw shellfish may be eaten in season as desired. (Shellfish are best from September through April, when they are not molting.) People with these problems are usually warned to avoid shellfish and organ meats because of the high cholesterol content they contain. As discussed in other parts of this book, however, the cholesterol content of foods is a red herring. Cholesterol-rich foods are good for you; cholesterol is simply not the cause of heart disease.

The consumption of organ meats and of several dozen oysters or clams a week, when in season, has been the rule for various individuals I have worked with during their recovery from heart disease. Recovery was adequate even in an individual who without fail consumed four to six ounces of liquor daily, though that is definitely not recommended.

Dairy products derived from grass-fed animals and meats from grass-fed animals are beneficial. Information presented earlier on seafood, fats, and protective nutrients should serve as a guide in food selection for people with a history of heart disease.

Calcium and the Heart

Abnormal deposits of calcium are present in both atherosclerosis (the buildup of plaque on arterial walls, particularly those of the coronary arteries) and arteriosclerosis (hardening of the arteries). In the former, calcium, cholesterol, and other fatty materials are involved; in the latter, the hardening is mainly calcification. In both cases, vitamin K_2 prevents the problems. Again, the MK4 type is preferred.

These two problems are generally concurrent and are often associated with arthritis; imbalances in calcium metabolism affect all three. Again, abnormal calcium metabolism traceable to the diet appears to be the major contributing factor in the deposition of calcium in both joints and arterial walls. Research over the course of the past twenty years or so indicates that a lack of vitamin K_2, in short supply in modern diets but richly supplied in grass-fed animal foods, is the predominant cause of this problem.

These abnormal deposits occur in a host of medical conditions.

Arteriosclerosis may lead to senility and stroke when arteries to the brain are affected, and it contributes to the poor circulation to the extremities common in old age. Kidney stones and gallstones usually contain large amounts of calcium. In multiple sclerosis, calcium is precipitated into muscles, and in arthritis deposits occur on bone surfaces and in joints. Calcium deposition may also relate to hypertension, for a gradual deposition of calcium contributes to a hardening of the arteries. Resultant inelasticity of these vessels raises blood pressure.

Blood Pressure, Cholesterol Levels, and the Thyroid Gland

High blood pressure usually accompanies heart disease and is often involved in its development. Both high blood cholesterol and high blood pressure are classic signs of hypothyroidism, low thyroid function, and a lack of optimal amounts of vitamin A and vitamin D. Recent research has demonstrated the importance of vitamin D. Extensive writings in the medical literature in the earlier part of this century detailed relationships between blood pressure, blood cholesterol, and the thyroid gland. Thyroid problems were then diagnosed symptomatically rather than through laboratory testing. Tests now used often indicate a normal condition despite the presence of overt symptoms of low thyroid function, and articles in medical journals frequently point out the limitations of these tests.

Thus many Americans have both high blood pressure and high blood cholesterol that are caused in part by undiagnosed low thyroid function. Thyroid hormones control the rate at which cholesterol and other fats are metabolized; their relative lack thus leads to higher levels of blood cholesterol. How a lack of thyroid hormones contributes to high blood pressure is not as clear, but in the 1920s physicians involved in the new field of endocrinology proposed the concept of cellular infiltration.

Because fats in cells throughout the body (including those in cells lining the blood vessels) are not burned up at a normal rate when thyroid function is low, they accumulate along with other waste products of incomplete cellular metabolism. Liken this to a wood fire getting insufficient oxygen—it smolders, and charcoal accumulates. The accumulation in cells lining blood vessel walls causes these cells to take on extra fluid and swell. As the vessels become less elastic, the blood pressure is slowly raised over the years. This is the concept of cellular infiltration, a physiologically sound theory to explain the observation that hypertension occurs in hypothyroidism.

Current standards for blood pressure reflect averages rather than what is healthy. Blood pressure measurements among the elderly in Vilcabamba and Georgian Russia as measurd in the 1970s were in the range of 100 over 60 to 120 over 80. Americans are considered to be doing well if the blood pressure stays under 140 over 90.

When people who do not have marked blood pressure problems begin a traditional diet, blood pressure usually slowly falls into the 110 over 70 to 120 over 80 range (if not there to begin with). Those with markedly elevated pressure at the start (higher than 140 over 90) usually experience gradual reductions until no medication is needed (under 140 over 90). Further reductions occur if a careful program is continued and, if weight is a problem, it is reduced into a reasonable range.

Caffeine and the Heart

Caffeine often increases blood pressure, which may drop twenty or more points within a few weeks of abstaining from coffee even if no other changes are made. Caffeine also may cause palpitations (alarmingly strong and rapid heartbeats) and influence arrhythmias (irregularities in the rhythm of the heartbeat). Sugar too may bring on these symptoms.

An example is a gentleman who "converted," as he puts it, to eating mostly natural food over the course of several years. Still, he maintained a fondness for sweets and coffee. He began mixing his regular drip coffee half and half with decaf; he drank twice as much. Once a week or so, he binged on rich desserts.

He occasionally began experiencing unnerving palpitations and arrhythmias during the night. Evaluation by a cardiologist revealed no serious problems, and he continued his regular program of jogging, tennis, and rowing; he was in quite good condition. The problem occurred only during the night.

Questioning revealed that the problem occurred two or three nights a week, sometimes after binging on sweets and sometimes on nights he ate no sweets. He concluded that coffee rather than sweets caused the trouble. His cardiologist, knowing caffeine can produce the symptoms, advised he cut down on, or give up, coffee.

He cut down to a cup or two a day, but the problem continued to occur. He seemed to think that such a small amount of coffee couldn't be responsible for his problem. He was persuaded to give up coffee entirely, which he nearly did (he still had a cup once or twice a week). But the problem still occurred once a week or so, sometimes on the nights he had coffee, sometimes on other nights.

We discovered in time that the symptoms often occurred on the nights he ate sweets. On nights he did drink coffee (with or without sweets), the symptoms might occur. Both coffee and sweets were capable of inducing his palpitations and his arrhythmia, though neither one did so every time; the occurrence of symptoms was apparently related to the dose. The combination of coffee and sweets was most likely to cause symptoms.

This case is typical of the potential effects of caffeine and sugar on the heart. It also illustrates the strong tendency toward denial of the possibility that favorite foods and drinks may cause problems. People tend to think that unless a food causes a readily identifiable symptom every time it is eaten in any quantity, it is not a likely cause of the symptom. This is not accurate. Though foods may act upon us in such an easily identified manner, the process is often more subtle. Our reactions depend upon the amount of the food ingested, when it was eaten last and in what quantity, what it was eaten with, and the overall status of the body at that time. An equal amount of a food causing no reaction once may cause a marked reaction the next time it's eaten.

In rotation diets, foods not known to cause allergic reactions are eaten once every three, four, or five days. Foods that do cause reactions are avoided for a time, after which one may attempt to introduce them on a rotational basis. Foods that previously caused allergic reactions may then cause no symptoms. As we have established, allergy symptoms are caused by malfunctioning of the immune system, which produces antibodies in response to the allergenic food. The allergic reaction may then be strong if the food is soon eaten again, causing marked symptoms. When the food is not eaten again for several days, antibodies causing the allergic reaction dissipate, and any reaction occurring tends to be milder.

The heart symptoms above were a response to both caffeine and allergens in foods. Changes in blood-sugar levels caused by sugar (caffeine affects this too) may interplay with these reactions. The acute heart symptoms, like acute symptoms that may occur in any system of the body, were directly caused by the foods.

The Importance of Exercise

Regular and controlled exercise is of particular benefit for problems with the heart and circulatory system; for full recovery it is essential. Although parameters vary for each person, the heart should be taxed slightly beyond its customary workload for (at first) a short time, and daily. Very short walks are a good beginning for most people, at a speed not so fast as to cause any shortness of breath. For a person unaccustomed to walking, only a distance causing no strain or fatigue should be covered. The keys to success are commitment and regularity. As one grows stronger, the length and intensity of the walk may be gradually increased. Moderate resistance exercise, beginning with light weights, is also extremely beneficial.

CANCER

People with cancer and seeking help usually feel a great deal of tension. Often pressure from different family members and physicians has been placed on the individual concerning the variety of possible treatments available. This dilemma can lead to confusion for the patient.

Controversy surrounding the treatment of cancer through alternative therapy adds to this difficulty. The medical establishment condemns alternative treatments of cancer. Surgery, chemotherapy, and radiation, the accepted treatments, usually alleviate symptoms of cancer for a time by destroying or removing cancer cells. But the underlying conditions that led to cancer are left unchanged, and cancer cells remaining continue to multiply.

Statistics concerning cancer survival are discouraging, but the actual situation is worse. Many of the people who survive for five or more years after the initial diagnosis end up in the later stages of cancer. Still they are counted as cures in the statistics; a cure by definition is anyone surviving five or more years. This makes the official statistics almost meaningless.

These people often seek alternative therapy. Having exhausted conventional treatments, they hope that an alternative may help them. Other people seek to use nutrition and other alternatives in support of their conventional treatments. This has become more popular as some individuals in conventional medicine have recognized that optimal nutrition strengthens the patient and allows him or her to withstand chemotherapy with fewer side effects. And some people decide from the start that their best chance of survival is to avoid conventional treatment and search for a natural approach that will work for them.

For those having had (or in the process of having) conventional treatment, anything done to improve nutrition is in support of that treatment; nutrition should not be considered the primary means of treatment. For the individual who has had chemotherapy or extensive radiation, nutrition may be of only limited benefit. This was Max Gerson's experience, as it has been mine. The basis of natural therapy is the strengthening of the immune system to enable it to reject the cancer. The capacity of the immune system to be so strengthened is compromised by the poisonous chemicals used in chemotherapy.

Whole-food diets and proper supplements reduce side effects of chemotherapy or radiation. Often individuals subsequently feel well for several months while continuing excellent nutritional programs.

Unfortunately, in many cases I have followed, tumors eventually reappear.

This is why the choice between conventional and alternative therapy should be made at the outset. It is difficult for a nutritional or any metabolic program to succeed after chemotherapy has failed.

The recent trend has been for more people to use nutrition as an adjunct to chemotherapy. This diminishes side effects and also often helps make the person in the later stages of cancer more comfortable. It may alter chances of survival. But although such cases are not a fair test of the value of nutrition as therapy for cancer, the failure of such programs to increase survival may increase established resistance against nutritional therapy for cancer.

An extensive review of the problems inherent in conventional cancer treatment may be found in Ralph Moss's book *The Cancer Industry* (originally titled *The Cancer Syndrome*). While working as assistant director of public affairs at Memorial Sloan Kettering Cancer Center in New York, Moss wrote anonymously for months in an in-house booklet titled *Second Opinion* about the efficacy of Laetrile in cancer treatment. Laetrile is an extract of apricot pits, which some Sloan Kettering researchers had found to have an anti-tumor effect in animal experiments. When he confessed at a press conference that he was the writer, he was fired the next day. The booklet expressed opinions that were contrary to those of his superiors. He subsequently wrote *The Cancer Syndrome*. The book is a revealing inside view of the cancer establishment and very helpful for anyone who may be questioning conventional therapy; propaganda and misinformation about cancer and its treatment abound.

Information about the realities of conventional treatment enables one to choose intelligently.

As with all diseases, no one treatment for cancer is best for everyone. For many people, conventional treatment is appropriate simply because they are unable to go against conventional medical advice. Nutritional therapy for cancer requires personal commitment, discipline, and hard work; well-meaning family members who believe it offers the best chances of recovery may not realize this. Unless the patient comes to understand and embrace a natural approach to disease and to cancer, nutritional therapy cannot succeed.

For the individual rejecting surgery, chemotherapy, and radiation, and willing to follow a rigorous nutritional course, nutrition-based therapies offer the best chance of survival. Some people die, but some survive for years with cancer—with no sign of it worsening. Others recover completely.

Physicians writing earlier in this century reported that people with cancer typically survived many years unless operated upon, in which case death often shortly followed. A tumor is the body's way of segregating a diseased area, and when cut, cancer cells may spread much more rapidly than when the tumor is left alone. But cancer may be legally diagnosed only by a biopsy, presenting a dilemma.

Most people want to know what a biopsy will show before choosing a course of therapy, despite the risk involved. Others, particularly those who are certain they would choose natural therapy whatever a biopsy showed, may choose to avoid it. A number of people I have worked with have rejected biopsy, in many cases with good results. These include women with breast lumps and men with lesions of the prostate gland, testicles, or breast. An individual choosing this course should be highly motivated to follow a careful and thorough nutritional program. Even if someone is not, however, we should recognize a person's right to choose to live out his or her life without being subjected to surgical dismemberment and an array of poisonous drugs.

One reason little is known with certainty about the best ways of approaching cancer is that few individuals with cancer find reasonable alternatives to conventional treatment. Until more people with cancer seek these alternatives, this problem will remain. The difficulty is increased by restrictions placed on medical doctors by the medical establishment about the ways they may treat cancer, making it difficult or impossible for them to use alternative therapies.

The person with cancer must look deep inside him- or herself and choose how he or she wishes to live the rest of their life, whether that be for one week or fifty years. The therapy or combination of therapies best for a person is that which is most attuned to judgments and emotions including (but perhaps going beyond) reason, common sense, and the conventional wisdom such a person may have accepted all of his or her life. The philosophy and ideas expressed in this book are intended to help clarify an understanding of why—perhaps most of all when death is threatening—a return to a more natural way of living and eating may provide a better chance of survival than conventional therapy does.

The course of cancer, when treated with the kind of nutrition discussed, varies according to several influences. Among them are the stage of the cancer, the condition of the individual when starting nutritional therapy, the type of cancer, and the thoroughness with which the individual applies the recommended therapy.

A Case of Malignant Melanoma

One case is that of a man named Konrad whom I initially saw a week after he was diagnosed with malignant melanoma. A small mole on his arm had been removed and the biopsy showed grade IV melanoma (deep penetration of a highly malignant tumor below the surface of the skin into the underlying dermal layer). This type of melanoma has a poor prognosis. The treatment his surgeon had recommended was excision of the tissue around the area of the melanoma and removal of all lymph nodes in the arm and armpit, followed by extensive chemotherapy. Five-year survival is less than 50 percent.

Konrad decided to have the surgical excision of the tissue around the area where the mole had been removed; a patch of skin about two inches square and half an inch thick was removed. He declined lymph node removal and chemotherapy and began a program of carefully planned nutritional therapy. His surgeon continued to see him monthly and, displeased with Konrad's decision to forgo more extensive surgery and chemotherapy, offered the opinion that he had little chance of survival.

Konrad's therapy included many elements. Fresh raw-vegetable juices were made twice daily, yielding at least two quarts a day. Fresh organic vegetables and some whole grains were consumed. Liver juice was made daily, and coffee enemas were taken twice daily. Most vegetables were eaten raw. Fish was regularly eaten. Since dairy products of sufficient quality were not available, we used none.

Konrad did well, to the surprise of his surgeon (who eventually grew curious about his diet), and the melanoma had not reappeared when I last heard from him some fifteen years after I had initially seen him. He had continued eating natural organic foods, including a considerable amount of liver and fish, and he regularly makes raw-vegetable juice. The liver juice, coffee enemas, and many of the supplements used in the earlier stages of his therapy had long since been reduced or stopped.

He considers himself recovered, but he shied away from using the word "cured," agreeing with me that he must remain vigilant to minimize chances of a recurrence. Some patients let their programs slide once cancer is no longer evident; too often the disease subsequently returns. In individuals fighting cancer, I have often seen tumors diminish and increase in size according to how thoroughly programs are followed.

I have met several people who recovered on the Gerson therapy in the 1950s, and have worked with several others who recovered in a similar manner, including a woman who recovered from breast cancer under the care of Max Warmbrand. He was a naturopathic physician and osteopath who practiced for many years in Connecticut and New York City until his death in 1976.

But by and large, cancer is difficult, and many people lose the battle. For the person who believes in it, natural therapy without the damaging effects of conventional treatments offers the best hope for recovery. I have seen many encouraging results, but in the later stages of cancer, even the most rigorous therapy may fail to halt the disease.

Many clinics have been established for alternative therapies for cancer, mostly in Mexico and Europe. A number of promising therapies have been developed, the best of which have integrated many of the methods discussed here.

Optimal diet for cancer varies for each person. Some people have recovered on mostly raw-food diets; others have used mostly a cooked-food program. Some do best on a regimen comprised of large amounts of animal protein and fat; others thrive on mostly vegetables and fruits. An individual's needs may evolve as he or she progresses through therapy. One size does not fit all.

While many nutritional regimens stress a low intake of animal protein and fat, I have found that in some individuals a great deal of animal-sourced foods of the proper quality to be of crucial importance. For many people, a substantial amount of their food should be eaten raw. The most important foods to choose from include sprouts, salad greens, parsley, and other raw vegetables, raw carrot and green juices, fruits, wild salmon and other seafood, grass-fed meats and organs, and raw dairy foods from grass-fed cows. The diet must be strict; it is critically important to avoid all industrial fats and oils and refined carbohydrates, particularly sugar.

A number of special foods and food supplements are useful when combatting cancer; some will be discussed later. The most useful and universally applicable supplement is bovine tracheal cartilage. Thoroughly researched for many years by John Prudden, M.D., this supplement has a proven record of helping many cancer patients recover.

The Work of Dr. John Prudden

Decades of research by Dr. Prudden has shown that bovine tracheal cartilage (BTC) can be an effective and safe anticancer agent. Prudden, a surgeon, authored sixty-six journal articles and other publications, including "The Treatment of Human Cancer with Agents Prepared from Bovine Cartilage" (*Journal of Biological Response Modifiers* 4, no. 6 [1985]: 551–84). With colleagues at Columbia Presbyterian Medical Center, he initially demonstrated that BTC dramatically accelerated the healing of wounds and reduces inflammation. This led Prudden to test it for other possible therapeutic applications.

Scores of his cancer patients benefited from the use of BTC, in addition to many patients with inflammatory diseases such as rheumatoid arthritis, osteoarthritis, and immunological skin disorders. Patients with shingles or mononucleosis often made rapid improvements when ingesting BTC, which works by stimulating and normalizing the immune system. Other physicians have written that it attacks cancer directly via anti-mitotic effects (preventing cell division). These effects and much more are described in Dr. Prudden's 1993 article, "Summary of Bovine Tracheal Cartilage Research Program."

Here are some of the most impressive individual results Prudden wrote about:

- The disappearance of a large rectal carcinoma in a fifty-four-year-old man, with demonstrated progressive normalization in the microscopic appearance of the cancer cells in sequential biopsies obtained during treatment.
- Remission of a prostatic cancer, metastatic to bones, with complete normalization of all blood values. At the time Prudden published, the man was well nineteen years after beginning therapy with BTC and was ninety-one years old.
- An eighteen-year remission of a carcinoma of the pancreas with nodal involvement in a sixty-nine-year-old woman.

Dr. Prudden supervised the investment of over $10 million in research on BTC, showing it to be effective in a wide range of conditions, using an optimal dosage of twelve 750 mg capsules daily. This is also the optimal dosage following wounds or injuries. To best facilitate healing after surgery, begin taking BTC one month prior, and continue for two to three months after.

A number of different BTC products of varying quality are available. The product I have recommended for over thirty years is manufactured by the same New Zealand company, using the same process, that produced this material for John Prudden. Freeze-drying freshly harvested cartilage preserves the unaltered proteins, enzymes, and fat-soluble activators present. The tissues are taken only from grass-fed, inspected animals, raised without the use of pesticides, hormones or antibiotics, in New Zealand—where mad cow disease has never occurred. (See www.drrons.com.)

Cancer Prevention

Prevention is the best way to deal with cancer. In many primitive societies, cancer was rare or perhaps even unknown; evidence indicates that food was the primary protector. Current research has focused on individual nutrients such as vitamins A, C, D, E, and selenium as cancer-inhibiting factors. Extensive research has been done on the nature of carcinogenic substances. Industrial fats and oils are extremely carcinogenic and they also enhance the effects of other carcinogens. They are a major reason for the worldwide epidemic of cancer.

For many people, two themes emerge. One is the idea that "everything is bad for you," and the other is the notion that large doses of nutrients thought protective against cancer are helpful. We all know people who attempt to avoid everything potentially carcinogenic or who dose up on the "anticancer" nutrients, or both. Others rationalize that since everything is bad for you and one can't avoid everything, why try—just eat whatever you want!

Avoiding carcinogens to the extent possible is reasonable, and native foods are rich in nutrients protective against cancer. Carcinogens are not the crucial issue, for if the immune system is sufficiently strong, one is protected. Primal nutrition provides that strength. Even a person who has for years eaten refined foods may avoid cancer. Of patients I have seen over the years, several hundred have been followed for at least six months; these were people who embraced in whole or in part diets of traditional foods. Among them, very rarely has anyone developed cancer during the time followed.

This is not coincidence. Cancer seems to be rare among people eating traditional, native-type diets, even in twentieth-century America.

GASTROINTESTINAL DISEASES

Colitis

Colitis is an inflammatory reaction in the colon, often autoimmune or infectious. An acute bout of colitis is nearly always best dealt with by fasting. If rectal bleeding occurs, a physician should be consulted to determine the cause. In ulcerative colitis, fasting until the bleeding stops allows the lesions to begin healing. Although this may take several days, usually a day or two suffices. Warm water enemas may be helpful; herbs may be used in the enemas to promote healing.

When one stops eating, peristalsis (the involuntary wave-like motion of the intestines that propels feces toward the anus) is greatly reduced, and feces may stagnate in the large bowel. As water is reabsorbed across the bowel wall, they become hard and impacted. Enemas remove them, and the bowel is left clean; healing of lesions may then occur much more easily.

Once rectal bleeding has stopped, a diet of well-cooked vegetables, broth, and fish may be very helpful. No other foods and no raw vegetables or fruits should be eaten. Chew foods well, and eat little at first. If no further rectal bleeding occurs, more food may be eaten. After a few days, slowly introduce other primal foods. Very small amounts of raw vegetables should be gradually introduced only if no symptoms occur; the amounts may then be slowly increased. Usually it is best to not consume any grains.

Gastritis (inflammation of the stomach) and ulcers are treated in much the same manner as colitis. If bleeding is present or suspected (dark stools are a cardinal sign), see a physician for a definitive diagnosis.

Coffee and alcohol increase secretions of gastric acid, aggravating nearly all gastrointestinal problems.

Hemorrhoids

Hemorrhoids are a common problem afflicting a large percentage of people. They may be either internal (inside the anal opening) or external, and occur as early as the teen years. A hemorrhoid is actually a dilated rectal vein, and if the blood within it clots, the hemorrhoid is said to be thrombosed. These are the large, dilated, painful, inflamed, sometimes incapacitating hemorrhoids often given surgical attention.

In office surgery, the thrombosed hemorrhoid is incised and an attempt is made to remove the clot. This is an extremely painful procedure usually giving little relief, temporary at best. A hemorrhoidectomy is the more extensive hospital procedure in which hemorrhoids are surgically removed.

Although an acutely inflamed hemorrhoid might ideally be treated by fasting, enemas are simply too painful to endure for long. And without enemas, pressure exerted by stagnant and hardening feces within the bowel makes hemorrhoids worse. Although bowel movements are somewhat painful during the three to five days required for a thrombosed hemorrhoid to resolve, the best course is to follow the dietary principles described in this book. Be sure to get plenty of fats and use coconut oil liberally, as well as daily cod-liver oil. Soft stools should result, keeping pressure exerted on the hemorrhoid by the large bowel to a minimum, since such stools may be easily passed without straining.

I have treated some severe cases of thrombosed hemorrhoids in this way. In one case, a thrombosed hemorrhoid with a diameter the size of a quarter took five days to resolve. The patient was uncomfortable being on his feet for more than a few minutes at a time and spent most of the five days on his back, after which he began moving around a bit more. Within two weeks he could function normally.

Conventional medicine gives little recognition to the role foods play in gastrointestinal disease. The digestive tract directly interfaces with food, and in many people is the part of the body first and most easily influenced *by* food. The gastrointestinal tract indicates which foods eaten are well received; a poor reception often indicates developing problems. Belching, intestinal gas, indigestion, and often diarrhea speak of problems with certain foods. If these early warning signals are ignored and not addressed, symptoms of more advanced gastrointestinal problems may result.

HYPOGLYCEMIA, DIABETES, AND WEIGHT PROBLEMS

The interrelated and often associated conditions of hypoglycemia, diabetes, and excess weight, to one degree or another, are due to problems with carbohydrate metabolism. Hypoglycemia may be an early stage of diabetes; both involve abnormalities in blood sugar. Avoidance of refined carbohydrates, fruits, fruit juices, and sweeteners lies at the heart of the dietary treatment for diabetes and hypoglycemia. Weight problems usually involve the excessive consumption of carbohydrates, especially refined carbohydrates. A sluggish thyroid gland, typically undiagnosed because of the inadequacy of standard thyroid tests, also often plays a role.

Whole-food diets featuring a lot of vegetables, good fats, and grains may control symptoms of hypoglycemia, but are improved by the addition of substantial amounts of high-quality animal foods. The latter will often reduce cravings for sweets, especially when sugar is completely avoided for a few weeks.

The same is true in diabetes. The diabetic condition is chronic; improvement comes more slowly. Eating whole foods with plenty of fats nearly always results in a reduction of the need for insulin in diabetics. Indeed, many individuals beginning a careful diet soon after a diagnosis of adult-onset diabetes have eliminated the need for insulin.

The main causes of excess weight are refined carbohydrates, poor quality and unnatural fats, and lack of exercise, all of which may depress the function of the thyroid gland. This in turn may make the weight problem worse. Not only do refined foods provide poor nutrition and excessive calories; they also displace foods needed for a fully active thyroid gland and thus a fully active metabolism.

Fats of proper quality need not be avoided by an overweight person.

Many people fail to lose weight eating unbalanced low-fat diets. This often leads to binge eating. A more reasonable approach uses the primal foods necessary for good health and utilizes necessary food supplements to achieve a well-balanced metabolism that allows weight to be lost naturally.

HEADACHES

Many people suffer regularly from at least an occasional headache. These headaches in nearly all cases disappear within the first few weeks of carefully following a carefully balanced primal diet.

The reason is simple: almost all headaches, including migraine, are food related. Many are direct expressions of allergies. Like other organs, the brain may react to constituents in certain foods by retaining fluid and swelling, causing a headache. Similar reactions in the nasal sinuses may also cause headaches. Eyestrain and fatigue may also play a role.

A persistent headache failing to end with careful dieting, or a headache following an injury, should be investigated by a physician, for headaches may be a sign of serious injury or disease. Much time and expense could be saved, however, by instituting a simple primal diet for a few days before an extensive work-up is done in an attempt to determine the cause of the headache. (Cheese is often suspected of precipitating migraines.)

One middle-aged patient of mine suffered from severe migraines once or twice a month for over thirty years before finding they ceased when she stopped drinking alcohol. She was not a heavy drinker, taking a drink or two a few times a week. And the drinks did not always precipitate a migraine. But they sometimes did, for when she stopped drinking entirely, the migraines stopped. In the years since, she has had headaches only on some days after the rare occasion when she has had a drink or two the night before. Other individuals have told me they are particularly susceptible to headaches after drinking red wine. Perhaps this is due to the pesticides used on many wine grapes. The grape skin is used in making red wine, but not in white.

ANXIETY, EMOTIONAL DISTURBANCES, AND MENTAL ILLNESS

Thinking is as biological as digestion. Disturbances of the mind must ultimately have a biochemical explanation, though we may be unable to provide it.

Nutrients profoundly affect some mentally disturbed states, and reactions to foods may cause such states. Sugar-induced hypoglycemia, for example, is often accompanied by depression, anxiety, or both. Deficiencies of vitamin B_{12}, vitamin D, and vitamin A often accompany depressed mental states.

In studies of inmates in American jails, reformatories, and mental institutions, Weston Price discovered that large majorities, often approaching 100 percent, had deformities of the dental arch and other marked abnormalities in the shape of the skull. His work paralleled that of other investigators—he was not the first to discover these correlations between changes in the shape of the skull and criminal behavior, mental backwardness, and abnormal mental states.

Price's work suggests that dietary changes have led to anatomical changes that have resulted in increased incidence of these problems. Given that anatomical changes have occurred in large segments of the population, we are left with the issue of how the foods eaten influence the mental state of an individual, whatever anatomical equipment the individual might have (this taken in terms of potential as dictated by the physical capacity of the brain).

In the experience of many clinicians working with natural food, including myself, the mental state of an individual may sometimes be profoundly influenced by dietary changes. Feelings of greater stability, calmness, and confidence are common in patients embracing a whole-food diet. Broth especially helps with this.

Many factors besides food affect the state of mind of individuals with marked mental and emotional problems, but, as we have discussed, food can be a profound and even a dominating influence. Some of the early proponents of megavitamin therapy were physicians using vitamin and mineral supplements for people suffering from schizophrenia and other mental illnesses. The use of traditional foods in a carefully controlled diet would significantly enhance the responses of individuals with these problems.

Among patients specifically seeking help for more deep-seated mental disturbances, however, results are mixed. Many are unable to follow the details of a thorough program. Among those who have, particularly those suffering from anxiety and depression, many have experienced relief, but a few have had no improvement. It is impossible to know who will or will not respond.

How does food affect future generations? The mental well-being of Western society requires us to abandon refined foods, which have led to degenerative changes in the shape of the human skull that often (perhaps usually) accompany mental disease. Though this may be difficult to believe, the evidence is difficult to ignore.

CANDIDIASIS

Candida albicans is a yeast microorganism found in the normal human organism; it is concentrated on the skin and mucous membranes. Antibiotics, sweet foods, and oral contraceptives are among the influences affecting the amount of *Candida* occurring in an individual; overgrowth of *Candida* is called candidiasis. The orthodox viewpoint holds that candidiasis occurs only as either a localized yeast infection (as in the vagina) or as a systemic illness that may occur when the immune system breaks down in debilitating chronic illness. However, a growing number of physicians believe that overgrowth of *Candida* may lead or contribute to a wide variety of symptoms and conditions, including most of those previously discussed in this chapter.

Chronic yeast infections are thought to be capable of affecting any system of the body. Because the drug nystatin has activity against *Candida* and seems to have little other effect, it is often prescribed for individuals thought to be suffering from candidiasis. Often a yeast-free and sugar-free diet is prescribed in conjunction.

In my experience, symptoms of candidiasis disappear without the use of nystatin when the dietary principles explained in this book are carefully followed. This usually occurs in spite of the consumption of small amounts of yeast-containing foods such as apple cider vinegar, beer and wine, and certain breads. Many people achieve best results when all concentrated starches, including grains, breads, and particularly extruded breakfast cereals are completely avoided. All yeast-containing foods are eliminated for a few weeks. Nystatin may give more rapid relief, however, it must be kept in mind that although nystatin has proved useful for many patients unwilling to follow a sufficiently careful natural food diet, the relief it gives often disappears when the drug is stopped.

SKIN PROBLEMS

Eczema is often an allergic skin reaction to certain foods, particularly dairy products and sweets. Improvements usually begin within days of eliminating these foods. Lasting improvement comes when following a primal diet.

Psoriasis is chronic and recurrent; often arthritic symptoms accompany the silvery, scaly skin lesions. More intensive therapy is needed to treat psoriasis than is needed for eczema. Elements of the Gerson therapy—raw-vegetable juices, enemas, and raw-liver juice—are helpful, for the juices and enemas cleanse the body of toxins that cause eruptions. Vitamin D is a particularly critical nutrient for most people with skin problems, who are advised to consume broth, bovine tracheal cartilage, and other carefully selected special foods and supplements containing this important vitamin. (Vitamin D is also especially important in healing the gut.)

Acne, too, may be chronic. It may take several months for the acne of an individual following a primal diet to clear up. As the healing gets underway, new eruptions become less marked and eventually no longer occur. Cysts still present slowly dissipate. Hormones influence acne, and symptoms often become worse at puberty and during menstruation. Most fruits and all sweets are best avoided. Grass-fed animal foods and wild seafood are highly beneficial when treating acne. Cod-liver oil should be used for its vitamin A content. Once again, broth and bovine tracheal cartilage supplements are also very helpful.

Lesser skin eruptions that many teenagers and young adults experience are mostly due to sweets, excessive fruits, processed fats and oils and milk products, and a lack of fat-soluble protective nutrients. Vegetable oils, especially when used for commercial frying, affect the body's ability to metabolize fats normally. As noted above, citrus fruits and juices may contribute to eruptions, as can tomatoes, which may also affect mucous membranes, causing sores inside the cheeks and on the tongue, which are more common during the late-summer tomato season.

It may be hard to believe that these common foods may cause these symptoms, but sometimes they do—and even many more. Understanding how the body reacts to foods is not a simple matter. Think of the body as a laboratory and food as the experimental variable in a continuous study. Take notes. There will be a test.

OTHER CONDITIONS

People sometimes ask about the nutritional treatment of uncommon and seldom seen conditions. They tend to think their problem will not respond to nutrition, despite evidence of successful cases. This thinking results in part from their believing that their own diet is quite good and thus can have little to do with their problem.

Even for these individuals, a committed effort to follow the program outlined in the pages of this book has usually led to significant improvement. This includes people with well-known conditions such as multiple sclerosis, muscular dystrophy, epilepsy, macular edema, cataracts, and glaucoma, as well as those with other, seldom seen, chronic and debilitating diseases. Even those with conditions typically believed to be entirely genetic, such as Down's syndrome, have shown some improvements in overall health and mental function.

Price's evidence indicates that the occurrence of such genetic conditions is profoundly influenced by the parents' nutrition and may be almost entirely prevented if their nutrition prior to pregnancy, and the woman's during pregnancy, was optimal. His observations are in conflict with the views of most geneticists, who have largely rejected the concept that nutrition affects the genes. Recent research and discoveries, however, have provided theoretical models for how the genetic material outside the nucleus of the fertilized egg may be directly affected by the mother's nutrition. This nonnuclear genetic material is now known to reside in the mitochondria, the energy-making part of the cell.

This research provides an explanation for Price's observations and indicates that the conventional thinking about nutrition in genetics has been erroneous. As with controversy in medical circles over the role of nutrition in health and disease, we may hope that what common sense, empirical observation, and traditional wisdom tell us is right will eventually be proved to the satisfaction of those who control policies affecting millions of lives.

The development of chronic disease is influenced by a person's genes, but the fundamental and underlying cause is the slow breakdown of the body as it is poisoned by foods for which it is not adapted. A host of other influences affects this process, particularly physical activity and one's mental and emotional state.

Treatment of all disease is thus accomplished in a similar manner. Recovery involves understanding natural laws governing human nutrition and the physical and psychological needs of each individual. To help oneself, these things must be well understood; to help others, they must be well communicated. For the physician, the foundation of such communication is best built by his own good health. This is the meaning of the ancient words, "Physician, heal thyself." Physicians should note, however, another ancient saying: "Only a fool has himself for a doctor."

PART 3

PRIMAL VERSUS MODERN FOODS

A Deeper Understanding of Primal Food Groups

One goes through three overlapping processes in learning to use primal foods as medicine. In the first, knowledge and understanding are acquired through study. Then one finds the desire and the will to put the information into practice. Finally, one must find sources for the foods one has decided are necessary. In this third part of the book we integrate these processes, examining primal foods and the production methods that make modern foods inferior to them. Understanding the differences between primal and modern foods helps provide the motivation to set and achieve health goals and serves as a guide to eating naturally. In our review of these foods and food groups, we continue to examine the differences between primal and modern foods, and the effects of their differences on human strength, resistance to disease, and longevity.

In traditional native cultures, fish and shellfish, animals (especially organ meats), and raw dairy products were considered of prime importance, as were vegetables and sometimes grains (albeit to a lesser degree). In the following pages, you'll discover why this is so, and you'll learn how to apply what you learn to part of a commonsense approach to your own primal diet that can prevent and usually reverse disease.

10
MEAT, FOWL, AND EGGS

Knowledge of primal foods used by our ancient ancestors, primitive cultures surviving into the twentieth century, and contemporary hunter-gatherers known to be free of chronic disease shows that meat, fowl, eggs, milk, and milk products should form a substantial part of an optimal diet, if of the proper quality. But differences between traditional and modern versions of these foods warrant close examination. In this chapter, the methods of the modern meat industry will be examined: the living conditions of animals; antibiotics, hormones, and feeds routinely used throughout the industry; and the inspection and regulatory systems for meat. Controversy about the meat industry centers on the use of antibiotics and carcinogenic hormones in particular, but perhaps even more significant is the effect of an animal's diet and exercise upon the composition of the meat produced. The products themselves will also be examined as we learn how the meat we consume has changed in the years since the end of World War II.

Naturally raised animals warrant an equally thorough examination. Increasing numbers of livestock producers raise animals out at pasture without using drugs, chemicals, pesticides, or hormones. Fats derived from wild ungulates have been shown by laboratory analysis to be significantly different from those of conventionally raised, grain-fed domestic cattle. Analysis has also shown similarities between fats from grass-fed domestic cattle and those from wild grazing animals. Fats of grain-fed animals are much higher in monounsaturated fats.

Saturated fats, omega-3, and omega-6 fats are about the same.

The quality of eggs, milk, and milk products is based on these same influences—animals must be well exercised, and range- and pasture-fed, if they are to produce top-quality food. The processes of pasteurization and homogenization also have profound effects on milk and milk products. Here again, comparing and contrasting information about conventional products and naturally produced counterparts provides a basis for making informed choices.

In recent years, many people have decided to eat less meat. Reports commonly appear in the media about antibiotics, chemical residues, and female hormones in animals, the dangers of cholesterol and fats, shoddy inspection procedures, and a host of other confirmed or possible problems with meat. Thus, meat consumption is down. But many people eating less meat would leap at the chance to have venison or other wild game, without thinking twice about the cholesterol content (which happens to be about the same in wild meat as in domestic). And though many others may not have a taste for it, most people intuitively know that wild game is healthy food as long as it is eaten with fat.

Several influences affect an animal's life and the composition and quality of its meat. Among them are its food, the use of drugs and toxic chemicals in its care and feeding, and its access to fresh air and exercise. An awareness of the connection between food and health takes us to the next step, to the realization that the composition of the meat we eat profoundly affects us.

THE CONVENTIONAL PRODUCTION OF MEAT

Commercial calves nurse from cows that have been fed hay grown with chemical fertilizers derived from petrochemicals and heavily sprayed with pesticides. Cows are usually fed a synthetic protein supplement.

When two months old, males are castrated and all calves are implanted with a growth-stimulating hormone (typically a female hormone). Because diarrhea is common at this age, many ranchers mass-treat calves with antibiotics; when calves are weaned at seven months of age, more antibiotics are used to control possible respiratory ailments. At that time, animals are again implanted with a hormonal growth promoter, wormed, and dipped in a toxic insecticide bath to kill lice that produce scabies. Farmers, by law, must dispose of residual liquids at licensed toxic-waste-disposal sites.

From this point on, low levels of antibiotics are constantly added to feed rations. For some undiscovered reason, this stimulates growth, as do hormonal implants.

Beef cattle typically weigh about six hundred pounds when fifteen months old, when another hormonal implant is made. Fly-control procedures are employed in grazing areas; insecticides are spread by tractor-driven sprayers or by aerial spraying of animals with crop-dusting aircraft. Ear tags impregnated with insecticide are often used. (The ears are the place of choice for hormone and insecticide implants because humans do not customarily eat an animal's ears.)

Animals go to feedlots for ninety days of fattening when about eighteen months old; again they are wormed, dipped, and implanted with a hormone. Fly-control insecticide procedures are intensified because of crowded quarters, and a larger dose of antibiotics is used in feed because of the great danger of infectious disease. Respiratory disease is especially difficult to control; dust kicked up by thousands of cattle is hard on the animals' lungs.

Because pregnancy in heifers in feedlots is highly undesirable development of a drug causing pregnant heifers to miscarry has been welcomed by feedlot operators; many routinely inject all incoming heifers. The drug, called Lutalyse, is a synthetic analogue of a naturally occurring prostaglandin that helps regulate the reproductive cycle. Specifically, Lutalyse brings on ovulation, which in a pregnant heifer induces miscarriage.

The active ingredient has the same effect on the human female reproductive tract. The label states: "Women of childbearing age . . . should exercise extreme caution when handling this product." A veterinarian wrote in a column in *Beef* magazine: "Pregnant women should not even handle the bottles as they could cause abortion and changes in the menstrual cycle . . . just from absorption through the skin." The manufacturer states that no residues of Lutalyse are ever found in beef. Can we be sure?

The Use of Antibiotics

Many millions of years ago certain microorganisms developed the ability to make compounds that can inhibit the growth of, or kill, competing organisms; we call these compounds antibiotics. Other organisms in response developed the capacity to resist the effects of the antibiotics; many resistance strategies were developed over the course of evolution.

With the development and increased use of antibiotics in the 1940s, resistant strains of microorganisms greatly increased, and doctors began finding that bacteria resistant to one or more antibiotics were causing disease in susceptible individuals. By the late 1960s, epidemics of such diseases, including typhoid and dysentery, had occurred in several places around the world.

This has been attributed in part to the overuse of antibiotics in humans. However, a large and growing number of scientists believe the use of very large quantities of antibiotics in domestic-animal production is a major cause of this worldwide increase in the number of disease-causing pathogens resistant to antibiotics. These scientists believe antibiotics added to animal feed are creating drug resistance in livestock bacteria that is transferable to human bacteria. As quoted by Orville Schell in *Modern Meat,* the Japanese microbiologist who discovered the mechanisms by which these "resistance factors" operate (and his work has been confirmed by a host of other researchers) wrote many years ago in *Scientific American* that the overuse of antibiotics might well make them useless. By all accounts, the problem has since become much worse.

In the late 1940s, researchers at Lederle Laboratories in Pearl River,

New York, accidentally discovered that animals grew more rapidly when their feed contained low levels of antibiotics. Publication of experimental results and marketing efforts followed shortly, and by 1954 nearly five hundred thousand pounds of antibiotics were added to livestock feed yearly; about nine million pounds a year were added by 1980. In 1980, American Cyanamid alone (the parent company of Lederle) sold drugs worth $120 million for animal use in this country, and drugs worth $265 million abroad. About half were tetracycline-based feed additives.

Money makes powerful lobbies; the drug and cattle industries have successfully blocked efforts of hundreds of scientists and physicians to prevail upon the government to stem the use of penicillin and tetracycline as feed additives. These efforts have been backed by an array of published documentation about the seriousness of the problem. The United States does not regulate the use of antibiotics on animals or in their feed.

The issue of residues of antibiotics and other drugs in meat is more difficult to track and measure than the resistance problem, for residues may only be discovered when tests are run, and by then the carcass has usually gone to market. Violative levels of antibiotics and sulfur drugs are often found in inspected animals. The continuous use of small amounts of antibiotics in feed, and the periodic use of large doses to control disease, assures that even if levels in excess of allowable amounts are *not* present, trace amounts of the drugs, their conjugates, and their metabolites will be present in the meat. (These conjugates and metabolites are compounds the drugs are converted to within the animal; they are little understood and are not measured.)

The Use of Hormones
A number of natural and synthetic sex hormones cause livestock and poultry to gain weight more rapidly and with greater feed efficiency. Used in increasing amounts since the early 1950s, these hormones have drastically changed the way animals are raised.

The endocrine system consists of tiny hormone-producing glands that, together with the nervous system, regulate metabolism. Active in minute amounts, hormones change delicate balances within the endocrine system by exciting cells in tissues sensitive to them. This excitation can be a trigger inducing the growth of cancer. Though we have evidence that the effects can be devastating, some of these substances have not been in use long enough to demonstrate the long-term effects of increased body loads.

Diethylstilbestrol (DES) was for many years the most widely used of these hormones in both livestock and humans. An inexpensive synthetic estrogen, it was extremely popular in the cattle industry. In tests with steers, DES increased weight gain 15 to 19 percent and feed efficiency 7 to 10 percent.

But in the late 1960s, physicians for the first time found clear-cell adenocarcinoma (cancer) of the vagina in girls and women under the age of twenty-five. Ensuing studies revealed that in the majority of cases, their mothers had been prescribed DES during pregnancy for the purpose of preventing miscarriage, a common treatment given an estimated three to six million women from 1941 to 1971.

Incredibly, DES therapy for pregnant women continued until 1971 even after DES had been shown to cause cancer in tests with laboratory animals, at levels close to those periodically detected in the inspection of meat from animals raised on DES. Detection methods do not reveal levels of various conjugates and metabolites of DES, which may be the substances doing the actual damage. This is a severe limitation of testing for residues of toxic substances used in raising animals; the problem of residues is likely much more severe than tests indicate.

Despite limitations, by the early 1960s testing procedures established that DES was present in meat, and it was to be banned under the Delaney Clause. This legislation, a 1958 amendment to the Federal Food, Drug, and Cosmetic Act of 1938, states that "no food additive shall be deemed safe if it is found to induce cancer when ingested by man or animal." However, in 1962 Congress passed another amendment specifically allowing continued use of DES in livestock. And it continued to be used to treat pregnant women at risk of miscarrying. Only upon publication of reports of cancer in young women as described above did pressure leading to the eventual banning of DES begin to mount, and it was finally banned in the 1970s.

Other incidents had occurred. For a time in the 1950s, DES implants were used in caponizing (castrating) male chickens. Dogs eating waste from the processing of these chickens, and some men and boys eating chicken necks, began showing signs of feminization (the implants were in the chickens' necks). The FDA then banned the use of implants for caponization (castration), and the USDA bought some ten million dollars' worth of contaminated chicken and destroyed it. Other reports in medical journals describe young children developing breast enlargement after exposure to DES in products accidentally contaminated with the substance.

In Puerto Rico, where DES continued to be used, a virtual epidemic of premature sexual development, with grossly enlarged breasts in young children of both sexes and ovarian cysts and precocious puberty in girls, occurred in the early 1980s. Hundreds of children were treated by physicians who eventually linked the problem to overuse of DES in locally produced chicken. The chicken producers in Puerto Rico had been selling over five hundred thousand pounds of chicken each year to the school lunch program. Then, while the plight of hundreds of sick children was being publicized, the weight of the chickens suddenly and mysteriously dropped from about four pounds each down to two to three pounds, presumably because the chicken producers stopped using DES. In Puerto Rico, drugs such as DES were also being sold over the counter for animal use with no veterinary prescription needed.

This story has a relatively happy ending, however. In the vast majority of children afflicted, symptoms largely disappeared once the ingestion of suspected products ceased. Those who drank a lot of milk were, to a degree, protected. Orville Schell's fine investigative account of this story, related in his book *Modern Meat* (much of the information in this section on the meat industry comes from Schell's research), paints a poignant picture of the pathos of the children and the callous unconcern of the industries and regulatory agencies involved. Whichever food producer was most to blame, the overuse of DES was almost certainly the cause of the problems.

In the United States, such problems have also been linked to soy formula; other evidence implicated meat and milk producers. The FDA and other regulatory agencies were uncooperative with attempts by physicians to convince the agency to investigate the suspect producers; nothing was ever proven. However, the FDA finally banned DES feed additives in 1972 and implants in 1973. But as a result of the livestock industry's legal maneuvering and appeals, the ban did not go into effect until July 13, 1979, when further sale and shipment of DES became illegal. Stocks on hand were to be usable until November 1, 1979, after which further use was illegal.

In March 1980, the FDA discovered that more than 50,000 head of cattle in Texas had been illegally implanted with DES after the ban. Throughout the spring, the count rose; the final tally showed 427,275 head of cattle in 318 feedlots in twenty states had been illegally implanted after the November 1 deadline. Illegal sales of DES had been made by forty-nine drug-distributing companies after the sale deadline date. How many cattle were illegally implanted and not discovered is unknown.

The FDA never prosecuted anyone for any of these violations of the law. Concepts of law and order are often rather selectively applied.

Since DES was banned, cattlemen have chosen from a variety of somewhat more expensive, similar drugs, including chemicals similar in structure to estrogens, and combinations of estradiol and progesterone (two hormones normally produced in minute amounts in the mammalian female body). The market is lucrative; more than 99 percent of conventional feedlot cattle are implanted. Because the substances now used are naturally occurring hormones, attempts to regulate and monitor use have become less restrictive; the drug and cattle industries are being left to monitor themselves.

The danger of these hormones is somewhat subtle. Only tiny amounts of residual substances in meat are ingested, amounts that may only be a small percentage of the same substance normally found in the female body itself. This may seem harmless enough, but the endocrine system is very delicate; fractional amounts of hormones may have profound and long-lasting effects. We are dealing with the unknown—the effect of small doses of hormones over extended periods of time has simply not been investigated. Given the track record of the drug and cattle industries and the federal regulatory agencies involved, the possibility that these substances will be irresponsibly overused seems likely.

The Toxic Diet of Modern Animals

Antibiotic additives in livestock and poultry feed, and the spraying of feedlots with insecticides to control flies, is not the end of the chemical infestation of meat production. Products called oral larvicides have been used to control flies. These organophosphate insecticides are added to feed, and pass through the animal's gastrointestinal tract, making the animal's manure toxic to fly larvae. The manufacturers admit that "small amounts" are absorbed, but claim they are metabolized and leave no residue exceeding the allowable levels in meat. Organophosphates are related to nerve gases; while some are thought to be relatively innocuous to mammals, others are deadly.

A partial list of substances that are fed to animals raised for food includes waste scraps and dust from plants manufacturing cardboard containers; waste matter from Frito-Lay plants; shredded cardboard, including the petroleum-based wax coating; waste paper, including additives such as ink, glue, clay, and plastic used in its manufacture; orange-peel pulp (rich in insecticide residues); and cooked garbage. (The cooked garbage was fed to pigs in many hog-producing states, and contained nearly anything one can imagine. Well into the 1980s, many pigs in northern New Jersey received New York City's garbage every morning.) A subindustry revolved around recycling these materials for animal feed. An array of synthetic flavoring and aroma agents were used to make many of these "foods" palatable to animals.

These products and a variety of mold inhibitors, flavoring agents, and bactericidal agents have been added to the list of nonfoods used to grow and fatten animals for human consumption.

The appearance in the media of these types of stories in addition to the red herring of the extended, extensive, and misleading cholesterol scare have been major causes of a decline in meat consumption in the United States. The real wonder is why consumption has remained as high as it has. While America may continue eating large amounts of meat in part because of a callous national indifference to our collective health, a greater influence may simply be that eating meat is very natural for most people. By and large we enjoy it; meat tastes good and feels satisfying. Humans have always been what some anthropologists call "opportunistic carnivores"—when meat is available, it is eaten. Modern-day hunter-gatherers go to great lengths to ensure a steady supply of meat, even when unlimited amounts of more easily obtained plant foods are available. The capture, sharing, and eating of meat is accorded almost mystical qualities.

Many people today may desire meat because they lack the nutrients provided by natural meat—not necessarily protein, but other fat-soluble nutrients, as discussed in previous chapters. Although modern commercial meat does not supply those nutrients, the desire for meat remains. When told meat is bad for health, we perhaps instinctively reason, "If meat is so bad, how did we make it this far as a species?"

The answer lies in the meat's quality, which in turn is a direct reflection on the quality of life of the animal consumed. The meat of modern mass-produced animals is not of the high quality that is found in the traditional diet. No private individual, stable, zoo, kennel, or even research facility may legally treat animals in the same way that they are commonly treated on factory farms. Thus individuals producing the nation's meat have complete control over the treatment and feeding of animals. Laws relating to the quality of meat as it affects the health of consumers are concerned only with preventing tainted meat from reaching consumers; they do not reflect any understanding of what constitutes natural meat with its attendant health benefits. Ironically, the interests of animals and consumers are coincident, for healthy, naturally fed, and humanely raised animals provide healthy food.

AN ALTERNATIVE EXISTS

Since early in the evolution of animal life, animals have utilized other animals in the struggle to survive. The earliest humans ate animals; as we evolved, the capture and consumption of animal life became increasingly important in the unfolding story of humanity. Ancient cave drawings and paintings, traditions surviving into the cultures of modern-day hunter-gatherers, and the rich folklore of a myriad of ethnic cultures all indicate that the killing of animals has always been done with the utmost respect and love for the animal to be eaten, be it wild or domestic. Native concepts of sacred foods and sacred meat discussed in chapter 1 underscore these traditions.

Most of modern production of meat, fowl, and dairy products is a travesty of this rich and uniquely human heritage. By eating these animals we unthinkingly participate in this travesty, perhaps because we believe that we have no choice. But an alternative does exist. Humanely raised healthy meat is available, for a growing number of people are raising food animals naturally. Healthy meat is good food for those who choose to eat meat. It is well worth the extra effort needed to secure it. Through its system of local chapters, the Weston A. Price Foundation (www.westonaprice.org) helps people locate local pasture-fed animal products.

Naturally raised meat, fowl, and eggs are what we will look at next.

PASTURED, NATURALLY RAISED
MEAT, FOWL, AND EGGS

Growing numbers of farmers and ranchers throughout America are carrying on a traditional American industry—the raising of animals out at pasture for much or all of the year, without using chemicals, hormones, or drugs. Others attempt this to the extent feasible; finding feed grown without pesticides or chemical fertilizers when adequate range is not available (winter in the north, summer in dry areas) can be difficult. Nevertheless, an increasing amount of meat, fowl, and eggs produced mostly or completely without chemicals, hormones, or drugs is becoming available.

Hormones and antibiotics aside, what distinguishes one animal from the next is exercise and what it eats. Meat, fowl, eggs, and dairy products are most beneficial when they derive from animals that have lived outdoors eating their natural diets. This means beef and lamb raised on grass, barnyard chickens and their eggs, and milk products from pasture-fed cows and goats. These foods (and seafoods) are rich in fat-soluble protective nutrients; their fat composition is in certain ways similar to that of wild game.

Grass-Fed Beef

Meat from 100 percent grass-fed cattle is becoming much more widely available, not only in specialty markets but also in many supermarkets. Cuts of such meat vary widely in tenderness and fattiness. Preferred are fatty cuts such as rib eye, and hamburger that is "75 percent lean," rather than the 85 percent and 90 percent one usually sees. When it comes to grass-fed beef, more fat is both healthier and tastier.

Organ Meats

Organs, particularly liver, have rich concentrations of many nutrients. But because the liver purifies the blood, it concentrates substances not naturally present in an animal. While the liver is one of the best parts of a naturally raised animal, liver from conventionally raised animals should be avoided.

Brain is seldom eaten in America today. In other cultures, and in North America in earlier times, it was a delicacy. Some physicians have made use of brain in therapeutic diets. It is now known to be a rich source of DHA (docosahexaenoic acid, very similar to EPA and likely involved in many of the same key metabolic pathways). Francis Pottenger, Jr. recommended brain in an eggnog recipe so it could be eaten raw; liver too was used raw, blended with juice. These foods may be used with excellent results, sometimes in these raw recipes but also lightly broiled. A practical way for many people to obtain these foods is in food supplements. Capsules of freeze-dried organs and glands from grass-fed New Zealand cattle are available.

Heart is extremely lean and muscular, but very tender when lightly cooked. The flavor is similar to that of steak. These and other organs are often available in stores carrying naturally raised meat and fowl, sometimes fresh but often frozen. Organs may be priced rather reasonably because of little demand. I have seen them advertised as pet food and sold cheaply, which seems ironic given that, in times past, Native Americans of the far north ate the organs and left the muscle meat for their dogs.

Lamb

Francis Pottenger, Jr. found lamb of particular value. Among his many publications was an article appearing in the *Journal of Applied Nutrition* in 1957 entitled "Therapeutic Effect of Lamb Fat in the Dietary." He notes that lamb fat, particularly lightly cooked or raw, is extremely beneficial for individuals suffering from dry skin or dry hair. Pottenger attributed lamb's benefits to polyunsaturated fats of animal origin, structurally different from those of vegetable origin. EPA had not yet been discovered; Pottenger empirically found that foods we now know are rich in EPA had great therapeutic benefit.

He wrote that the nutritional value of animal fats depended on various influences: the species of animal, whether or not it had been castrated, the age at slaughter, and the feeding methods used to rear the animal, including the use of hormones and the chemicals used in feed. Precisely because lamb is quite fatty and was ideally raised according to all of the above-referenced counts, it was well suited for individuals with problems related to deficiencies of unsaturated fats of animal origin. Pottenger did not observe the same benefits when beef was substituted for lamb. Lamb was cooked rare, no more than two minutes on a side at 450 degrees Fahrenheit for a one-inch chop. Lamb is very fatty so this will provide substantial, very lightly cooked fat.

Pottenger also wrote that in using substantial portions of lamb and of brain—both very fatty—even in people with initially high cholesterol and triglycerides, he never encountered increases. Instead, levels invariably went down. Parallels with recent discoveries by physicians working with fish oils are striking, and further demonstrate why animals raised on their natural diets provide food for building strength, resistance to disease, and longevity.

Fowl and Eggs

While chickens sold as "organic" or "naturally raised" may indeed be free of chemicals and drugs, most are raised in henhouses. Conditions there are roomier than for conventionally raised chickens, and the diet may be organic grains, but the animals still have little or no exercise and are not eating their natural diet.

Free-range chickens, on the other hand, eat greens, insects, and worms. Free-range chickens have skins that are a golden yellow color due to the rich supply of carotenes in fresh greens. They are a bit tougher and have a gamier taste than conventionally raised chickens. Their eggs have far more omega-3 fats.

Some fertile and organic eggs are from confined chickens. While superior to conventional supermarket eggs, they do not compare with eggs from free-range chickens. The latter have a bright yellow-orange yolk, a noticeably thicker and stronger shell, and a distinctly enhanced flavor.

Now that we have discussed the consumption of meat, fowl, and eggs—what to incorporate and what to avoid, and why—let us now turn our attention to fish and shellfish and put it under the same microscope of critical examination.

11
FRESH AND SALTWATER SEAFOOD AND THE ENVIRONMENT

As wild creatures, fish and shellfish live in their native environment, consume their natural diets, and are among the foods we are best adapted to eat. But because environmental pollutants may contaminate them, they should be selected with care. This chapter provides an overview of the water pollution problem and of influences affecting the quality and flavor of seafood in general. A more thorough guide to understanding and selecting fish and shellfish for both enjoyment and maximal health benefits is provided in appendix 2, where particular attention is paid to the issue of how one may determine which species are likely to have been least affected by water pollution as well as specific nutrient characteristics.

WATER POLLUTION

Many highly toxic pollutants contaminate coastal waters and even the deep oceans. These chemical compounds and heavy metals accumulate in the fats of fish. Many shellfish particularly concentrate pollutants because they constantly filter water. Thus fatty fish and shellfish are often avoided by many people; in recent years, a misbegotten fear of cholesterol and all animal-sourced fats has added to concerns. Fears about pollutants in fish and shellfish are more reasonable.

People have always used waterways for waste disposal. In earlier times, fewer people used fewer chemicals and created less sewage; many chemicals now widely used did not even exist back then. Today sewage, industrial wastes, detergents, and other pollutants (many highly toxic) are discharged into rivers, lakes, and oceans.

Treatment of sewage fails to adequately remove nitrates and inorganic phosphates. These major pollutants lead to eutrophication, an excessive growth of algae that decays in slow-moving estuaries, rivers, and bays. The resultant foul-smelling substances are toxic to fish, shellfish, and other wildlife that live in these coastal areas or must pass through en route to breeding grounds.

Agricultural fertilizers and spray residues include chlorinated hydrocarbons such as DDT and organophosphates such as parathion and malathion. Organophosphates are related to nerve gases developed in Nazi Germany during World War II. These substances all reach water via seepage and runoff. Wind carries mercury and other poisons in dust that is blown from chemical factories near waterways. Discharge of wash water and industrial wastes, dumping of trash and highly toxic chemicals, and oil spills are the other principal modes of contamination of coastal areas.

The principal industries contributing to this are the paper industry in the Pacific Northwest, Alabama, and Mississippi; chemical plants in the Gulf and mid-Atlantic states; and the oil industries in New Jersey, Louisiana, Texas, and California. All are concentrated at seashores or on large rivers, and much of the wastes discharged do not receive any type of treatment. Mercury, nickel, fluoride, oil, cement, white lime, caustic soda, hydrocyanic acid, and lactonitrile are among the many items discharged in large quantities.

Drums containing highly toxic materials, especially chlorinated hydrocarbons, have been dumped a few miles offshore from major coastal cities. They eventually leak.

Millions of tons of oil have been spilled into the world's oceans, mostly in coastal areas. The resulting oil-laden sediments move considerable distances with bottom currents. For as many as seven years after a spill, oil has been shown to be incorporated into the body tissues of crabs in sufficient quantities to drastically affect their behavior, reproductive capacity, and ability to survive.

Mercury and PCBs (polychlorinated biphenyls) are two industrial pollutants of particular concern because of their ubiquitous presence in the environment. Mercury is also used in agriculture; millions of pounds of mercury marketed yearly in the United States wind up in croplands. Although the Food and Drug Administration prohibits the sale of foods containing mercury, tests show grains, apples, eggs, milk, and other products contain levels in the range of 0.01 to 0.1 ppm. The World Health Organization suggests a maximum of 0.05 ppm.

Once in waterways and the sea, mercury is absorbed into plankton and moves up the food chain. Highly carnivorous species that live for several years and grow large acquire the densest concentrations of it. Although living in open ocean, tuna and swordfish are especially susceptible; the metal concentrates in the fats of these large fatty carnivorous fish.

PCBs are used in transformers and capacitors, as hydraulic and heat-transfer fluids, as plasticizers and solvents in adhesives, and as sealants. In the 1970s, four thousand tons entered waterways yearly, largely through sewage, leaching of industrial fluids, and from landfills and dumps. An outbreak of illness in 1968 in Japan was called *yusho,* or rice-oil disease, because the patients had eaten rice oil contaminated with tetrachlorobiphenyl (a PCB), which had leaked from the pipe of a heat exchanger during manufacture of the oil.

The patients numbered about one thousand. They developed darkened skin, a cheese-like discharge from the eyes, severe acne, numbness, nerve pains, swollen joints, edema, and jaundice. Among the eleven live and two stillborn babies born of these patients, all but one showed at least some of these symptoms. The disease lasted in many cases for more than three years. Shortly before these people became ill, seven hundred thousand chickens had been contaminated and died of the disease.

The patients had each consumed from 0.5 to 2.0 grams of the PCB; fat tissue from the skin contained from 13.1 to 75.5 ppm of the substance. (One-tenth of a teaspoon equals 0.5 grams.) Thus great harm may be done by small amounts of PCBs. Concentrations may vary widely within the same area. While apparently some PCBs and mercury are found in seafood from even the most remote waters, a dramatic difference in the concentration of poisons is based on the life history of the seafood consumed.

Species spending most of their lives in deep waters far out at sea are most likely to be least contaminated; coastal species living in polluted waters are most contaminated. Shellfish and fatty fish especially should be from relatively unpolluted waters.

Also, as we have mentioned, pollutants become more concentrated in fish that are higher up the food chain, making smaller species more desirable. Smaller, deep-water fish include herring, sardines, and anchovies; the smaller salmon such as pink, coho and sockeye; some members of the cod family, including scrod, hake, haddock, and pollock; and mackerel, pompano, red and yellowtail snapper, striped bass, butterfish, squid, octopus, and tilefish, among others. Tuna, bluefish, swordfish, and king salmon are best eaten when taken from waters off coastlines in unindustrialized areas. A wide variety of anadromous fish (oceangoing species returning to rivers to breed) are best eaten when taken in the unpolluted bays and rivers of unindustrialized and lightly populated areas, as are freshwater fish from similarly located lakes and streams.

The habitat of most commonly eaten shellfish is coastal waters. Since all are bottom dwellers, and since bivalves such as oysters and clams constantly pass water through their systems to filter nutrients, shellfish in contaminated waters concentrate undesirable substances. A knowledge of the waters shellfish are taken from is thus imperative when judging their desirability. Good fish merchants know where their stock is from.

GUIDELINES FOR PURCHASING SEAFOOD

I remember a small fish market I once frequented many years ago on the docks of the fishing village of Menemsha on the island of Martha's Vineyard off the coast of Massachusetts. The cement floors were always wet from a recent rinsing, a sea breeze blew through open windows, and out the back door one saw fishing boats tied up at docks. Fish eyes shined and scales glistened; fish on ice in glass cases were so fresh they looked almost alive, and all one could smell was the ocean and the faint sweet fragrance of prime seafood.

That is quality.

When examining a whole fish, first look at the eyes, which should be clear and full. If milky and sunken, look no further; this fish is not fresh. The flesh when pressed should be firm, rather than soft—one's fingers should leave no indentation. A clean fragrance, unblemished skin color, and bright red gills confirm the diagnosis of fresh fish. Fillets or steaks should appear clean, crisp, moist, and firm. Yellowing, a dried out appearance, or any strong odor indicate lack of freshness.

Less oily species generally keep well longer than those with a high oil content. Few species have more than about 15 percent fat content; those that do include herring, mackerel, and some varieties of salmon at certain times. The fat content varies greatly with both the diet of the fish and the season, most species being prime in fat and flavor in autumn. The seasonal variation is greatest among larger fish.

Any species may be excellent in one area and poor in another. The presence of pollutants in the water; various types of algae; the foods available to the fish in the locale; seasonal variations in fat content, freshness, seasoning, and method and amount of cooking all combine to determine whether a given fish lives up to the potential for the species.

The species with the most health benefits may be those found in more northern waters, perhaps because of their higher EPA content, and I generally recommend seafood from northern waters over tropical and subtropical species. However, I've never found any problems with eating the tropical and subtropical species as well. Avoid farm-raised fish because of the use of chemicals and artificial feed.

Seafood has been central to the lives of all traditional people who lived near the ocean. In many native cultures, fish and other animals of the hunt were in a very real sense worshipped—considered to be sacred food. Procuring and eating the wild creatures of the sea and the land was a sacrament, a sacred and ritualistic series of acts of great spiritual as well as physical significance. This sense of the sanctity of all life, of the essential oneness of the hunter and the hunted, of human and animal, is totally lost on most modern people. Ultimately, this loss of sanctity in our lives, of spirit—of love, if you will—is the reason we suffer, first emotionally and eventually physically. As we consider the constituents of an ideally healthy native diet, I believe we must give equal consideration to the spiritual aspects of food and eating—indeed, of living—which were an integral part of native cultures everywhere. If we do not, our efforts to attain health through diet alone will ring hollow and, I believe, ultimately fail.

Next we will turn to dairy foods, first conventionally produced products that are best avoided. Modern mass production methods unfortunately have taken much that was good out of these foods. As with meat, however, a growing number of producers are making grass-fed, high-quality dairy foods available. In the following pages, in our ongoing quest for enhanced health, we will examine conventionally and alternatively produced milk and milk products.

12
MILK AND
MILK PRODUCTS

Not everyone agrees that milk and milk products should be part of the human diet after infancy. While human milk is designed by nature as the perfect food for human babies, the argument has been made that just as no other species drink milk after weaning, neither should we.

Many adults have difficulty digesting pasteurized milk. Many others develop chronic allergies from using milk products. While this lends credence to arguments against milk, such physiological reactions are usually due to the poor quality of conventionally produced milk and milk products. While for some individuals genetic influences play a role, for most the body's reaction to milk depends largely upon the quality and state of the particular milk used.

MILK'S ROLE IN MANKIND'S EVOLUTION

Domesticated animals are generally thought to have first been used to produce milk eight to ten thousand years ago, though some archaeological evidence in recent years indicates that some humans may have secured milk from animals as long as thirty thousand years ago; until then, the only milk humans used was from the mother's breast. This proved adequate through millions of years of evolution. While humans, once weaned, could no doubt live in health without milk today, quality grass-fed raw milk is generally an outstanding addition to a healthy primal diet. Indeed, milk gave a considerable evolutionary advantage to those of our ancestors who were able to digest it beyond infancy.

The Swiss of the Loetschental Valley were among the few native groups Weston Price studied who used milk products (the others were certain African tribes, including the Masai). The native Swiss group used raw, whole milk (both fresh and cultured), cheese, and butter, all in substantial quantities. Milk was from healthy, grass-fed animals and was used unpasteurized and unhomogenized. Such foods clearly can play a major role in a health-enhancing program for the individual who is genetically enabled to utilize these foods well.

As beneficial as high-quality dairy products may be to the human diet, we could attain optimal health without them. Dr. Weston Price discovered groups who consumed no dairy food but had complete resistance to dental decay and chronic disease. Their diets invariably included other rich sources of calcium and other minerals. The soft ends of long bones were commonly chewed, and the shafts and other bones were used in soups. Bones of small animals were ground up and added to food.

Modern medicine is discovering the importance of a substantial intake of calcium. For example, several recent studies have linked high blood pressure and other problems with chronic subclinical calcium deficiency. Paradoxically, other problems are associated with high consumption of conventionally produced dairy foods. This has not gone unnoticed by researchers, nutritionists, and physicians. The importance of the quality and freshness of milk products lies behind the paradox. This concept has not been considered in attempts by the medical community to explain the health effects of dairy foods.

Milk from domesticated animals became important as a human food several thousand years ago. With domestication and settlement, fewer wild animals were available, and as groups of people roamed less, they hunted less, and ate more grains and vegetables. Milk replaced animal bones as the chief source of calcium and some other minerals. Adaptations in evolution are always the effects of particular causes. Humans developing the ability to digest milk into adulthood possessed a survival advantage; such change is the basis of evolution.

TODAY'S PROCESSED DAIRY PRODUCTS

Conventional dairy products of today are capable of doing much harm to the human body. However, they are considered healthy foods, and most people consume them habitually, finding it difficult to give them up. Be this as it may, many people today often experience symptoms of fatigue, nasal congestion, colds, and allergy as a direct result of consuming dairy products. These symptoms disappear rapidly when dairy consumption is reduced or eliminated. Other symptoms are subtly and indirectly related to these foods, and a host of other chronic problems developing over the years are greatly influenced by them.

For the full story on conventional versus traditional, primal grass-fed dairy foods, please see my book *The Untold Story of Milk*. Let's now examine a few salient and pertinent facts about homogenization, synthetic vitamin D, and pasteurization. Following that, we will discuss raw dairy products and the best way to begin incorporating them into the diet.

Homogenization

Homogenization breaks down fat globules in milk, causing them to remain dispersed. This is done so the cream in milk will not rise to the top. Homogenization on a commercial scale was introduced over a period of years in the 1930s so that large volumes of milk could be shipped in trucks without the milk churning into butter, (which naturally happened without homogenization). Consumers resisted the new homogenized product because they were used to judging the quality of milk by the amount and color of the cream at the top of a milk bottle. More cream and deeper yellow color meant more fat and flavor and vitamins A and D, all of which were known to be good. It took many years of indoctrination of the public via advertising dollars to dispel this truth from people's minds and replace it with whatever it is that makes many people today accept the white liquid in markets that passes for milk.

Homogenization produces a substance in homogenized milk that damages arterial walls, according to a controversial theory of Kurt Oster, M.D., former chief of cardiology at Park City Hospital in Bridgeport, Connecticut. Oster wrote extensively about this. His thesis was that the enzyme xanthine oxidase (XO), found in milk fat, is normally not absorbed into the bloodstream from the intestines when unhomogenized milk is drunk. The homogenization process emulsifies fats in milk, releasing the XO and making it available for absorption. Individuals using homogenized milk have high levels of XO in the blood, while those using only unhomogenized milk, skim milk, or no milk have very low levels. The theory is that XO acts chemically to scar arterial walls, with a subsequent deposition of fatty material on the scars contributing to the development of atherosclerosis. Oster and many other physicians, including Dr. Kurt Esselbacher, chairman of the Department of Medicine of the Harvard Medical School (at the time that he publicly expressed his full support of Oster's overall concept), believe homogenized milk is a major cause of heart disease in the United States.

Mary Enig, Ph.D., a renowned expert in the biochemistry of fats and oils and their effects in the human body, and many other experts disputed Oster's theory, saying that his chemical explanation did not make sense. The theory never gained widespread acceptance.

Homogenization occurred at the same time as widespread pasteurization was mandated—the subsequent rise in heart disease would be attributed to both processes.

The Past Use of Synthetic Vitamin D₂— Irradiated Ergosterol

Vitamin D_2 (irradiated ergosterol) was for many years added to most commercial dairy products and many other processed foods; it was also commonly used in multivitamins. Years ago, when cows spent most of the year outdoors eating grass, cows made natural vitamin D. Carotenes that the cows consumed gave butter, particularly summer-made butter, a naturally bright-yellow color. Such butter, however, did not store and ship as well as a lower-vitamin, paler butter. Over the years the quality and vitamin content of butter dropped as the color faded—as cows came to spend less time outdoors eating grass and more time indoors eating grains. Eventually, yellow dye was added to most butters.

Vitamin D is a complex of several vitamins existing in certain animal fats. There are over 800 isomers of vitamin D. One such isomer of the complex, vitamin D_3, is produced by the action of sunlight on skin. Irradiated ergosterol is a synthesized approximation of vitamin D_3, with a slightly different biochemical structure than its natural counterpart. Studies have shown that this D_2 is more active than vitamin D_3 and overstimulates calcium metabolism. Clinical experience with arthritis patients and others with problems involving calcium utilization indicate that vitamin D_2, whether in milk, other foods, or vitamins, contributed to health problems, especially calcification of the soft tissues. As a result, it is no longer as widely used as it once was. Failure to include adequate sources in the diet of natural vitamin D, and the fat-soluble nutrients vitamin A and vitamin K_2 that are associated with it in nature, further contributes to problems with calcium utilization.

In the 1930s, several studies linked irradiated ergosterol with calcification of the placenta and other problems in pregnancy. Results published in medical journals caused some concern at the time, but these warnings and those of Weston Price and others about the dangers of synthetic vitamin D_2 went largely unheeded.

Grossly abnormal calcium metabolism led to the death of at least one infant in England, when for a short time the amount of irradiated ergosterol added to milk was increased from 400 I.U. (international units) to 1,000 I.U. per quart. The infant dying from this highly unusual abnormality was the first reported death due to "idiopathic hypercalcemia of infancy" (high levels of serum calcium due to an unknown reason). The addition of irradiated ergosterol to milk in England was subsequently stopped.

Pasteurization

Pasteurization is done for both sanitary and commercial reasons. Pasteurization usually kills most pathogens—which thrive in conventional dairies—rendering raw milk free of them. The milk is usually shipped long distances in tanker trucks and packaged for sale or made into various milk products on a commercial scale. The modern dairy industry is huge and would not be possible without the processes of pasteurization and homogenization.

Pasteurization denatures all enzymes and heat-labile nutrients, changing the chemical structures of proteins and fats in the milk. As small farmers were forced off their farms and into cities by the commercial realities of post–World War II modern farming, raw milk gradually began disappearing from the American scene. Many health issues became much more prevalent. Heat-processed milk, cheese, and yogurt create allergies in consumers, though the symptoms may not be recognized as allergies. Reactions to pollens, molds, dust, and other environmental substances are usually linked to these and other dietary influences. Modern confinement cows are routinely fed antibiotics and soy feed grown, usually GMO, with pesticides. They are subjected to insecticides, drugs, and other chemicals. These substances may appear in their milk.

Commercial interests dictating food production have joined with regulatory authorities to make raw milk difficult to obtain in many parts of the country. Scare tactics have been used to convince the public that all raw milk is dangerous. Pasteurization and homogenization enables quantities of milk to be collected, shipped long distances, and stored. This is impossible with raw milk, which traditionally has often been made into soured milk products. Thus raw milk has always been locally produced.

Concern for consumers' health appears in milk advertisements, but the production of food is a business, whether the food is milk, meat, cereals, vegetables, fruits, or candy bars. Profits are placed before concerns about consumers' health. As a result, modern milk is not fit for consumption. Raw milk from grass-fed, chemical-free animals is truly an entirely different, highly desirable primal food.

In indigenous cultures where adults consume milk, often the product is cultured or clabbered milk. Both are similar to homemade raw yogurt, and are partially predigested—much of the lactose (milk sugar) has been broken down by bacterial action. This process must be accomplished over a period of several hours in the stomach when one drinks fresh milk; yogurt or clabbered milk is much more easily and quickly digested than fresh milk.

Many people with a history of allergic reactions to milk, even raw milk, can use and enjoy cultured raw milk. Similarly, though pasteurized cheeses may cause problems, small amounts of raw-milk cheeses often do not. Considerable individual differences exist; some people are much more adapted for these foods than others. Milk products from pasture-fed animals almost never cause allergic reactions and are superior to those from animals fed mostly grains.

RAW DAIRY FOODS

Sometimes change must necessarily proceed rather slowly in early stages of dietary adjustments. Food preferences result from a lifetime of likes and dislikes, habits, and culturally ingrained responses to foods available in different situations; though much needed, change may come with difficulty. This is all true when one is considering the elimination of conventional dairy products in one's diet and the introduction of raw-milk products instead. The following guidelines for the use of dairy products are suggested:

- If you are using commercial dairy foods, eat none for a few days before introducing raw milk. This gives the body an opportunity to clear itself of antibodies causing allergic reactions to milk products, allowing the best chance to react well to high-quality raw-milk foods.

- Then try some raw milk or homemade raw yogurt. Sip a small amount, at room temperature. In some adults, any milk causes allergic reactions—nasal congestion, postnasal drip, or diarrhea or loose stools several hours later. Raw milk available in many places is produced neither organically nor from grassfed animals. Individuals reacting poorly to such raw milk may react more favorably to organic raw milk or raw milk from grass-fed animals. In many cases, one is best off using no milk, or very little, if milk from grass-fed animals is unavailable. In the more northern parts of the United States, fresh grass is unavailable in the winter and cows in viable raw-milk dairies live on some combination of hay and grain. Milk from cows fed very little or no grain produce superior milk.

- Cultured raw milk or homemade raw yogurt may be made from raw milk; allergic reactions to these foods are much less marked than to the milk itself. Cultured milk is made by adding a buttermilk or kefir culture to raw milk and allowing it to stand in a warm room for forty-eight to seventy-two hours. Fermentation increases with time, and more curds separate as the taste becomes stronger. Initial addition of a culture viable enough to grow in unheated raw milk results in a more yogurt-like consistency and flavor.

- Butter rarely if ever causes allergic reactions. The best butter, made from grass-fed animals, is a darker yellow to orange color.

- Raw-milk cheeses too are marvelous foods and may be an important part of the diet. The feeding of the animals is paramount, with the best-made cheeses derived from raw milk from grass-fed animals, with animal rennet.

Raw goat's-milk and sheep's-milk cheeses may also be excellent. Compared to cow's milk, goat's milk is more similar biochemically to human's milk. Sheep's-milk and goat's-milk cheeses are sometimes produced organically, and these ruminants naturally feed on grasses, weeds, and shrubs. (Use the Weston A. Price Foundation Shopping Guide in selecting quality cheeses: www.westonaprice.org/about-the-foundation/shopping-guide.)

Many cheeses labeled "raw" are heated to 150 degrees Fahrenheit; however, raw-milk cheese should not have been heated to over 105 degrees Fahrenheit. Natural cheeses are not ground, melted, or mixed with anti-mold chemicals, preservatives, and a variety of food additives, as are most conventionally produced cheeses. An organic cheese is made from milk from organically fed animals, though not necessarily pasture-fed, and should be free of pesticide residues; some producers order laboratory tests periodically to ensure this is the case. Raw-milk cheeses are required by law to be aged for at least sixty days. Since this reduces the risk of harmful microorganisms in the cheese, aged raw-milk cheeses may be sold even in states where raw milk may not legally be sold for human consumption.

Availability and Safety of Raw-Milk Products

The availability of these raw-milk products varies from region to region because of restrictive laws; many states prevent the sale of raw milk and most forbid the sale of raw butter for human use. Laws prohibiting the sale of these foods hide under the cloak of public safety but are actually the result of lobbying by the dairy industry to protect commercial interests. Raw milk of a quality suitable for market cannot be mass-produced on huge farms by cows that are little more than milk machines, living far from the land that nature intended grazing animals to feed upon. Raw milk cannot be shipped in tanker trucks, processed in plants, and distributed in supermarkets far from where it is produced, as can commercial milk. Nor will raw milk keep for weeks on a shelf.

Raw milk from healthy animals is outstanding food for many people, particularly for growing children. In states where raw milk is inspected and tested by government agencies, this may help assure that animals are healthy and milk is produced under sanitary conditions (although too often regulations are used by authorities to harass and attempt to drive out of business farmers producing and selling top-quality, grass-fed raw milk). State government regulations and enforcement are stringent about the production of raw milk, which is allowed bacteria counts only a fraction of those allowed in milk to be pasteurized. Such raw milk is safer than conventionally produced milk, for any problem in the pasteurization process—they occasionally occur—leads to contaminated milk.

The Superiority of Raw Milk

Studies by eminent physicians and scientists, including Francis Pottenger, Jr., have clearly demonstrated the superiority of raw milk as compared with pasteurized. Raw milk contains vital heat-labile nutrients not found in pasteurized milk. The medical establishment and public health authorities have failed to recognize evidence that a deficiency of these nutrients has substantially contributed to the development of the epidemic of diseases plaguing modern civilization.

Poorly produced raw milk can lead to disease, particularly in susceptible individuals. But many state health agencies, under political pressure from the dairy industry, have simply categorically prohibited the sale of raw milk and raw butter, claiming all such products are dangerous to the public. This is not true; the history of raw milk in this country shows raw milk and raw-milk products are not dangerous or harmful when these foods are conscientiously produced. The public has been robbed of the right to good food, and the industry and government agencies responsible have convinced us they are the protectors of public health. The dairy industry meanwhile counts profits (much of which comes from government subsidies, that is, our taxes) as national health deteriorates.

Food is big business. The interest groups profiting from the food business have deliberately made it difficult to eat simply and naturally; traditionally produced milk, cheese, and butter can be hard to find. Only if we support the few dairy farmers producing natural products of the highest quality will this change. Like organic vegetable farmers (discussed in the next chapter), organic dairy farmers remain a minority. But good quality raw-milk cheeses are available in many stores, and many states allow sales of raw milk and a few of raw butter. By educating legislators and demanding the highest-quality foods for ourselves and our children, more and more states will follow the lead of those with laws allowing the sale of raw milk and raw-milk products; demand in California is such that these foods are available in many supermarkets.

The adulteration of milk has made a liability out of this delicious traditional, primal food. Professionals in the fields of medicine and nutrition are evenly split between the pros and cons of drinking conventional milk; resulting confusion makes it difficult for the lay person to choose foods wisely and is cause for concern in light of the problems to which adulterated milk contributes. Sadly, the public cannot win; avoiding conventional milk and milk products may contribute to calcium deficiency, while using them contributes to the problems detailed in this chapter.

The use of other calcium-rich foods, such as green salads and green vegetables, and food supplements such as calcium hydroxyapatite derived from the bones of grass-fed animals, or both—by those avoiding milk and milk products—is one viable alternative. Another is the use of whole, grass-fed raw milk, and butter and cheese made from raw milk, where available, and butter, yogurt, cream, cheese, and kefir made from pasteurized grass-fed milk. Ideally both sources are used. The raw versions of these dairy foods are best, but when those are not available, the pasteurized versions may be integrated into a modern primal diet.

13
VEGETABLES, WHOLE-GRAIN FOODS, FRUITS, NUTS, AND SEEDS

In this chapter we will examine more closely the part of our diet that is plant-based, comprised as it is of vegetables, whole grains, fruits, nuts, and seeds. Before we do that, however, it's important to put a spotlight on the processes by which these foods are grown, given that *how* our food is grown is often just as important as *what we eat*. For starters, let's look at the practice of organic farming versus that of chemical agriculture. Following that we will detail other important considerations pertaining to the role of plant-based foods in the modern primal diet.

CHEMICAL VERSUS ORGANIC FARMING

People often ask if there is really much difference between most produce available in supermarkets and produce sold as "organically grown." The answer, quite simply, is yes. But only when some details are understood does the answer have much meaning. An examination of how food is conventionally produced today and how food has traditionally been grown makes the difference clear.

Chemical Agriculture
Imagine driving on back roads through America's heartland, seeing thousands of square miles of midwestern farmland. Travel in the mind's eye

through the cattle, vegetable, and citrus country of Florida, the apple and cherry groves of upstate New York and New England, the fields of vegetables in valleys of Oregon and Washington, and everywhere in between along backcountry roads where farmers grow our food. A picture of great beauty emerges; rural America remains very lovely.

But the loveliness is tinged with a lingering sadness, for hundreds of millions of pounds of poisonous pesticides are sprayed on the land every year. And though this land is vast, one realizes it is nonetheless finite and perishable.

Many of these poisons work systemically and become part both of the soil and of plant tissues. Farmers consider this advantageous because they need not reapply them after a heavy rain. Some, like DDT, have been banned, but a wide variety of others continue to be used in varying amounts. While allowable amounts vary, the maximum allowances of minute amounts provides testimony as to the toxicity of these substances. No one will argue these agents are not incredibly toxic in tiny amounts. Given the documented performance of the FDA in enforcement (consider the DES affair) and the agency's admitted lack of manpower to test adequately both the pesticides and the foods themselves for residues, the established limits on concentrations are not particularly reassuring.

In the United States, production of food was once the province of small farms owned by families. Now it is big business. In a land once producing food with considerable love, care, and attention to concerns of consumers, little thought is now given beyond the expedient and the maximally profitable. One need not elaborate on the obvious.

Consider, however, the results. The land lies essentially raped. Once-abundant wildlife is in many areas scarce or gone entirely. Insects have grown increasingly resistant to pesticides; larger amounts of toxic chemicals are used, killing insect predators and thus destroying natural checks. Meanwhile, more and more petrochemically derived fertilizers are used in attempts to maintain high yields. Humus reserves have been depleted; the living organisms of the soil have been killed. This circle has made most farms as dependent on chemical fertilizers and pesticides as an addict is on drugs.

Herbicides are used on weeds; fungicides are used in fields to control fungus diseases and in storage and transport to control rot. Fumigants are sprayed on stored foods to kill insects. Thousands of additional chemicals are added to foods when they are processed.

Tests of these substances, when they are tested, are made individually. But interactions of two or more chemicals have unpredictable results, often resulting in greater toxicity than results from the use of one alone. Effects of potential carcinogenic agents are equally unpredictable; the development of cancer often takes many years or even decades from the time of the initial exposure to carcinogenic agents.

Organic Farming and Living Soil

An organic agriculture is more than the absence of negative and harmful influences. In the early 1900s, a man whose work changed the shape and substance of many buildings Americans live and work in wrote of the need for an organic quality in architecture. He borrowed a word from agriculture because he envisioned an architecture in touch and in scale with nature, as the living soil is with the plants it nurtures. The man was Frank Lloyd Wright. He called his vision for buildings and the spaces they define "organic" architecture. To be in one of his buildings is to know why. Many are integrated with the landscape in a quite remarkable way, which many people find beautiful.

An organic agriculture truly lives and breathes. The soil teems with microorganisms that give vigor and resistance to plants, with worms to aerate the soil, and insect predators to control pests. High in humus and nurtured with natural fertilizers, a living soil provides plants that, when consumed as food, offer superior taste and nutritional value.

More farmers are realizing that their own interests are no more served by chemical agriculture than are the public's, and as they change to organic methods, more naturally grown foods will become available. Conversion of chemically overworked soils is not easy; such soils are often reduced to a state not conducive to organic growing. This is one reason organic foods initially may cost more to produce. Prices have come down in recent years, however, and are in many areas competitive with conventionally grown crops. Healthy native and so-called primitive cultures ate plant foods that were nourished by virgin soils or a carefully and naturally maintained traditional agricultural system. This was an integral part of their success. Naturally grown foods are one of the primitive influences needed to solve modern problems. There is a growing awareness of this reality, even in mainstream American agriculture. I once heard a report on the production of grapes in California, on National Public Radio's evening news program, *All Things Considered.*

The report focused on Gallo wines. It turns out that Gallo was quietly converting their grape farms to organic methods. In fact, Gallo had become the biggest organic grower—not just of grapes, but of anything—in all of California. Over 6,000 of their 10,000 acres of grapes were under organic cultivation. The reason? Economics. Organic works better. It's more efficient and it saves Gallo money. Modern culture generally treats Earth and its creatures kindly only when it benefits our pocketbooks.

Organically grown vegetables are becoming more and more available in natural-food stores and supermarkets; optimally, they are bought seasonally, directly from growers. They may complement the conventionally grown vegetables many of us often must settle for because of the difficulty and expense of obtaining organically grown vegetables. Another important consideration is the use of indigenous foods in a context other than its original one. This we will consider next.

USING INDIGENOUS FOODS

Foods most suited to any given individual may be those indigenous to the type of climate in which one's ancestors evolved and lived. People of European ancestry may not be biologically equipped to utilize foods indigenous to the tropics and the subtropics in any substantial quantity. People of European descent evolved and developed under the influence of foods native to northern and temperate parts of the world.

Adverse effects from foods in the vegetable kingdom that are of tropical origin are commonly seen clinically. I have not seen similar effects from animal foods. Many very popular foods are not indigenous to northern and temperate climates. These include citrus and other tropical fruits and their juices; the nightshade (Solanaceae) family of vegetables, including tomatoes, potatoes, eggplants, and green peppers; and some nuts, including cashews. For some people, these foods may constitute a major portion of the diet, and a variety of symptoms and clinical problems may result from ingesting them. Improvement often results when use of the offending food or foods is reduced sufficiently or discontinued.

Now let's take a look at the role of vegetables, whole-grain foods, and fruits, nuts, and seeds, and examine how they fit into our primal-diet picture.

VEGETABLES

Primal Weston Price–type diets place considerable emphasis on animal foods. These foods have always provided certain essential nutrients unavailable in foods in the vegetable kingdom. Traditional cultures and contemporary hunter-gatherer societies invariably have customs and rituals surrounding the use of certain animal foods.

This is not to deny, however, the importance of *plant* foods in native diets. In all regions except the northernmost Arctic, plant foods, either cultivated or gathered, play a vital role. Generally, the closer the country in question is to the equator, the more enhanced role plants will play in the diet, particularly in terms of calories consumed. For many people in the temperate zones of North America, a diet in which a substantial portion of the calories consumed are provided by plant foods may be appropriate. The precise proportion varies with individual genetics, tastes, and needs, and indeed tends to vary with the individual, seasonally and throughout one's life. Vegetables, however, are used in indigenous diets everywhere except for far northern climates. Although animal fats should provide us with a majority of calories, for most of us vegetables have a very important role to play in a modern primal diet as well.

Salad Greens and Cooked Greens

Salad greens all year long are something of a modern luxury. I find a green salad with blue cheese an invigorating prelude to heartier fare, especially in summer when the size of the salad might grow larger. If one suffers from gastrointestinal disease, one should use raw greens with caution, if at all, in the early stages of dietary treatment. Others may begin eating small salads and slowly increase the size. Body and mind may then gradually adapt to larger amounts of raw greens. Use desired varieties of lettuce and sprouts, celery, parsley, and other palatable greens.

Dressing helps make a salad enjoyable; extra-virgin olive oil and raw apple cider vinegar are preferred ingredients. Balsamic vinegar may provide additional flavor. Canned sardines packed in water or extra-virgin oil are an excellent addition to salads, with outstanding health benefits.

Cooked greens also provide many nutrients. Broccoli, kale, beet greens, and sometimes dandelion and other greens are readily available, and should be well cooked and eaten with fat. Regular use of large quantities of vegetables containing oxalic acid is discouraged; these include spinach, swiss chard, and rhubarb, which should all be cooked. Oxalic acid is found in most kidney stones. Although it is a normal metabolite, its presence in stones indicates a disorder in its metabolism and excretion.

Dulse and Nori

Edible seaweeds are incredibly dense in nutrients. Rich in many vitamins and minerals, they especially concentrate iodine, critical in thyroid-gland function and lacking in the diet of many Americans. An excellent source of trace minerals, sea vegetables have always been widely utilized by native coastal cultures and even inland people, who bartered for them.

Dulse and nori are the most easily used edible seaweeds now sold commercially; both are customarily eaten uncooked, either alone or in salads. Nori is also used in traditional Japanese sushi, rolled with rice, vegetables, and raw fish. Other edible seaweeds are generally well cooked, otherwise they are hard to digest. They also should be organic because many chemicals may be used in drying seaweed.

Dulse sold in natural-food stores is harvested off the coast of Canada from the cold waters of the northern Atlantic, dried, and packed. It is very thin, and a little goes a long way; a fraction of a bag may be cut up or pulled apart and sprinkled into a salad.

Like dulse, nori is not processed with heat. Japanese people have farmed the ocean for nori for centuries by seeding rope nets, which are stretched between buoys just below the ocean's surface. In a few months, the ropes are pulled aboard ships and the nori is sucked into machines. The mash is slowly dried on shore at low temperatures in flat, square forms. The paper-thin sheets that result are sold throughout the world.

Nori is grown in coastal Japanese waters, while the dulse available comes from northern Canadian waters far from major population and industrial centers; the latter seems preferable. The flavor of seaweed may seem a little strange at first, but dulse for many people quickly becomes a welcome addition to raw vegetable salads. Nori is easily used in sushi and other traditional Japanese dishes, but also makes a tasty snack eaten alone.

The Nightshades

Foods from the nightshade family (Solanaceae—tomatoes, peppers, egg-plants, and potatoes) may be occasionally enjoyed, but problems often occur with regular overuse of these foods. Garden-ripe tomatoes in late summer taste good, but when eaten in quantity they cause many people to develop small sores in the mouth and on the tongue, and often skin problems as well. Like all minor symptoms, these should not be ignored; they yield clues about how foods affect the body. Hypersensitive reactions to the nightshades often reflect a deficiency of vitamin K_2.

Tomatoes, like citrus fruit, tend also to aggravate gastrointestinal problems. Potatoes may cause gas, and some people note indigestion after eating green peppers.

It may seem an overreaction to minimize the use of these foods because such symptoms occur in some people. But the green parts of the nightshade plants are poisonous—everyone knows not to eat tomato vines, for example. Centuries ago, the tomato itself was also considered poisonous; only in the past few hundred years has it been used as food. Plants from the Solanaceae family contain a glycosidic compound similar to a metabolite of vitamin D_3. Vitamin D_3 is a prime regulator of calcium absorption and utilization. When grazing on these plants, animals develop stiff legs and a number of symptoms indicative of calcium problems. The compound appears to detrimentally influence their calcium metabolism. Literature about animal husbandry from all over the world reveals that each culture has a name for these symptoms in animals, and in each case, their cause is the same—grazing on plants from the nightshade family.

Avoiding the nightshades is not the sole solution for arthritis or any other serious problem. But evidence indicates these foods play a role in arthritic and other diseases. The nightshades are indigenous to tropical and subtropical climates. They are a recent introduction to the diet— our ancient ancestors did not have these foods. A prudent diet emphasizes other foods and limits tomatoes, eggplants, peppers, and potatoes to occasional use. Adequate vitamin K_2 intake is protective and often allows for moderate intake of nightshades without adverse effects.

Raw-Vegetable Juices

Fresh raw-vegetable juices have their place in therapeutic diets for some people in certain situations, and may be an occasional adjunct in a primal traditional diet. They are best prepared from mostly greens and a little carrot. A piece of apple may be juiced to sweeten the mixture a bit. Raw green juice was an important part of Dr. Max Gerson's therapy for cancer. Juices are best freshly prepared and drunk at least thirty minutes before meals to avoid interfering with the digestion of solid foods. Our ancestors did not have juice machines, however, and juices are best seen as optional, not for everyone, and not for everyday use.

WHOLE-GRAIN FOODS

Whole grains should be properly prepared—soaked for at least six to eight hours in an acid medium before use—and they should always be cooked. Whole grains contain phytic acid in the bran of the grain, which combines with key minerals and prevents their absorption in the intestinal tract. Soaking the grain before cooking neutralizes the phytic acid, breaks down complex starches, lessens allergic reactions to grains, and makes grains less difficult to digest properly. Acid mediums include cultured buttermilk, milk kefir, coconut kefir, water kefir, cultured yogurt, whey, lemon juice, or apple cider vinegar. Use one tablespoon of acid medium per cup of pure water.

The History and Role of Whole Grains in the Diet

Essential in the diets of some historical and contemporary native agricultural cultures, whole grains were at the heart of the natural food movement that spread throughout America in the 1960s. For many people interested in natural food, vegetables and whole grains became a substantial part of the diet as they moved away from conventionally produced meat and dairy products. We have seen that other foods, particularly seafood and grass-fed domestic animal meat and dairy products, are, along with vegetables, the most natural candidates to be dietary staples. What about whole-grain foods though? What role should they play in a contemporary primal diet?

Among people Weston Price studied in the 1930s and found immune to dental decay, only those in the Loetschental Valley of

Switzerland and on the islands of the Outer Hebrides off the coast of Scotland used whole grains (rye in the Loetschental, oats in the Outer Hebrides) as an essential part of the native diet. Grains were also staples in a number of African diets and in parts of Peru. The people of Georgian Russia, Vilcabamba, and Hunza also used substantial quantities of whole grains. Evidence presented in chapter 4, however, indicates grains may have played too large a role in the diet of many people in Vilcabamba and Hunza.

The place of whole grains in the diet, even those carefully grown without pesticides and chemical fertilizers and properly prepared, has been debated for many years by people interested in anthropology and nutrition. Domesticated grains became a staple in the diet of some humans beginning only about fifteen thousand years ago, when settlements first appeared around the edges of wild grain fields and people first learned to domesticate these plants. Many of us are descendants of ancestors who first used grains fewer than two thousand years ago. Anthropologists tell us that humans are biologically the same as we were at least forty thousand years ago. We all thus evolved to our present biological state on a diet that did not include grains.

As noted above, a majority of the cultures Weston Price found to have immunity to dental and chronic disease used no grains. A number of other cultures he studied used considerably more grains than those two cultures did, and suffered from a small but significant amount of dental decay and other indications of less than nearly perfect health. Grains have become a staple over the past fifteen thousand years in agrarian societies the world over—yet Price's work showed clearly that hunter-fisher-gatherer societies enjoyed greater strength and immunity than their grain-eating agricultural contemporaries and in many cases dominated them.

Anthropologists have demonstrated that the introduction of grains into the human diet coincided with a marked reduction in the size and strength of humans. We cannot escape the importance of the question about what role grains should play in our diets today.

Recommendations Pertaining to the Use of Whole Grains in the Diet

My answer is to use and recommend whole-grain foods only as an option for a small part of the diet. A truly primal diet leaves them out. Grains are convenient—they store and travel easily, and they are relatively inexpensive. Their inclusion in the daily diet is satisfying for many people, who nevertheless often pay the price for consuming them, usually in excess weight and less than optimal health. Grains are not essential for a healthy diet, and their use at the expense of grass-fed animal foods and vegetables is detrimental. But properly prepared, small amounts are a reasonable and enjoyable indulgence.

The grain most easily prepared with the least amount of cooking is toasted buckwheat, or kasha. The inedible outer hull of the buckwheat groat has been mechanically removed and the raw groat lightly toasted. Indigenous to northern Russia, kasha is a hearty food, rich in a more complete protein than any other grain, and considered the most strengthening of the grains.

Because the toasting process has partially cooked the kasha, it may be prepared in a few minutes—simply mix one part kasha to one part hot or boiling water and let stand a few minutes. Kasha is convenient when traveling; it is not perishable and can be prepared by simply adding hot tap water. Lots of butter and a little Celtic salt are good on buckwheat, and I have occasionally enjoyed it with eggs.

Brown rice is the most commonly used whole grain. Available in both short-grain and long-grain varieties, short grain is traditionally considered more strengthening. Mixing in a wild rice (gathered largely in northern Minnesota and Canada, where it grows in shallow lake bottoms) adds a distinctive flavor. Brown rice is subject to oxidation at high temperatures and is best kept airtight and refrigerated or in a cool place.

Foods Made from Whole Grains

In addition to whole grains, which remain fresh and in their natural state until cooked and eaten, a host of foods made from whole grains are available. These include breads, flours, pastas, and pastries.

When grain is made into flour, its nutrients are exposed to oxygen. Certain nutrients, particularly vitamin E, are very much susceptible to destruction through oxidation. Other, little understood effects result in loss of vital nutrients. Many animal experiments have demonstrated a great difference between the effects of fresh whole grains or freshly ground flour and those of flour not completely fresh. If flour is to be used, it should be ground fresh, at home.

Visitors to Hunza many years ago observed that when traveling about the country, natives carried small hand mills for grinding wheat to make fresh chapattis—the small loaves of bread that are a dietary staple. They did this rather than grinding flour at home and making chapattis before leaving, or even rather than carrying flour with them. Food was scarce, and the Hunzas recognized the need to utilize their grains in the most efficient possible manner: completely fresh.

Breads made from sprouts without the use of flour are available in natural-food stores, but unfortunately most contain gluten. Sprouted grains are less subject to oxidation than flour and are rich in nutrients. Various grains are sprouted and made into loaves, either plain or with small amounts of sea salt, lecithin, yeast, and other natural ingredients. The finest are slowly baked at low temperatures to ensure minimal destruction of heat-labile nutrients.

Scores of sizes and shapes of whole-grain pastas are available, most made from whole-wheat flour and, in some products, spinach or artichoke flour. Like whole-grain breads and sprouted whole-grain breads, these foods may be useful, especially for individuals and families making a transition from refined foods and becoming accustomed to the taste of natural food. Simply cooked whole grains day after day may prove unpalatable; whole-grain products provide an important alternative for those who choose to include whole-grain foods regularly in the diet.

In the next section, we will consider the role of fruit in a primal traditional diet. Fruit, like grains, is thought of by most people as a dietary necessity, but the amount and kind of fruit most beneficial depends very much on individual circumstances.

FRUIT, NUTS, AND SEEDS

Fruit

America loves fruit—orange juice for breakfast, fruit at lunch and for snacks, fruit for dessert. Especially for many health-conscious people, fresh fruits and fruit juices are considered important foods and are eaten daily all year round.

Fresh fruit supplies raw enzymes, vitamin C, and potassium, but only tropical fruits are truly rich in enzymes. Vitamin C is partially destroyed by cooking, and fresh fruit is an important source of it for many people, though it may be equally well supplied by other raw foods, especially vegetables, raw milk, and organ meats. Potassium too is abundant in vegetables. Because many people eat few vegetables and little raw food, fruit has become a major source of vitamin C, potassium, and vital heat-labile nutrients. As a result, some people feel better eating fruit and eat substantial amounts of it.

The question, however, is whether raw-food nutrients might be best supplied by other foods, and if so, what then should be the role of fruit in the diet? Could excessive fruit be contributing to the development of problems? What about fruit juices?

Consider the place of fruit in the diet of our ancestors. *Homo erectus,* considered to be the ancestral human species preceding and leading to the development of *Homo sapiens,* is thought to have developed in Africa and then migrated throughout Europe and Asia around one million years ago. By the time this migration took place, men were hunting cooperatively, and meat played an important if not dominant role in the diet. Food gathering was also important in the mixed economy of early humans, and in Africa fruit undoubtedly was an important food. But as migrations spread north, fruit must have played a diminishing role. For hunter-gatherers of Europe and northern and central Asia, fruit came to be a small part of the diet. Even among modern-day African hunter-gatherer and herdsmen tribes, fruit generally plays a role secondary to that of animal foods, wild vegetables, and in some tribes, grains.

For our European ancestors, berries were available in summer, and other temperate-zone fruits were available in fall. Seasonal patterns are much the same in most of North America. But now many people use tropical and subtropical fruit all year long, often in substantial quantities. Heat-processed juices, devoid of the nutrients found in fresh fruit, also are often consumed in substantial quantities.

Quantities of fruit are not part of the diet we are genetically programmed to eat, and this includes those of us who are of Asian, Hispanic, or African descent. None of our ancestors consumed a great deal of fruit, or fruit juice of any kind. In the South Seas, coconut (which is a fruit), palm fruit, and bananas were consumed, but in moderate quantities. The African tribes discussed earlier in this book favored animal foods, fish, and wild vegetables as dietary staples. Our physiological responses to food are simply not adapted to handling large quantities of fruit, especially sweet fruits, and juices, which may particularly contribute to the development of such serious problems as diabetes.

Gastrointestinal diseases, including ulcers and colitis (particularly the acute phases), are aggravated by excessive fruit and juices, as are skin diseases. Also, many arthritic patients are aware that their symptoms are worsened by these foods.

Symptoms due to hypoglycemia—low blood sugar—are aggravated by fruit juice, dried fruit, and sometimes fresh fruit. An eight-ounce glass of fruit juice has the fruit sugar of several pieces of fruit and is rapidly absorbed; the body must immediately metabolize this sugar. Dried fruits have much the same effect. Extracted fruit juice does not appear in nature, and the body has no effective way of handling any substantial amount of it.

In whole fruits, the fruit sugar is much more dilute and more slowly absorbed. Fruit is digested over some time, enabling the body to have a much more measured and controlled response to it. When ripe and fresh fruits are eaten in moderation, the metabolic response is good. Even quite a large amount of some fruits may be eaten occasionally without problems by people in good health. Berries, low in fruit sugar, are well tolerated on a regular basis by most people. Wild berries are best because they are lowest in natural sugars.

Fruit may cause gas and indigestion in some people, even in small quantities. Excessive gas is a clear sign the body is reacting poorly to foods.

Generally, those recovering from health problems are wisest to avoid excessive fruit. Those in good health usually tolerate fruit more easily. Those of us living in southern parts of America are no more prepared genetically to consume excessive amounts of fruits than are people living in the north; a few years, or even generations, do not change one's genetic predisposition and physiology.

Once accustomed to a primal diet, one has little desire for excessive amounts of fruit. Animal fats are far more satisfying. When an abundance of raw-food nutrients are supplied by grass-fed animal foods and vegetables, there is no need for much fruit, and cravings for it seem to disappear. Modest amounts of fruit are enjoyable, and even wild blueberries (available frozen in many natural food stores and some supermarkets) taste somewhat sweet, even though they are tart compared to domestic varieties. If you want fruit juice, squeeze an orange or half a grapefruit into a glass, then fill it with sparkling water.

In traditional Chinese medicine, all fruits are yin; tropical fruits and fruit juices are extremely yin. Excess yin may result in discharges and eruptions—diarrhea or inflammation of the bowels, acne and other eruptive skin diseases, rashes, colds, and many other problems. Yin foods of good quality are most appropriate at the most yang time of the year—summer—for yang is hot, and yin foods help balance the heat. In considering the place of fruit in the diet, this rather inexact concept of yin and yang is a useful tool; my clinical and personal experience has confirmed this traditional wisdom. Let fruit consumption ebb and flow with the seasons. Foods that are sometimes beneficial may at other times be harmful.

Nuts and Seeds

Though often thought of as protein foods, most nuts and seeds supply far more calories from fats than from proteins. Their high oil content makes them subject to oxidation and rancidity. Walnuts are high in omega-3 fats, are especially subject to rancidity, and should be stored in the refrigerator or freezer. But many other nuts—including almonds, pecans, and cashews—are high in oleic acid and are not prone to rancidity.

Eaten in substantial amounts, nuts and seeds may cause considerable intestinal gas. Nuts need to be properly prepared by soaking in salt water and then dehydrated. Many unsuspecting people suffering with this embarrassing problem of gas, and fond of snacking on nuts and seeds, have discovered that it was not due to "nerves" or some other undefinable cause. The problem disappears if the nuts are properly prepared by soaking in water and eaten in modest quantities.

A more serious problem occurs in people with herpes. Symptoms of genital herpes may be controlled by avoiding refined food and following a primal diet. Minor symptoms—a few tiny spots with some itching, lasting only a day or two—may occur with occasional dietary transgressions. Major outbreaks may be triggered, however, by eating nuts. The amino acid arginine, prevalent in all nuts, has been implicated; but some nuts, including cashews and peanuts, are especially likely to aggravate herpes. Almonds, on the other hand, are usually well tolerated.

Nuts have been a part of the food supply of many native cultures. As for seeds, pumpkin, sunflower, and sesame seeds are tasty and healthy snacks or additions to salads.

Many nuts and seeds are used to make edible oils, many of which are useful in a modern primal diet. A discussion of these and other oils is the subject of the next chapter.

14
EXTRAS

Oils, Condiments, Seasonings, Beverages, and Refined Products

The extent to which one might incorporate the recommendations of this chapter depends on how committed one is to eating mostly unrefined food, how simple one wishes to keep the diet, and how serious one's health problems may be. These suggestions can be useful in adding variety and flavor to basic foods. Individuals with chronic health problems should employ many of them minimally or not at all, while those in good health might embrace some of the suggestions without a problem. For everyone concerned, however, caffeine, refined flour, sugar, and even natural sweeteners like honey and maple syrup are best consumed only occasionally at most and, at times, not at all.

Let's now turn our attention to edible oils and the processes by which they are created.

MANUFACTURING METHODS OF THE OILS WE EAT

Two general methods of oil extraction are used in the production of commercially available edible oils: industrial processing—which uses both heat and chemicals—and pressed (expeller extracted). Conventionally produced industrial oils are heavily used in most prepared and restaurant foods and in condiments such as salad dressings. Biochemically, they are strikingly different from carefully made, unrefined oils, and they do the body harm.

Industrial Processing

The industrial process that is employed to create oils is an undesirable method in which the solvent is subsequently separated from the extracted oil. The solvent commonly used is hexane, a petrochemical. The oil is then bleached and saponified (treated with an alkaline agent to produce soap). The soap is then taken off, and the residue processed further. Resulting oil has been subjected to high temperatures many times during these processes. The last series of steps involves up to forty to fifty filtrations to deodorize the oil and remove impurities from it.

The resulting oil is devoid of the natural substances found in more naturally made oils. Such substances include chlorophyll, lecithin, carotenoids (occurring in most plants, which may be converted into vitamin A in the body), vitamins, and minerals. Vitamin E is found in plants from which oils are extracted; it protects the oils from oxidation. Removal during refinement results in oils highly subject to rancidity, which is why petrochemically derived preservatives such as BHT (butylhydroxytoluene) are added. While some claim BHT helps preserve us and delays the aging process, safer methods are available, for animal studies show that BHT has a wide range of toxic effects and is a suspected human carcinogen.

Pressing

The second method of oil extraction is known as pressing. Oils initially extracted by pressing may also subsequently be solvent-extracted and go through industrial bleaching, saponification, and filtration processes. Despite this, they may still be labeled cold-pressed, a term with no legal definition. Without clarification it is meaningless. What *is* helpful is the presence of a label stating an absence of preservatives. This shows that *some* vitamin E is present, indicating that a simpler refinement process than that used for most supermarket oils has transpired in the creation of the oil.

The pressing method may be used to produce an unrefined and

truly cold-pressed oil. Any heat produced during this process tends to be minimal when the pressing is done slowly and carefully. An unrefined oil is clear and shows sediment in the bottom of the container. Such oils contain the full complement of substances natural to them, and again, the label may state the vitamin E content.

TYPES OF OILS AND GUIDELINES
REGARDING THEIR USE

The following are general guidelines on oils to use and avoid:

Minimal Use: cold-pressed sesame and sunflower oils

Moderate Use: cold-pressed extra-virgin olive oil, pumpkin seed oil, macadamia nut oil, avocado oil, and coconut oil (which is so beneficial that one may use as much as is desired)

Never Use: soy, corn, canola, and cottonseed oils

Coconut Oil

Coconut oil is a marvelous oil with many health benefits. Coconuts have nourished cultures around the world for thousands of years. On many tropical islands, coconut is an essential dietary staple and among these cultures, it is revered.

Coconut oil is of special interest because of its healing properties and its extensive use in traditional medicine among Asian and Pacific populations. Pacific Islanders have always considered coconut oil to be the cure for all illness, and the coconut palm is called "the tree of life." It has also been called "the healthiest oil on Earth." In traditional medicine around the world coconut is used to alleviate the symptoms of a wide variety of health problems.

In recent years, science has unlocked the secrets to the coconut's amazing healing powers. Once mistakenly believed to be unhealthy because of its high saturated fat content, we now know that saturated fats are good for us and that coconut oil is a uniquely healthy food.

What makes coconut oil so beneficial? Simply, it is the high concentration of medium-chain fatty acids (MCFAs) found in it.

MCFAs are unique fat molecules, and by far the best source of MCFAs is unrefined, virgin coconut oil. The vast majority of fats and oils, whether saturated or unsaturated, from animals or plants, are composed of long-chain fatty acids (LCFAs). The size of fatty acids is extremely important, because the human body responds to and metabolizes fatty acids differently depending on their size. MCFAs have uniquely beneficial physiological effects.

I use coconut oil when cooking meat, seafood, fowl, eggs, vegetables—just about anything that I cook. Heat one or two tablespoons in an iron skillet and cook in it, using ghee as well if desired. Juices coming off the food create a tasty mix. Cook with coconut oil over a low flame; the oil should not be overheated.

Olive Oil

The vegetable oil most suited for salad dressing is olive oil. The oil of the olive, used for thousands of years, has returned to its place as a healthy, traditional salad oil.

The first pressing of olives is done with gentle pressure, and temperatures produced are not much above room temperature. Oil thus extracted is sold as "extra virgin"; that from the next pressing is sold as "virgin." Oil from subsequent pressings of pulp and pits is processed with high heat and chemical solvents and is sold as "pure" olive oil. Like coconut oil, olive oil should not be overheated when used in frying and sautéing.

Olive oil and vinegar dressing is excellent on salads. Because vinegar is so acidic, it does not spoil and requires no preservatives. Organic varieties of both balsamic vinegar and raw apple cider vinegar are available. Balsamic vinegar and other nut and seed oils may be used to enhance flavor. In making soup with bones, vinegar lends acidity to help leach calcium into the broth.

HONEY AND OTHER SWEETENERS

Because honey is a naturally occurring sweetener, many people believe that eating substantial quantities of it is beneficial, or at least harmless. The same belief extends to maple syrup, though what one buys has been concentrated by boiling the sap that flowed from the maple tree. Sweeteners such as molasses, brown sugar, corn syrup, dextrose, turbinado sugar, fructose (also called levulose, or fruit sugar), and others are often represented as being less harmful than sugar itself, but they all have similar effects. In recent years, high-fructose corn syrup, a particularly destructive sweetener, has been widely introduced into processed foods. Sucanat (dehydrated cane sugar), maple sugar, and coconut sugar are also similar to sugar in their effects on metabolism, and should be used only occasionally by most people, and in small amounts.

Only honey is not concentrated. Honeycomb, bee pollen, and royal jelly all contain many vitamins, minerals, and other natural substances. Much has been written about the qualities of honey and these other products of bees, and one hears tales of Russian beekeepers living to advanced age. Folklore and the inherent appeal of honey's sweet taste combine to make it a most attractive food.

Honey contains the simple sugars fructose and glucose, and a sizable amount of sucrose. (White sugar is nearly pure sucrose. Sucrose is rapidly broken down in the body to glucose and fructose.) Glucose is the form of sugar circulating in the blood and used by cells of the body to produce energy; glucose and sucrose in foods both cause a rapid rise in blood sugar. If consumed alone without fats, fructose is utilized in a slightly different manner and is thought to cause a somewhat less rapid rise in blood sugar (fructose, however, causes a more rapid increase in serum triglycerides and perhaps in uric acid, and it must be processed in the liver, putting a strain on the organ).

In many people, particularly those using sweeteners habitually, a pronounced rise in blood sugar leads to a subsequent drop to below the normal fasting level. This condition is known as hypoglycemia, or low blood sugar. Weakness, fatigue, and a variety of other physical and mental symptoms may result.

All sweeteners, honey included, are more or less equally capable of causing low blood sugar. Furthermore, all usually exacerbate symptoms of whatever conditions may be present. Put simply, whatever is wrong, sweets and sweeteners usually make it worse.

I have not seen exceptions—substantial amounts of these concentrated sweets invariably seem to create problems. In relatively healthy individuals, a teaspoonful of honey—or sugar—or a baked sweet good ("natural" or otherwise) is harmless on occasion. In individuals with chronic conditions, even seemingly small amounts often cause a flare-up of symptoms. This may well be related to overgrowth of *Candida* (the yeast microorganism discussed in chapter 9) in many individuals with chronic diseases. Because of the addictive nature of sweets, small amounts usually lead to larger amounts before long, further ensuring the provocation of symptoms.

The work of Dr. Melvin Page showed that even small amounts of sweeteners have dramatic effects on the blood. Page, a dentist very knowledgeable in the field of nutrition, kept careful records of thousands of patients for many years. He studied relationships between dental decay, the ratio of calcium to phosphorous in the blood, and the ingestion of sweets. He found that even a one-ounce dose of honey, fructose, or sucrose had a pronounced effect on the ratio of calcium to phosphorus in the blood. Sucrose had the most pronounced effect (fructose—fruit sugar—had the least). He found this ratio was invariably elevated in individuals developing dental decay.

This is interesting in light of Weston Price's discovery that the saliva in the mouths of decay-free native people had certain consistent characteristics relating to the ability to keep calcium and phosphorous in the saliva in solution—characteristics not found in the mouths of individuals eating refined foods. (The calcium and phosphorous content of the saliva, of course, is directly influenced by the content of these two elements in the blood.) Page's work thus directly complemented Price's—both men showed that disturbances of calcium and phosphorous metabolism occur in tooth decay. We may infer that these same disturbances affect the condition of the entire body. Francis Pottenger, Jr.'s work demonstrated that gross skeletal changes occurred in cats fed sweetened foods—again we see disturbances of calcium and phosphorous metabolism.

Thus, the reasonable work of these three men has given indications as to why the human body reacts so poorly to sweets.

What of the argument that honey is a natural food enjoyed by humans since the dawn of mankind? This is probably true, but wild honey was generally a rare treat available in limited quantities, especially in more northern climates. The compulsion for sweets largely disappears in individuals not consuming them. Our primal ancestors likely had neither the desire nor the opportunity to use much honey.

HERBS AND SEASONINGS

Many organically grown fresh and dried herbs, seasonings, and spices are available, most ground and packaged as convenient powders. Conventionally grown and produced ground herbs, seasonings, and spices are irradiated and contain some or all of the following: fillers, anticaking agents, artificial coloring, preservatives, monosodium glutamate (MSG), and pesticide residues. Reactions to these various extraneous substances often occur.

Culinary herbs go well with natural foods. Many commonly used herbs also have medicinal properties useful in helping alleviate symptoms of acute or chronic disease.

Black pepper is a great seasoning and is best enjoyed fresh ground from peppercorns.

Salt

The most commonly used and widely misunderstood seasoning is salt. Salt restriction is often advised for those with high blood pressure; this benefits some people and not others. High blood pressure has many causes, and excessive salt is simply one contributory factor in some individuals. The foods eaten play an important role in the sodium content of the diet. Processed foods of all kinds almost invariably have large amounts of salt added in production. Different natural foods vary widely in sodium content. Salt added to natural food should be unrefined sea salt, which contains all of the trace minerals, essential for life, that are found in the sea. I prefer traditional Celtic salt, raked off the sea in salt flats on the coast of France.

Foods of animal origin have more sodium than vegetables, grains, and fruits. Humans have a requirement for sodium, thought to be at least two to five grams per day (a teaspoonful is five grams). If too little is supplied in food, some must be added to maintain normal sodium balance; this biological necessity did much to determine where early agriculturists settled. A diet with a substantial amount of animal foods includes adequate sodium, but added salt makes many foods tastier and for the vast majority of people is perfectly healthy.

Few inland areas have readily accessible salt; the earliest farming villages tended to grow up around places that did. People often went to great lengths to get salt. Some Chinese drilled deep into mountains and with bamboo pipes brought up brine from salt deposits. Inland farmers in many places relied on riverboats and caravans to bring them salt. Salt in ancient times was the most valuable single commodity in commerce. At least one writer has pointed out that where salt was plentiful, democratic and independent societies tended to develop, and where it was scarce, those who controlled the salt, controlled the people.

So salt has a history as old as mankind, and it is not an evil substance. The problem now is its refinement and high usage in processed foods. Canned vegetables, for example, have hundreds of times more sodium than fresh unsalted vegetables. Salt is added to nearly all processed foods; the taste buds grow used to it, and unsalted food comes to taste plain.

The standard American diet (SAD) contains more salt than typical hunter-gatherer, primal diets, which often had no added salt. But in many hunter-gatherer and fishing cultures, lots of salt was used in drying and smoking game animals and fish, with no associated problems. Individuals eating moderate to substantial amounts of animal foods do fine with added salt. The less animal-sourced foods that are eaten, the more salt is needed. Salt content in smoked fish and other salted foods varies greatly from product to product. In smoked fish, the subtler, more time-consuming smoking methods use considerably less salt.

Traditionally, soy sauce (also called tamari or shoyu) is made by allowing soybeans, and often wheat, to ferment in water and salt (in wooden barrels, often cedar). Organic brands are free of the additives, pesticide residues, and sugar found in conventionally produced soy sauce. Soy sauce may be used to add flavor. Because I prefer minimizing the use of grain-based foods and legumes, I prefer to use sea salt. I recommend in general using salt to taste, and not worrying about restricting its use.

BEVERAGES

Alcohol

A Few Words about Alcoholism

In considering the health effects of liquor, wine, and beer, one should remember that they may act as drugs. For many individuals, some combination of genetic and environmental influences makes alcohol in any form dangerous. The physical ravages of alcohol abuse are well known. More insidious are the mental processes involved, the ways in which addiction plays on the mind.

Alcoholism perhaps begins in the mind, though genetic and physiological idiosyncrasies appear to predispose some individuals. Over time alcohol may take over not only the mind but the body as well. The inclination for this particular form of self-abuse is stronger in some than others, but anyone drinking enough can become addicted to alcohol.

Recovery involves a commitment not only to stop drinking, but also to change certain aspects of personality that lead to drinking. If such commitments are not made, the individual sooner or later drinks again. Actively seeking help through Alcoholics Anonymous provides a good chance of rehabilitation for many. Members tend to drink a lot of coffee, eat a lot of sugar, and smoke a lot of cigarettes—but this beats drinking oneself to death.

The fermented drink kombucha, by the way, has helped many alcoholics with their cravings. Though there is debate, the majority of recovered alcoholics and counselors working with alcoholics believe that once an individual has been physically addicted to alcohol and they stop, he or she can never drink again without eventually drinking heavily once more. Acceptance of this is the first step for many people in recovering from an acutely addicted state.

Most alcoholics deny to themselves and others that they have any problem with alcohol. And if it's not a problem, why seek help? An anecdote popular among drinkers sums up the attitude: "Who says I have a problem with alcohol? I get drunk, I fall down, I get up. No problem."

Nothing in this section on alcoholic beverages should be taken to mean that those recovering from alcohol abuse should consider using small amounts of alcohol. I wish also to warn of the fine line that for many separates the regular use of small amounts of alcohol—as a tasty beverage, relaxant, and mild mood enhancer—from the beginnings of dependence and eventual abuse.

If alcohol in any way prevents the achievement of goals and one's full potential to live happily, the line has been crossed. Addiction per se may not be present, but allowing a damaging drug to replace positive things in life reveals a weakness. It is a very human weakness—the simple desire to slip into a drug-induced state of relaxation, rather than using one's time to pursue active goals and find more positive ways to relax.

If alcohol plays a significant role in one's life, an honest examination of attitudes may be helpful. An experiment many people find enlightening involves abstinence from alcohol for a month. It is normal for even a light and occasional drinker to miss alcohol the first week or two. But the individual missing it more and more into the third and fourth weeks, and anxious for the month to pass, discovers that alcohol apparently is quite important. Those without dependence issues generally do not miss alcohol by the end of the month and subsequently experience no particular desire to drink on other than special occasions.

Health Considerations Pertaining to Alcohol

Some medical studies suggest people having a drink or two a day enjoy better health and live longer than those abstaining. Some enjoy citing this information while drinking two double scotches a night, with three or four ounces of whiskey in each. The studies, however, refer to standard one-ounce drinks, or the equivalent in beer or wine (a small glass of wine or a bottle of beer each contains less than one ounce of alcohol). Other studies, however, indicate that no measurable health benefits are derived from alcohol.

It may be that the ability to occasionally or even regularly imbibe small amounts of alcohol and let it go at that is associated with character traits that favor a long and healthy life. Centenarians studied in Georgian Russia in the 1970s enjoyed homemade vodka and wine. Both are made from unheated grapes and are rich in enzymes and minerals, while low in alcohol content. This was a healthy way to enjoy alcoholic beverages, and one might note that in America today, microbreweries produce draft beers and some bottled beers that are unpasteurized. Moderate use of alcohol is not incompatible with a healthy and long life.

Though not recommended, even an immoderate use of alcohol may exist without extreme consequences. A case in point involves the lifelong story of a gentleman always fond of strong drink. In middle age, he suffered considerably with repeated attacks of angina pectoris, chest pains thought to relate to spasms of the coronary arteries and relieved by nitroglycerine. He then began following many of the suggestions found in this book, eating seafood several times a week, taking cod-liver oil daily, and walking several miles most days (he gradually built up the walking). By no means a model patient, he ate a fair amount of refined foods. Daily, during the first ten years after the angina began, and for at least twenty-five before, he had at least two or three and an average of five or six ounces of liquor—and sometimes more—every night. He cut back somewhat in his later years, though he drank rather more heavily at times. He lived to be ninety.

Medical textbooks state that on the average, a heart attack, often fatal, occurs within five years of the first symptoms of angina. This gentleman certainly beat those odds. Despite the limitations of his diet and the stress of excess alcohol, protective nutrients and regular exercise enabled him not only to escape a heart attack but also to lead a fairly vigorous and active life. He was no genetic miracle, for his father died of a heart attack in his early sixties, and he himself while in his thirties suffered a mild and nearly symptomless stroke, from which he fully recovered. The point is that however one chooses to live, learning and applying a few age-old nutritional principles may enhance health and lengthen life. Most people who choose to live the way he did do not live to ninety. My guess is that he is perhaps the one in a hundred that did. We don't meet the other ninety-nine. They're dead.

Regular use of hard liquor is not a wise practice; the weight of physiological evidence indicates that, in all but the smallest amounts, alcohol acts as a poison. An individual not regularly drinking liquor notices a marked effect upon ingesting even an ounce or two, and continues to feel sluggish the next morning. Because alcoholic beverages are not regulated by the FDA, a wide variety of toxic ingredients found in liquor and in most wines and beers are not listed on the labels. These substances include ammonia, asbestos residues, coloring and flavoring agents, glycerin, hydrogen peroxide, lead residues, mineral oil, methylene chloride, plastic, pesticide residues, and sulfur compounds.

Many people enjoy an occasional beer, especially in hot weather. German law allows only the use of hops, malt, and water in the brewing process; imported German beers are thus pure. Some other imported beers (and now many American microbrew beers) are made from only natural ingredients without the use of chemicals or preservatives, as are some American and imported wines.

Coffee and Other Caffeinated Beverages

Caffeine is found in coffee, cola drinks, and a number of nonprescription drugs. Closely related compounds include theobromine, found in chocolate and cocoa, and theophylline, found in tea. A twelve-ounce can of Coca-Cola contains about the same amount of caffeine as a cup of instant coffee (about sixty-five milligrams), and a chocolate bar contains nearly half that amount of theobromine.

Intake of caffeine and related compounds above one's individual limit causes caffeinism. Extreme nervousness, poor sleep, abnormalities of the functioning of the heart, intestinal and stomach upset, and irritability are among possible symptoms, which are indistinguishable from those of anxiety neurosis. These symptoms may be evoked in adults by doses of caffeine and related compounds beginning at about two hundred milligrams a day—the amount found in three cups of instant coffee or two cups of percolated coffee.

A seventy-pound child drinking one Coke and eating one candy bar ingests nearly one hundred milligrams of caffeine and theobromine. By weight, his dose is equal to or greater than that of many adults consuming two hundred milligrams. Many children suffer from caffeinism, which may manifest as hyperactivity or other behavioral problems. Effects of caffeine and related compounds depend on the dose and on the weight and tolerance of the individual user.

Withdrawal symptoms occurring when frequent users stop ingesting caffeine include headaches and drowsiness. Nearly everyone stopping caffeine experiences these symptoms, often for as long as a month. Headaches usually begin within twenty-four hours of the last dose. Caffeine is a potent and highly addictive drug.

Caffeine aggravates ulcers (and other stomach and intestinal conditions) by increasing stomach acid secretions. Marked effects on the heart and circulatory system explain why studies have shown coffee drinkers are at increased risk for heart attacks. Other studies have shown increased risks of pancreatic cancer and cancer of the bladder. Pregnant women are urged to curb caffeine consumption because caffeine enters the placenta and affects the growth and development of the fetus; several studies have linked birth defects with caffeine consumption.

Methylene chloride, commonly used to remove caffeine to make decaffeinated coffee, was found by government researchers to cause liver cancer in mice when given in high doses. An alternative method (the water-drip Swiss process) decaffeinates without use of methylene chloride or other carcinogenic chemicals.

Coffee is stimulating and imparts an alert and pleasant feeling. Caffeine stimulates the adrenal glands to release adrenaline, providing energy via the "fight or flight" mechanism. Constant overstimulation by caffeine weakens the adrenals, resulting in adrenal exhaustion and associated symptoms—fatigue, reduced immunity, and eventually chronic disease.

Driving on a long trip may be an occasion to use coffee to keep alert and avoid drowsiness; if driving all day, one might have three or four cups. Coffee in this situation has survival value—it makes one a better driver when attention to the road is required for several hours. One using coffee only on such occasions may find that the next day the "high" feeling imparted by caffeine is missed, and one longs for a cup of coffee. The feeling passes within a day or so, but the experience helps one understand how people become addicted to caffeine.

By and large, coffee and caffeine are best avoided. Caffeine aggravates a wide variety of medical problems and is likely involved in the development of these problems as well.

REFINED FLOUR AND SUGAR

How white flour and sugar adversely affect the human body has been detailed in many excellent books. The issue of why we go on using them long after we're fully aware of their effects is more difficult to understand.

The need to conform is real; we tend to be influenced by friends and social norms. We rationalize by calling foods that we know weaken us "a treat," then saying that a little bit won't hurt. We realize that regular use of all but the smallest amounts of liquor and food containing refined flour and sugar is harmful; still we want them. Perhaps too many lives lack the meaningful and exciting activities that human beings have traditionally enjoyed, and as a substitute food and drink become irrational entertainment. Though this is natural enough on occasion, there is little doubt we overdo it.

Life is change. Eating primal foods consistently causes changes, among them a marked decrease in the desire for strong drink and foods containing white flour and sugar. The reasons are physiological—the well-balanced body and mind seem to have less desire for poor foods.

Many people find it easiest to entirely avoid sweets. When constantly eating small amounts, one is always attempting to decide how much is too much. Memory of the sweet taste constantly lingers. A decision simply to be done with it ends daily decisions and mind games. Within a month or two one stops thinking about sweets, as memory of the taste fades a bit. At this early stage, even a little taste usually augments one's desire. Success comes only with continued abstinence; with time the taste for sweets is lost. Some even eventually find it possible to eat sweets occasionally with no thought of them the next day—if one still wants them at all. But for most, sweets are like Pandora's box—best not opened by mere mortals unless prepared for difficulty.

Meaningful and enjoyable activities—family life, time spent with friends, sports, hobbies, challenging work, gardening, fishing, a thousand other things—may replace the entertainment value often demanded of foods. Food is both a fuel and a pleasure, and the highest octane is necessary for maximum pleasure, not only in eating, but in all elements of life. One may love the foods one consumes and yet not hesitate to modify the diet as new things are learned. And a sweet treat now and then may give so much pleasure that we might best think of this as something we should occasionally indulge in.

Tastes grow accustomed to simple foods over time; the natural flavors of primal foods become more satisfactory. The eating is enjoyable, but a greater pleasure lies in the performance of the body. Securing the best foods for self and family is the most basic and primitive element of life, the one from which all other functions derive. If this were a priority in modern living, it would be a different world indeed.

One eating well need not be preoccupied with food; securing the finest foods becomes a reflex and a necessity. A number of things may be enjoyed as much as eating, and a few considerably more.

Everyone trying to eat a more natural diet goes through a process of learning not to want refined foods. Commitment and time are needed— along with the realization that the products of factories and a poisoned agriculture are halfway foods, macabre and twisted perversions of the living foods that nature designed the human body to thrive on.

Because we all have eaten so many of these halfway foods for much of our lives, the subject of the next chapter—special foods, vitamins, minerals, and food supplements—is of importance to many of us. Recognizing that modern foods are lacking, we take supplements. Many of the most helpful supplements are concentrates of superior foods. Supplemental vitamins and minerals may often be of additional benefit, particularly when prescribed in conjunction with dietary changes.

15
SPECIAL FOODS AND FOOD SUPPLEMENTS

The most important thing to understand about supplements is that they can be wonderful foods that complement even the best diets. It is next to impossible in the modern world to find the incredible array of outstanding foods that were routinely available to our primal ancestors daily, as a matter of course. The right carefully prepared supplements can to a great degree make up for this. There is no question but that properly selected supplements can enhance health and longevity. As with most things in life, successful use of supplements depends on knowledge and discipline.

Over forty years ago, I read a little book called *Vitamin E for Ailing and Healthy Hearts*. It's still a good read. The Shute brothers, who were Canadian medical doctors, presented the case for vitamin E supplements. I began taking vitamin E and researching the usefulness of vitamins, minerals, herbs, and special foods in the treatment of health problems, eventually going on to become a naturopathic physician. Many of these substances are helpful to anyone interested in optimizing their health, while others are appropriate for people who develop various health problems typical of modernized cultures. The question is really not whether to take supplements. Rather, the questions are which ones, when, and how much.

These are hard questions, and because the answers are different for each of us and depend on individual needs, they can't be fully answered here. However, some general information can help us make informed decisions. I'll address the sources, types, and effectiveness of various nutritional supplements, many of which are best thought of as special foods, as well as the relationships between supplements and foods.

SOURCES AND FORMS OF VITAMINS

One of the significant factors in choosing a supplement is the source of the nutrients it contains. Vitamins may be extracted from foods or synthesized in biochemical or biological processes. It can sometimes be challenging to determine the source of the vitamin from reading its product label. For example, vitamins made in laboratories may be labeled "natural" because they are made from "natural" precursors. Moreover, these synthesized vitamins may not be biochemically identical to their counterparts in nature. When selecting fat-soluble vitamins, it is important to choose ones extracted from natural sources (such as vitamin E derived from vegetable oil).

And although fat-soluble vitamins should always come from natural sources, this is not strictly the case for water-soluble ones. There are natural sources that can provide small amounts of water-soluble vitamins for general use—acerola powder for vitamin C, for example, and low-temperature-dried yeast flakes grown on an appropriate medium for B complex. However, for larger therapeutic doses, it is necessary to use synthetic vitamins. How these vitamins are formulated makes a big difference in how well they are absorbed and tolerated.

Vitamins A and D

Decades ago, researchers definitively established the benefits and safety of reasonable doses of natural vitamins A and D. The synthetic versions appear to cause the same problems the natural vitamins can cause in excessive doses, but can do so when taken in much smaller amounts. Traditional diets are rich in these nutrients and typically contain upward of ten times the recommended dietary allowances (RDA) the government now tells us are adequate. Natural vitamins A and D are beneficial, and are particularly important for pregnant women. In fact, foods rich in these vitamins were emphasized in virtually all of the traditional cultures studied by Dr. Price.

Vitamins A and D are present in fish oils. Synthetic forms of vitamins A and D frequently used in supplements should be avoided. An example is vitamin D_2, or irradiated ergosterol, which we discussed at some length in chapter 12. Vitamin D_2 is produced by irradiation of primary grown yeast with ultraviolet light. It is added to a variety of foods, as well as vitamin supplements, particularly those formulated without the use of animal products. Irradiated ergosterol has significant biological differences from vitamin D_3, which is produced in the body when ultraviolet light strikes the skin and is also richly supplied in fish oils, milk fats from animals feeding on fresh greens, and liver. Vitamin D_3 may also be naturally derived from lamb's wool.

Relatively small amounts of the synthetic forms of fat-soluble vitamins may be toxic. This toxicity has contributed to the media frenzy about the dangers of vitamins A and D. Unfortunately, both the mainstream media and the medical establishment fail to distinguish between the synthetic forms and natural vitamins A and D as found in or derived from animal fats.

Vitamin E

Vitamin E is another nutrient for which it is very important to select the proper form. Synthetic vitamin E, labeled "dl-alpha," is biochemically different from natural vitamin E, labeled "d-alpha." Like synthetic vitamin D, synthetic vitamin E has detrimental effects. It is incompletely metabolized in the body and may even disrupt the metabolism of natural vitamin E in the liver. The most beneficial natural vitamin E products come as mixtures of the alpha, beta, gamma, and delta tocopherol fractions. I use and recommend a mixed tocopherols product that is extracted from soybean oil and purified through distillation to be completely free of all traces of soy.

Vitamin C

Almost all of the vitamin C in supplements is made in a laboratory, despite labeling that implies otherwise. For example, the label might say "ascorbic acid from sago palm." In this case, dextrose, a form of sugar that contains no vitamin C, is extracted from sago palm. This is used as the base molecular material for a complex laboratory process that synthesizes the vitamin. In another instance, the label might say "vitamin C derived from the finest natural sources." This could be true, but the vitamin C still was likely synthesized. The label might also say "with rose hips and acerola," which would mean that these substances are used as the base material for the tablet or capsule. However, a tablet of rose hips or acerola can contain only about 40 mg of truly natural vitamin C; the rest was synthesized.

Another significant factor pertaining to vitamin C is buffering. This process complexes a mineral (typically calcium, magnesium, or potassium) with ascorbic acid. Buffered vitamin C is gentler on the stomach than regular vitamin C, which because of its acidity often causes gas, bloating, and upset stomach. Buffered C offers superior absorption, as well.

The B Vitamins

As with vitamin C, the labeling of B vitamins may be misleading. Labels often proclaim that the products contain "natural" B vitamins derived from yeast. However, manufacturers almost always add laboratory-synthesized B vitamins (with the exception of B_{12}, which may be chemically refined from bacteria) to the food fed to the yeast during its growth, and then fortify the yeast with additional synthetic B vitamins once it has grown. This allows for the production of yeast at any B-vitamin potency desired. Ammonia is also generally added to the growth medium of the yeast, just as it is used in chemical farming—as a nitrogen fertilizer to increase protein content in the product. The only truly natural B-vitamin supplements are freeze-dried liver, and yeast grown without the addition of B vitamins.

SOURCES AND FORMS OF MINERALS

Unlike vitamins, which are organic compounds, minerals are elements and as such cannot be synthesized; whatever the source, calcium is calcium. However, the way in which minerals are biochemically arranged with other molecules is of considerable importance. In both foods and supplements, minerals exist as complexes with other substances, and the substances with which they are complexed affect the degree to which they are absorbed and utilized. Some mineral supplements are extracted from foods (for example, calcium hydroxyapatite), while others are complexed in the laboratory (for example, amino acid complexes of calcium) or found in nature (for example, calcium carbonate). Those extracted from foods are ideal.

Calcium

Calcium is the most commonly used mineral supplement, and it is available in many different forms. However, only one is a food extract—calcium hydroxyapatite, the form of calcium that naturally occurs in bone. In manufacturing this type of calcium supplement, low-temperature processing techniques are used to extract microcrystalline hydroxyapatite concentrate (MCHC) from raw bovine bone. MCHC is a complex crystalline compound composed of calcium, phosphorous, delicate organic factors (thus the importance of low-temperature processing), protein matrix, and the full spectrum of minerals that naturally comprise healthy bone.

Look for a calcium supplement in which the only source of calcium is MCHC. Many supplements say "MCHC" or "calcium hydroxyapatite" on the label, but when you read the ingredients carefully, you discover that a secondary source, typically dicalcium phosphate—an inexpensive, poorly absorbed form of calcium—contributes an unstated percentage of the calcium.

The best calcium formulas contain magnesium and the trace minerals manganese and boron, which are important in the absorption and utilization of calcium. The magnesium-containing compounds that are the most efficiently absorbed include magnesium taurate, magnesium glycinate, and magnesium citrate. Magnesium oxide is somewhat less absorbable, but it has a much smaller molecular size than many other forms of magnesium and so is frequently used with MCHC because it is much easier to fit in a capsule together with MCHC.

USP NUTRIENTS AND "FOOD VITAMINS"

Understanding the labeling of vitamin and mineral supplements can also be a bit tricky in another way. In order to make informed decisions regarding specific products it is important to understand some of the differences between USP grade (or USP purity) supplements and three categories of "food vitamins"—food-based supplements, food form supplements, and food concentrates.

USP Grade Supplements
When a product is listed as USP grade, the nutrient(s) have been manufactured in laboratories by biochemical processes and meet the strict purity and potency standards of the United States Pharmacopeia. These are the quality standards used in almost all nutritional research. In other words, virtually all the published research on the benefits of vitamins and minerals has been conducted using USP grade nutrients.

Food-Based Supplements
These are made by taking standard USP nutrients and putting them in tablets or occasionally capsules with dried foods and herbs (along with fillers and other additives). Taking these vitamins and minerals is no different from taking standard USP vitamins and minerals with a meal (but a lot more expensive).

"Food-Grown" or "Food-Form" Supplements
The process of making this type of product involves proprietary methods that add standard USP vitamins to a liquid broth containing yeast.

As the yeast grows, the vitamins and minerals incorporate into its cell structure. The yeast is killed in a drying process, and the residue is pressed into tablets, typically with herbs, binders, and manufacturing additives. Because of the amount of space taken up by the yeast, products made this way are very low in potency. Even if absorption is superior, the low potency and high cost make them very cost inefficient for anyone wishing to take, say, 500 mg of vitamin C or 400 IU of vitamin E, on a daily basis. Another problem I've encountered in my naturopathic practice is that many people taking these yeast-based supplements for any length of time develop yeast sensitivities. This is particularly true for those with a history of *Candida* problems, which are common in our carbohydrate-addicted culture.

Food Concentrates

These products are actually dried foods, often organic, that have been encapsulated or pressed into tablets, frequently with the aid of manufacturing additives. Because of size constraints, these products are necessarily of very low potency in terms of the amount of vitamins and minerals present, although they may have potent effects. Taking these supplements is comparable to eating good foods, in very small quantities.

POTENCY, PURITY, AND ADDITIVES

How potent a given supplement will be depends on what forms the nutrients are in and how much of the product is actually absorbed and utilized. Forms identical or close to those found in foods are generally better absorbed and utilized.

There are two issues relating to purity. The first is whether the raw materials are pure. Reputable manufacturers insure that each batch of raw materials is laboratory tested for purity, and they can provide users with copies of certificates of analysis. The other issue concerns the additives nearly all manufacturers use in the production of supplements.

Tablets may contain potentially allergenic binders, fillers, and coloring agents. They must be coated with shellac (an insect resin, usually listed in the ingredients as "natural glaze") or vegetable coating (derived from corn, to which many people are sensitive). Other potentially allergenic fillers such as lactose are used to top off capsules. Even small amounts of additives may cause allergic reactions in sensitive individuals. This is a major reason why so many people have adverse reactions to supplements or fail to receive the significant benefits pure supplements can offer.

The vast majority of supplements also contain stearates, manufacturing agents used as lubricants to speed up production. Most capsules and tablets are produced by "jobbers" in mass-production plants, which churn out a multitude of formulas for various companies. Magnesium stearate and stearic acid are lubricants added to the raw materials so that production machinery will run at maximum speeds.

These additives have a number of effects, including decreased absorption. In a study published in *Pharmaceutical Technology* in April 1986, the percent dissolution for capsules after twenty minutes in solution went from 90 percent without stearates to 25 percent with stearates. These substances clearly affect the dissolution and rapid absorption of nutrients.

Hydrogenated oils are a common source for the magnesium stearate used in pharmaceuticals and supplements. Stearates are made by hydrogenating cottonseed or palm oil. Cottonseed oil has the highest content of pesticide residues of all commercial oils. In the hydrogenation process, the oil is subjected to high heat and pressure in the presence of a metal catalyst for several hours, creating a hydrogenated saturated fat. Hydrogenated vegetable fats contain altered molecules derived from fatty acids. The metal catalyst used in the hydrogenation process may also contaminate the stearates produced.

In December 2011 the World Health Organization reported that several batches of magnesium stearate were contaminated with silicate, zeolinte, calcium hydroxide, dibenzoylmethane, bisphenol A and Irganox 1010. While some of these substances may not be harmful, as is the case with zeolite, others are, such as bisphenol A (BPA). The industrial chemical BPA is an endocrine disruptor found to have other harmful effects. The European Union has banned its use in baby bottles, and several consumer groups in the United States have petitioned the FDA to ban its use in food containers. Whether or not the contaminants found in the magnesium stearate are benign or harmful is not the issue. The issue is contamination.

While we don't know the percentage of supplements in the United States that are contaminated, according to a *New York Times* article, nearly all of the herbal dietary supplements tested in a congressional investigation contained trace amounts of lead and other contaminants. There have also been news stories over the years about contaminated supplements, such as heavy metals in 20 percent of Ayurvedic herbal products tested in the Boston area in 2004. Clearly, contamination is an issue of concern.

While magnesium stearate is certainly not the only supplement ingredient ever found to be contaminated, the potential for contamination is just one more reason to avoid it. If you do wish to consume supplements containing magnesium stearate, it would be a good idea to ask the manufacturer if they batch-test the supplement for purity. If not, then you really do not know what you are putting into your mouth.

While contamination is a concern, I do not support stricter government regulations on dietary supplements due to contamination issues. These issues are best addressed by batch testing. Even when the most reliable ingredient suppliers are used—those in the United States, Europe, and New Zealand—raw materials going into supplements should be independently analyzed. No additives are used in the purest products, as attested by the manufacturers' certificates of analysis. For these reasons, I recommend additive-free supplements.

Because the supplements industry routinely uses additives in their products, manufacturers and distributors always deny that the presence of these substances is in any way detrimental. Nevertheless, it seems to me a simple matter of common sense that the most desirable products would not contain non-nutrient substances added solely to expedite the manufacturing process.

NUTRIENTS PRESENT IN ANCESTRAL DIETS

Consider ancestral diets, which are invariably rich in animal fats from grass-fed wild or domestic animals, organ meats, and seafood. The following is a partial list of nutrients richly supplied in those foods, nutrients often marginally supplied in most modern diets, even the diets of those following Dr. Price's teachings.

Fat-Soluble Nutrients
Vitamins A, D, and K_2, and the omega-3 fatty acids EPA (eicosapentaenoic acid) and DHA (docosahexaenoic acid), are available from raw butter, cheese, and whole milk from grass-fed animals; egg yolks; organ meats; and seafood. Cod-liver oil is a fine supplemental source of A and D, and a small amount of K_2, but most of the cod-liver oils sold today have had the majority of the natural vitamin A and D content removed. I recommend from one-half to one teaspoon daily of cod-liver oil which is unadulterated and contains the full complement of naturally occurring vitamins.

Another useful fish-oil supplement containing vitamins A and D and omega-3 fatty acids is krill oil. A small amount of krill oil daily has been shown to have a host of benefits. This is true also of supplemental vitamin E. Good food sources of vitamin E are liver, unrefined vegetable oils, nuts, and seeds.

Minerals
Calcium, magnesium, and trace minerals (including iodine, zinc, selenium, and chromium) are typically found in abundant supply in ancestral diets. They are available from whole raw milk, bone broths, unrefined sea salt, and sea vegetables such as kelp and dulse. However,

supplementing with calcium hydroxyapatite can be good insurance for men and women alike against osteoporosis. As previously noted but bears repeating here, the trace minerals manganese and boron are important in the absorption and utilization of calcium, thus the most beneficial calcium formulas contain these minerals.

Most people, especially individuals with low thyroid function (usually undiagnosed because of the inadequacy of standard thyroid tests), benefit from extra iodine in the form of a supplement. This may be a sea vegetable extract or, if larger doses of iodine are appropriate, as they often are, a combination of iodine and iodide extracted from kelp. In fact, moderate doses of a balanced iodine-iodide formula benefit most people in many ways besides improving thyroid function, because most diets are deficient in iodine.

Zinc, selenium and chromium are other commonly supplemented trace minerals. Zinc is important for a healthy prostate. Selenium has antioxidant properties and functions together with vitamin E in many biochemical processes. Poorly supplied in modern foods, selenium is especially important as a supplement in areas of the country where the soil is deficient in selenium since such areas statistically correlate with higher incidences of cancer. Chromium helps regulate blood sugar and is particularly important for people with poor glucose metabolism.

Therapeutic doses of chromium and selenium may be considerably higher than is generally thought, based on therapies now used at cutting-edge alternative-medicine clinics. Quality multivitamin-mineral supplements, designed to be taken in a dosage of anywhere from one to six capsules daily, typically supply 30 mg of zinc and 200 mcg each of chromium and selenium when taken at the full dosage.

Antioxidants

Vitamin E, vitamin C, coenzyme Q_{10} (CoQ_{10}), alpha lipoic acid, and other antioxidants are featured in the primal diet. They are richly supplied in organ meats such as the heart and the liver. There is ample evidence that antioxidants help retard the aging process, thus many researchers think this is a critical area to supplement. Ironically, the foods richest in many antioxidants—organ meats—are among those most vilified by the medical establishment for their cholesterol content. I have long found freeze-dried supplements made from the organs and glands of grass-fed animals to be a wonderful complement to the diet (more on this below).

Vitamin E is among the most important antioxidants. How much supplemental vitamin E is ideal is difficult to determine. The RDA of 11 to 15 IU (for people age nine and older) was arrived at by averaging the amount found in the diets of several thousand people surveyed; it reflects the modern norm rather than an optimal intake. The native groups with high immunity that were studied by Dr. Price consumed at least ten times the amount of both fat-soluble and water-soluble vitamins provided by modern diets, and ten times the RDA should prudently be considered a minimal intake. Higher amounts may be important for women during menopause and in many other situations.

Vitamin C, too, often is a useful supplement, even if the diet is rich in vegetables. Hunter-gatherer diets provided an estimated 400 mg daily. A supplement is useful for many people, even in amounts up to several thousand milligrams a day under special circumstances.

I also recommend that CoQ_{10} be supplemented by many people, in a dosage of anywhere from 25 mg to 1200 mg per day. This natural antioxidant is found in many foods and is synthesized by the body. Some people experience increased energy on CoQ_{10} and endurance athletes may perform better. CoQ_{10} is best absorbed with fats. The richest food source is heart.

Supplementing with alpha lipoic acid, from 25 mg to 600 mg per day, can also be useful for many people. Benefits to athletes include enhanced energy production in muscle tissues, decreased glucose uptake by fat cells, and improved muscle recovery. Alpha lipoic acid helps regenerate damaged nerves, and is a standard prescription by doctors throughout Europe for this problem and for neuropathies in general. Organs and glands are a rich natural source of alpha lipoic acid.

SPECIAL FOODS

By "special foods" I mean supplements that are clearly foods, but that in small quantities may have great potency. Cod-liver oil, described above, is a good example of a supplement that is a special food. Quality cod-liver oil provides critical nutrients in a concentrated dose.

Other special foods available as supplements, such as freeze-dried organs and glands or colostrum, may be used in much larger quantities.

Colostrum is a marvelous special food, providing a wide variety of health enhancing and therapeutic benefits. The most potent colostrum is available as a freeze-dried powder made from the first milking of cows that have just given birth.

Bovine tracheal cartilage, freeze-dried from tissues taken from New Zealand cattle and then encapsulated, is another supplement that is a special food with a rich history of therapeutic usage. John Prudden, M.D., whose work with bovine tracheal cartilage was detailed in chapter 9, studied this substance extensively for decades and published many articles about its benefits in a wide variety of conditions, including auto-immune diseases, cancer, and wound healing.

Other special foods I include in my diet are freeze-dried powders prepared from a wide variety of vegetables, fruits and herbs, including wheat grass, barley grass, berries, carrots, and beets. These special foods in small amounts supplement a range of very important nutrients. A number of other herbs and food-derived supplements belong in the special foods category, along with freeze-dried organs and glands, discussed below. These essential primal traditional foods are useful in even the best diets.

Organs and Glands

Individual organs and glands, including liver, heart, brain, thymus, kidney, pancreas, adrenal, spleen, ovary, and testicle, are available as food supplements. Multi-gland combinations are also available. The best products are from freshly harvested organs and glands from grass-fed

New Zealand cattle, which are raised without the use of pesticides, hormones, or antibiotics.

The organs and glands are freeze-dried at 40 to 60 degrees below zero (Fahrenheit). Freeze-drying tissues preserves the unaltered proteins, the enzymes, and the fat-soluble activators so important in traditional diets. The freeze-dried powders are encapsulated, providing a convenient way to include organs and glands in your regular diet. (See Dr. Ron's Ultra-Pure at www.drrons.com.)

Herbal Supplements

The potency of herbal supplements depends on the quality and potency of the raw herb used, the care taken in manufacturing, and the concentration of the finished product. A tremendously wide range of quality is found in different products. A poor-quality product may have no effect whatsoever, while the same dosage of a superior one may be very effective. The quality and potency of herbal extracts, as well as correct dosing, are of critical importance in achieving good results.

Hawthorn

Hawthorn has historically been a key herb in the support of heart and cardiovascular health. Double-blind studies by teams of European medical doctors over the past twenty years have demonstrated dramatic benefits to the heart, even in cases of advanced heart disease, from the use of properly prepared and dosed hawthorn extract, as well as from berberine extracted from the herb goldenseal.

Milk Thistle

Milk thistle regenerates liver cells and helps protect from chemicals and toxins to which we all are exposed. Milk thistle dramatically enhances liver health by protecting the outer membrane of liver cells and acting as a powerful antioxidant. It can help reverse the liver damage caused by toxins, including alcohol.

Dandelion

Dandelion, too, has a marked benefit on the liver, and it acts as a cleansing agent for the entire system. Dandelion used in sufficient quantity is also an effective diuretic.

Grape Seed Extract

Another useful supplement for many people is grape seed extract. In addition to their potent antioxidant action, the oligo-proanthocyanidins (OPCs) in grape seed extract strengthen the blood vessels and capillaries in the eyes, thus helping to maintain vision. One study of 805 men showed that the higher the intake of OPCs, the lower the risk of heart disease.

LIVING BETTER AND LONGER

Whole foods have always formed the core of my approach to health. In the early 1970s, I belonged to one of the first food co-ops in western Massachusetts. From there, I went on to naturopathic medical school, believing that if I learned enough about how food affects people, I could help them recover from most medical problems. That turned out to be even truer than I realized, once I discovered the work of Dr. Price and other pioneers of nutritional therapy.

My studies and years in practice have shown me that certain high-quality nutritional supplements and special foods can play a critical role in optimizing health and longevity. Supplements work best in conjunction with proper diet and, properly understood, these nutrients, herbs, concentrates, special foods, and extracts complement even the best diets. If the diet is less than optimal, an individual may achieve marked relief from particular symptoms, but unless the diet is corrected, other imbalances will soon occur, and with them, other problems. A deeper and more lasting healing occurs when recovery is based on providing multiple factors present in proper foods rather than just a particular substance the body is obviously lacking.

Our knowledge about the body's needs is growing rapidly, and just as we embrace the wonderful health-giving qualities of traditional whole foods, we should embrace the best of what modern science has given us. Although we must be cautious of marketing campaigns that claim every new supplement is a magical elixir, scientists and clinicians have clearly demonstrated the efficacy of a wide range of these products. The challenge and realistic goal is to separate the wheat from the chaff and apply this knowledge so we can live healthier, happier, and longer lives.

TOWARD A PHILOSOPHY OF NATURAL LIVING

As a child, I loved animal stories, especially those by a turn-of-the-century chronicler of the Indians and wildlife of North America, Ernest Thompson Seton. Years later, as a young adult, I rediscovered these words of Seton in a little book entitled *The Gospel of the Red Man:* "The culture of the Red man is fundamentally spiritual; his measure of success is, 'How much service have I rendered my people.'" I've tried to keep those few words in mind over the years.

My studies of the work of Carl Jung, the great Swiss psychiatrist, scholar, and founder of analytical or depth psychology, have been at the heart of my efforts toward self-knowledge and personal growth. Psychotherapy is part of the training of naturopathic physicians, and I have always incorporated psychotherapeutic work into my practice. In the words of Jung, the work of psychotherapy is "the healing of souls."

And what is this "healing of souls"? No less than coming to satisfactory terms with the vastness of the unconscious forces that drive our lives from within. The depth psychology of Carl Jung and the men and women who have followed his pioneering path provides us with the means for understanding this undertaking.

The lives and work of Carl Jung and Weston Price parallel and complement each other in an extraordinary way. Both men were born in the 1870s and spent their lives seeking to understand fundamental forces that operate in the lives of people everywhere to determine health

273

and well-being. Price, as we have seen, sought an understanding of the biological laws that determine physical development and health. Jung, meanwhile, by combining his encyclopedic knowledge of anthropology, history, religion, philosophy, and mythology with his understanding of psychotherapeutic processes, investigated and ultimately discovered forces in the human psyche that make us the individual psychic beings we are. His discoveries in the psychic realm were equally as profound and far-reaching as Price's in the physical—and as little understood and appreciated.

Together, the work of these two great men provides a basis for understanding how a person must be if one is to find health of both body and spirit and truly make the most of one's time on Earth. Price and Jung have given us blueprints for living and specific recommendations based on a marvelous understanding of all that has come before us.

People of earlier cultures developed highly accurate prescriptions for living satisfying and healthy lives, lives generally untroubled by the depression, loneliness, and personal turmoil that mark so many lives today. From native people, from men and women who studied and lived among them, and from healers who have understood, followed, and taught nature's laws, we have had passed on to us certain truths about food, attitudes, and ways of life. This wisdom, some of which I have tried to incorporate into this book, may help us to live in relative health and happiness, despite the turmoil we see about us.

"Most men," Winston Churchill once wrote, "occasionally stumble over the Truth, but most pick themselves up and continue on as if nothing had happened."

Information is of little value until and unless it leads to action. Developing one's own philosophy of natural living can only come with attempts to live by principles judged reasonable. Choice must be followed by commitment and by a willingness to work hard on our inner lives and learn from others. The reward may be the development of one's sense of being, of one's own unique and satisfying way of coping with the complexities of this often chaotic modern world in which we sometimes find ourselves lost.

It is this search for understanding—of myself and my world, of my gods and my demons, both within and without—that I live for; and out of the understanding comes a capacity for love, for relatedness. Carl Jung called the search the quest for individuation—that process by which the unconscious is integrated into the conscious personality, enabling a person to become a separate, indivisible unity or "whole," a single, homogeneous being, self-realized, able to embrace his or her "innermost, last, and incomparable uniqueness."

In the spirit that all's well that ends with a light-hearted smile, I offer up my top ten health secrets.

10. Exercise is overrated. My favorite workout is a thirty-minute walk, preferably in the sun, so I can then say, "Hey, I worked up a sweat!"

9. Take up a sport that's fun and gets you outside. I love tennis. My second favorite workout is a set or two of doubles, followed by a nap.

8. Sometimes just the nap will do. A nap is a beautiful thing, especially on a weekday.

7. Want to lose weight? Eat animals and plants. Give up grains and legumes.

6. Dogs and cats make you feel good. Bigger animals make you work hard, and sometimes step on your feet.

5. Speaking of animals, whenever you start thinking you're the cat's meow, watch out for the Rottweiler about to bite your butt.

4. Whatever Mom and Dad did right, love them for it. Whatever they did wrong, get over it. You're the boss now.

3. Your great-grandmother knew more about health and nutrition than your doctor. Start channeling her.

2. Wisdom may come with years, but that's not a lock. Humility

is the beginning of wisdom. There's no fool like an old fool. Change now before it's too late.

1. Nobody ever said on their deathbed, "I shoulda worked more." Make friends, have fun. You only go through once, and you can't take it with you.

THE ALL-MEAT DIET OF ARTIC ADVENTURER VILHJALMUR STEFANSSON

An experiment that was carried out in the early years of the twentieth century in New York City demonstrates the viability of an all-meat diet. It involves a character we have encountered previously in the pages of this book: the Arctic adventurer Vilhjalmur Stefansson. We now return to the geographical and gastronomic adventures of this particularly carnivorous early-twentieth-century man to see what he can teach us about traditional meat.

VILHJALMUR STEFANSSON'S 1928 EXPERIMENT

In his Arctic explorations, Vilhjalmur Stefansson and his men succeeded in living for months at a time in good health, free of scurvy, on a diet of nothing but seal and occasionally polar bear. During many other extended visits to the Arctic between 1906 and 1918, Stefansson lived on nothing but fatty meat, fish, and water for an aggregate of more than five years. This diet is estimated to provide about 80 percent of its calories from fat.

The prevailing view then as now among dietitians and medical people is that a mixed diet of animal and vegetable foods is necessary for health. Stefansson's revolutionary views and the narrative of his experience were viewed with skepticism. As he put it, many people expressed opinions amounting to "you are likelier to meet a thousand liars than one miracle."

Stefansson was quite well known for his Arctic exploits, and when a group of doctors asked to examine him extensively for evidence of ill effects from his years of living on an all-meat and all-fish diet, he agreed. This committee failed to find any of the supposed harmful effects, and published its findings in the *Journal of the American Medical Association* in 1926 under the title "The Effects of an Exclusive Long-Continued Meat Diet."

An experiment was subsequently organized whereby Stefansson and a colleague from his Arctic days were to live exclusively on meat and fish for one year in New York City. The organization administering the experiment was the Russell Sage Institute of Pathology. The committee in charge included physicians, professors, and administrators from Harvard, Cornell, and Johns Hopkins Universities; from the American Museum of Natural History; and from several other institutions. The research work, including several weeks of full-time monitoring of the men in Bellevue Hospital (at the beginning and end of the year), was done by a team of physicians headed by the medical director of the Russell Sage Institute of Pathology. During the intervening months, Stefansson and his colleague came daily to the hospital for analysis of blood and excretions, ensuring that if the men cheated on the diet the physicians likely would detect it.

The experiment was concluded in January 1929. Both men came through the year in excellent health. All tests for any detrimental changes detectable by physical or laboratory examination were negative. The only problem Stefansson had was during the early days of the experiment, when physicians asked him to eat only completely lean meat (chopped fatless muscle). Within two days, he became ill with diarrhea and "a general feeling of baffling discomfort."

This had also occurred in the Arctic once, when for three weeks he ate only caribou so thin there was no appreciable fat behind the eyes or in the marrow (caribou are normally about 5 percent fat). Still, he had consumed some fat then by eating tendons and the soft ends of bones, and he assumed that was why symptoms did not occur until the end of that three-week period. They appeared much sooner in New York because there was almost no measurable fat in the chopped fatless muscle. Noteworthy is the fact that Weston Price, Stefansson, and others had observed that native Alaskans typically preferred to eat the older, fattiest ruminants.

Stefansson's symptoms disappeared within three days of introducing fats—the sirloin steaks, brains and other organs, fish, and other meats constituting the diet for the year. Fish bones and rib ends were eaten for calcium. This diet was not really high in protein, for just as Stefansson's diet in the Arctic had provided some 80 percent of the calories from fat, so too did this diet.

Stefansson did not get scurvy, either in the Arctic or in New York. Confirmation of his explanation for this appeared in a 1977 article in *American Anthropologist* entitled "The Aboriginal Eskimo Diet in Modern Perspective." The authors state that Stefansson's appraisal, forty years earlier, of the vitamin C nutriture of those Eskimos living in the far north was accurate: "If you have some fresh meat in your diet every day, and don't overcook it, there will be enough C from that source alone to prevent scurvy." These Eskimos had no plant foods available most of the year.

One may surmise that Stefansson's years in the Arctic led him to prefer much of his meat very rare; parts of many cuts may well have been essentially raw, as the center of a rare steak is. Raw food, particularly raw meat, contains enzymes, vitamin C, vitamin B_6, and perhaps other health-building elements not found in thoroughly cooked foods.

The 1977 article in *American Anthropologist* reported that after careful analysis, the aboriginal diet of Arctic Eskimos (consisting mainly of land and sea mammals and fish, and virtually lacking plant foods) was found "capable of furnishing all the essential nutritional elements when prepared and consumed according to traditional customs. . . . There is no history among Eskimos of the epidemic vitamin-deficiency diseases which afflicted some cereal-based food cultures."

Stefansson wrote about the New York experiment and some of his Arctic experience in a three-part article called "Adventures in Diet" that appeared in *Harper's* magazine in November and December 1935 and January 1936. This fascinating account provides a lucid example of the need to avoid preconceived notions about diet, and does much to dispel the idea that meat and animal fats are necessarily unhealthy.

These accounts of the adequacy of an all-meat-and-fish diet for Stefansson and for primitive Eskimo groups are not meant to suggest an all-meat-and-fish diet would be appropriate for the reader. Genetics undoubtedly play an important role in these accounts; some individuals are likely much more suited than others to metabolize large quantities of animal food. The point rather is that for some individuals, large quantities of meat and fish are compatible with excellent health.

Meat that Stefansson ate in New York City in the 1920s was in many respects more similar to the wild game he ate in the Arctic than to conventionally raised meat generally available today. Beef cattle were to a much greater extent grass-fed, hormones and pesticides were not used in animal production, and antibiotics were yet to be discovered. The innovations of modern meat production described earlier have since taken place. Most cuts of meat that Stefansson ate during the experiment were fatty, and the fats were of a different composition and quality than those in today's conventional meats.

AN IN-DEPTH
LOOK AT
SEAFOOD SELECTION

The following information about seafood may be useful in understanding and selecting fish and shellfish for both enjoyment and maximal health benefits.* Particular attention is paid to the issue of how one may determine which species, and individuals within a species, are likely to have been least affected by water pollution. Consideration also is given to the relative amount of fats found in different species, to aid in judging which may be richest in eicosapentaenoic acid (EPA) and other marine lipids.

This material is divided into three sections: one on saltwater fish, one on shellfish, and a third on freshwater fish, with listings in each arranged alphabetically. The topics of raw fish, smoked fish, roe, stocks, and preservatives sometimes used on fresh fish and shellfish are examined in the closing part of the discussion.

---

*Editor's Note: Much of the information in this section is distilled from A. J. McClane's *The Encyclopedia of Fish Cookery,* a beautifully photographed and written reference work by one of the world's true experts on seafood.

SALTWATER FISH

Anchovies

Anchovies are often seen along the seashore traveling with other small fish, including silversides and small herring. The canned product is heavily salted, packed in oil, and sometimes smoked. A rich and distinct flavor is characteristic.

Bluefish

Like tuna, swordfish, and striped bass, bluefish is a fatty Atlantic Ocean species known to concentrate pollutants in its fatty tissues; polychlorinated biphenols (PCBs) have been found in blues. An oceangoing species, bluefish also spend considerable time close to shore. Accounts written 100 years ago describe multitudes of bluefish in inlets and harbors of New York and New Jersey, and even today they arrive in coastal northeastern waters in numbers every fall.

But the life habits of bluefish are such that for several months of the year on the East Coast, uncontaminated bluefish are available. Blues migrate from south to north in spring and summer, and reverse direction in fall and winter, ranging from Florida to New England.

Bluefish may be strongly flavored; small young fish are less so. Like all highly predacious fish, blues contain enzymes that spoil the meat rapidly if the fish is left ungutted without ice for a few hours. And their high oil content necessitates particular care when they are shipped. When well cared for, these fish cook to a soft texture, with a long flake and an unmistakably distinct flavor.

Broil bluefish enough to flake cleanly; broiling one side for a few minutes in a hot oven suffices for small fish, while larger fish require baking or broiling both sides a few minutes each. Blues also sauté nicely; try this with butter, onions, or garlic, white wine, tamari (soy) sauce, and seasonings.

Butterfish

So-called because of their high fat content, butterfish are found in both the Atlantic and Pacific Oceans and the Gulf of Mexico. Butterfish is reasonably priced, and when taken in clean waters is an excellent find. The flesh is firm, large-flaked, and sweet. A mixture of oil and water rich in fatty acids comes off in cooking; it may be used on rice or vegetables or in soup. The Pacific species is sometimes marketed as Pacific pompano. Butterfish are small, generally under twelve inches, and are sold as fillets.

The Cod Family

An extension of the Continental Shelf, the Grand Banks are a series of shoals running about four hundred miles from the southeast coast of Newfoundland to Georges Bank east of Massachusetts. Warm Gulf Stream waters meet the cold Labrador Current along the banks; the resulting plankton growth forms the basis of the ocean ecology that has supplied countless fish for hundreds of years. Atlantic cod, haddock, pollock, and halibut form the bulk of the fish taken; all but halibut are members of the cod family. The Atlantic cod is by far the most numerous, and the one most commonly referred to as cod.

A constant fog is created by the meeting of the warm and cold water currents, and the shallowness of the banks (average depth two hundred feet) builds huge seas. Many men have died catching cod for the world's dinner tables. For centuries, cod was a staple throughout the northern rim of the Atlantic, cooked fresh every conceivable way, made into chowders, cakes, and puddings, or salt-preserved for months. The entire fish was used; the roe, cheeks, tongue, and air bladder were considered delicacies. The liver and its oil have for centuries been used medicinally.

Cod was so important economically that for centuries it was found on coins, corporate seals, letterheads, legal documents, stamps, and even wind vanes. And, of course, we have Cape Cod.

Cod is a lean fish. The flesh is firm and white and will flake cleanly apart along lines of cleavage as soon as it has been cooked through. The head, liver, and roe all make excellent food.

The largest cod ever recorded weighed more than two hundred pounds, and was caught in 1895 off the Massachusetts coast. Today, cod over ten pounds are graded large. Those weighing one and a half to two and a half pounds are called scrod; their mild flavor makes scrod broiled with butter and lemon juice one of the easiest fish for an unenthusiastic fish-eater to enjoy. Broil fillets in a very hot oven for only a few minutes, until the flesh just flakes apart with the touch of a fork. Small fillets need not be turned over. The flesh is delicate and tender; the flavor is mild with a touch of sweetness. There is not a hint of the strong fishy taste that oilier species may have when not completely fresh and properly prepared.

Haddock is similar in both appearance and taste to cod, but is generally smaller, usually weighing from two to five pounds. Like cod, it is a deep-water species. Hake, another member of the cod family, is even smaller, generally less than two pounds; the flesh is coarser and somewhat stronger tasting. Pollock has a similar taste and generally weighs four to five pounds; it is sometimes called Boston bluefish.

Atlantic cod and these other members of the cod family fulfill my criteria for healthy eating—they are of moderate size and thus fairly low on the food chain, and they spend most or all of their lives far out at sea. Two members of the cod family not recommended are ling cod (burbot), a freshwater fish found mainly in deep lakes and in some rivers, and tomcod, a small shallow-water coastal fish caught mainly in brackish estuaries and rivers.

Dolphin (Mahimahi)

Not to be confused with the fascinating and often entertaining mammalian dolphin (a member of the porpoise family), this fish has a magnificence of its own. I remember well watching them caught on a fishing boat off the coast of Florida when I was a boy. Leaping high above the ocean's surface when hooked, the dolphin, often three to four feet long, flashed brilliant greens, yellows, and shades of red as they fought for freedom. Occasionally one would escape, throwing the hook; for these beautiful fish, one could not help but feel glad. Most, though, were drawn inexorably to the side of the vessel where a waiting crewman would pierce the loin with a gaff and toss the fish unceremoniously on the deck. Writhing, thrashing, slowly losing the rainbow colors that are displayed when dolphin are feeding or excited, the dolphin died on the deck.

When it comes to the eating, dolphin meat is wonderful—white, firm, moist, and sweet. A wide-ranging species found in tropical and subtropical seas the world over, dolphin was almost never seen in markets until appearing on the West Coast in the 1970s. Now it is shipped in from Hawaii and other locales and called mahimahi. Market fish, however, have never matched the beauty or the freshness of those caught on that Florida boat. Dolphin is unique; try it if it is good and fresh.

Halibut

The four species of commercial importance in America are actually members of the flounder family. The best are the Atlantic and the Pacific halibut, similar fish with firm, delicately flavored white meat.

These flatfish can grow to more than six hundred pounds, but today halibut more than three hundred pounds are rarely caught. The Atlantic halibut ranges from waters off New Jersey northward; the Pacific species from central California northward. Cool deep ocean is their habitat; seldom do they enter waters shallower than two hundred feet.

The Greenland halibut is inferior in texture and flavor to Atlantic and Pacific halibut. The dense musculature is not bad when cooked slowly in a fish soup, but it becomes dry and tough under direct heat. Sometimes inaccurately sold as "turbot," the Greenland halibut ranges over Arctic and sub-Arctic regions of the Atlantic and the Pacific, going no farther south than Cape Cod in the East and southern California in the West.

The California halibut is found from central California to northern Mexico. The meat is similar to the Pacific halibut, but it is less tasty. It is much smaller, usually weighing between four and twelve pounds.

Herring (See Also Sardines)

Herring is one of the richest sources of vitamin D. Vegetarians that feed on tiny plankton and migrate widely in huge schools far out at sea, herring were once the world's most abundant food fish. So great was their commercial importance that wars were fought over control of the Baltic Sea's herring grounds. The Hanseatic League, formed by merchants from the Hansa towns of northern Germany, controlled these grounds in the late 1300s. Some forty thousand boats fished the Baltic then, until the herring population center moved to the North Sea, likely because of depletion. Well into the nineteenth century, much of the history of northern Europe, England, Newfoundland, Spain, and Portugal was influenced by conflicts over the herring trade. More recently, conflict over exploitation by fleets of ships from the Soviet Union and other Communist countries led the United States in 1977 to extend coastal control of fishing rights to two hundred miles.

Two species of herring are of prime commercial importance. The Atlantic herring is found on both sides of the North Atlantic and as far south as North Carolina. The Pacific herring is found throughout the northern Pacific, and as far south as northern California. Typical length seen at market is ten inches, though herring grow to about eighteen inches and a weight of a pound and a half. The Pacific species spawns in shallow bay waters, while the Atlantic spawns offshore at depths down to one hundred feet.

Fresh herring is relished in Europe, but in the United States there is little demand, and usually it is seen pickled in wine sauce or sour cream. Fresh herring is prime when fat content is highest, about 15 percent in peak season, which varies in different seas. Herring sold in markets here has often been imported frozen from Iceland.

Two other types of herring that enter rivers and streams in eastern

America to spawn in spring and summer are the alewife and the blue-back herring. Although otherwise very similar, they are not nearly as tasty as Atlantic and Pacific herring. In New England, smoked alewives are sold as corned alewives when packed in brine and as pickled alewives when packed in vinegar cure.

Herring have been packed in metal containers for well over 100 years. Herring two to three inches long are referred to as sardines; many brands packed in olive oil are imported from southern Europe, but may be heavily salted. The olive oil is usually not of the highest quality.

Mackerel

Many mackerel species occur in both the Atlantic and Pacific oceans. Mackerel rapidly lose flavor if not iced immediately upon being caught. Quite oily, they are rich in the fatty acids DHA and EPA. Fat content varies with species and is highest in autumn.

Mackerel has in common with tuna distinctly separate red and white musculature. The outer lateral band of red meat is composed primarily of slow-twitch muscle fibers that sustain continuous swimming; these pelagic species never stop. The inner portion of lighter-colored meat is composed primarily of fast-twitch fibers that provide bursts of speed. The red and white layers correspond respectively with the fibers in a human being's muscles that adapt to endurance exercises such as long-distance running and to power exercises such as weight lifting or sprinting; but in humans the fibers are intermixed.

Atlantic mackerel, found from Newfoundland to Cape Hatteras, is the most common northern species. Atlantic and king mackerel have more red muscle, are fattier, and are more strongly flavored than other popular species. King mackerel, commonly called kingfish, ranges from North Carolina to Brazil, and reaches 100 pounds. Twenty- to forty-pound fish are commonly caught off party boats in southern waters; great fighters, big kings are quite a thrill to land.

Kings are good eating. Their southern range keeps them clear of more polluted northeastern coastal waters. They may be filleted or cut into steaks. To minimize their oil flavor, marinate in lime juice and a little tamari for a few hours and then broil with butter.

More delicately flavored mackerel include cero, Spanish mackerel, and wahoo. All are leaner and have less red muscle than Atlantic and king. Cero and Spanish mackerel range north to Cape Cod. Cero are generally marketed in the five- to ten-pound range, Spanish, in the two- to four-pound range.

Wahoo is leanest of the three and the largest, averaging thirty pounds when caught. Known in Hawaii as *ono,* which means "sweet," wahoo are found in all tropical and subtropical seas and have white, softly textured flesh. Seldom caught in adequate numbers for marketing, wahoo is considered by gourmets to be among the finest eating fish in the world.

Pompano

Pompano is considered by some connoisseurs to be the tastiest saltwater fish. Seldom weighing more than two pounds, with firm, delicate white flesh, they range as far north as Massachusetts, but are most popular along the southern Atlantic and the Gulf Coast. A larger but very similar fish called the permit is sometimes seen in northeastern markets; when weighing less than about eight pounds, they are similar in taste to pompano.

Salmon

Sculpted in the floor of the Grotte du Poisson near Les Eyzies, France, is a carefully detailed bas-relief of a salmon done by an ancient cave dweller. Salmon bones have been found in caves that were used by humans during the Stone Age twenty-five thousand years ago. North American Indians of the Columbia River basin in prehistoric Oregon thirteen thousand years ago had ceremonies honoring the salmon; the fish played an important role in their mythology. The people of these disparate cultures did not need the discovery of EPA to make salmon central in their nutrition and their lives.

There are seven distinct species of salmon. Born in rivers, all spend most of their lives at sea before returning to their river of birth to spawn. Salmon do not eat during the trip upriver, and the flesh becomes pale and waterlogged. Fish caught and eaten fresh—or canned—near the end of this trip are distinctly less flavorful than those caught in open sea or earlier on the upriver journey.

Only Atlantic salmon are native to the Atlantic Ocean. Once abundant in rivers of the northeastern United States, Canada, and Europe, the Connecticut River salmon had been eliminated by dams and pollution from sewage and textile mills by 1815. Fisheries throughout New England followed, and by the 1870s even the rivers of northern Maine had been suffocated in sawdust and effluents of the lumber industry. The Atlantic salmon was largely gone from America; only a few remain in rivers in northeastern Maine. Industrialized Europe suffered the same fate. Wild Atlantic salmon in American markets, now a rarity, are mostly from Canada and rural areas of Europe. But the Atlantic salmon most commonly found in northeastern United States is pen-raised, and chinook salmon is reared in seawater net pens in western British Columbia. Marine farming of salmon is growing rapidly in Norway and Scotland, on both coasts of Canada, and in many other countries of the North Atlantic. Because fish diseases have become one of the biggest obstacles for this new industry, drugs in rapidly growing numbers, particularly antibiotics, are being used in the aquaculture industry.

I advise against eating pen-raised and farm-raised fish because of this widespread and growing use of drugs in aquaculture. Residues invariably will be present in the fish. These fish are fed commercial feed; they do not eat their natural diets.

There are five North American Pacific salmon. Chinook or king is the largest (recorded up to 120 pounds), the fattiest (about 16 percent fat when prime), and the tastiest. When ocean caught, the flesh is deep red, rich in oil, and soft in texture. Coho or silver salmon is much smaller, often caught in the five- to ten-pound range. Their flesh is pink to red, but always lighter and less oily than that of king, though their flavors are comparable. Sockeye or red salmon, also called blue-back, usually has deep orange-red flesh nearly as oily as that of king, and a delicate flavor. Sockeye and king are the most expensive salmon; coho is a little less so.

Chum and pink salmon are the lowest in fat content, most reasonably priced, and least flavorful. There is a dramatic difference between their taste and that of king, coho, or sockeye. Unspecified canned salmon invariably is chum or pink. The quality of canned salmon varies widely with the time of year that the fish is caught, and this is usually reflected by price.

Gonads of the male (white roe) and the bright orange roe of the female may be lightly poached, eaten raw, or made into a caviar substitute. Rich in iodine and enzymes, roe were a staple of Native Americans, especially children and pregnant women. The bones, head, and skin may be used to make fish soup or stock. If the fish is baked or grilled whole, a smallish piece of meat just beneath the gill cover may be eaten; it has a delicate, slightly sweet, unique flavor.

Salmon is as rich in eicosapentaenoic acid (EPA) as any fish readily available. Most of its life is spent far out in northern seas, away from areas of coastal pollution. Smaller salmon, five to ten pounds, are quite low on the food chain and not as likely to concentrate pollutants as the larger king salmon. Fresh coho (silver) and small king salmon are available throughout the Pacific Northwest and are widely shipped. Except in the Pacific Northwest, fresh sockeye is seldom seen. Both coho and sockeye are generally good canned, though canned salmon does not compare with fresh. Fresh Alaskan salmon is available seasonally in most parts of the United States.

Sardines

Sardines are small fish from any of several species, including two- to three-inch-long herring, pilchards, and sprat. Sprat is also called brisling sardines.

The Maine coast is a major source of sardines in America, where in most places they are found only canned and packed in soybean oil, low quality olive oil, or mustard sauce. An imported variety packed in *sild* (the Scandinavian word for herring) sardine oil is found in some markets, lightly smoked and salted. Sild oil is not too strong and is tasty on salads with vinegar and a little olive oil, and it is rich in the unsaturated fatty acids concentrated in fish oils. Sardines may also be found packed in water and in 100 percent extra-virgin olive oil.

As is often the case with herring, whitebait, smelts, and alewives, when one eats sardines, one eats internal organs, skin, and bones; they are thus rich in certain nutrients, especially nucleic acids, found only in small quantities in most other foods. Raw shellfish also provide such nutrition, and additionally provide enzymes found only in raw foods.

Sardines were a major item in Dr. Benjamin Frank's "No-Aging Diet," popularized in his book of that title many years ago. His thesis is that sardines and other foods rich in nucleic acids—shellfish and organ meats in particular—help slow down the aging process.

Sea Trout

Sea trout are brown trout that spend most of their lives at sea. More numerous in northern Europe, small numbers of them breed in Canadian and American rivers, and fish in the three- to ten-pound range occasionally appear in New England markets. Most sea trout found in markets nowadays, however, have been pen-raised. The meat is similar to salmon—pink to red, quite fatty, and very tasty. The name is not to be confused with seatrout (one word), which refers to several members of an entirely different family of fish, the drum family.

Shad

Shad enter coastal rivers and bays seasonally on both coasts. Native to the East Coast, shad run there from December in the south to May in the north. This member of the herring family has been introduced on the West Coast and now thrives from central California into British

Columbia. The Columbia River run supplies a large market in May and June.

Shad typically weigh one to three pounds. The meat is white, sweet, and tasty, and the roe are considered a delicacy. As with all anadromous fish, the quality of the river water in which these fish are born and spend much of their lives affects the quality of the fish.

Shark

Shark and swordfish taste similar; mako shark is often substituted for swordfish. While the flavor and texture are similar, the flesh of mako is more whitish than the pinkish gray of sword. Both the blacktip shark of semitropical waters and the blue shark have snow-white meat. The dogfish shark has been likened to halibut, and indeed the dogfish is called harbor halibut along the coast of Maine.

England's famous fish-and-chips is most commonly made with shark, often the spiny dogfish or the porbeagle. Shark has always been popular in most parts of the world and remains so today, though not in the United States. Even in North America, however, prices have risen, indicating increased demand. But at less than half the price of swordfish, mako remains a bargain.

Soaking the flesh in either an acid or a salt solution before cooking is the key to enjoying shark. The flesh has a high concentration of urea; this is one reason the meat, which overlies a skeleton of cartilage, does not keep long. Enzymes convert urea to ammonia, which strongly flavors the fish if it is allowed to remain—soaking steaks or fillets in a salt or vinegar solution leaches out the ammonia. Use half a pound of salt to a gallon of water to submerge a large fillet or several steaks, and soak for several hours. Alternatively, lemon or lime juice, or vinegar with water, may be used to marinate small pieces for several hours prior to cooking, or consumption as sushi or sashimi. Like swordfish, the meat is firm and excellent raw; when cooked, it is best broiled.

Smelt

Like salmon and striped bass, smelt once entered hundreds of rivers and bays on both coasts, coming seasonally in legion numbers each year to breed. To a lesser extent, these small anadromous fish still do, though they no longer abound in waters along the shores of Manhattan and Boston's Back Bay as they did in the second half of the nineteenth century.

In many of the rivers where smelt still run, the waters are heavily polluted.

Rainbow smelt is most common in North American waters. Found on both coasts, populations exist also in the Great Lakes and in lakes across New England, New York, and southeastern Canada. Oceangoing fish enter rivers and bays in the spring.

The eulachon is the variety of smelt important in the Pacific Northwest, from Oregon to Alaska. The Kwakiutl Indians of coastal British Columbia, said to have been a strong and healthy people, used eulachon in some manner at every meal. In winter, the fish and its oil were mixed with summer-cut greens as a fishcake. Eulachon is also called candlefish; it is so oily the Indians dried the fish and, with a cedar-bark wick, used them as candles.

Eulachon is marketed both fresh and smoked. On the West Coast, the surf smelt, a smaller and less oily fish, and several other varieties of smelt sold as whitebait, are also marketed.

Smelt is usually sold in the six- to eight-inch range, frozen or fresh. They are easily cooked and eaten ungutted, with heads, tails, and organs; cook as with whitebait. The uninitiated will find this is most easily done with the smaller fish.

Snapper

Fifteen snapper species are found in American waters from North Carolina to Texas. Red snapper, the most popular, is found in the Pacific as well. The habitat of snapper is coastal waters sixty to two hundred feet deep. Fish seen at market usually weigh four to six pounds.

Red snapper is quite lean. Texture and fat content are similar to that of small cod. The flavor, though stronger than cod, is still quite mild.

Yellowtail is considered by many the most finely flavored snapper. Distinctively different from other snapper (it is of a different genus), the meat is white, sweet, and finely flaked. Freshly caught yellowtail—it loses its flavor quickly—is a favorite in many fine restaurants on Florida's Atlantic coast and on the Gulf from Key West to Texas.

Sole and Flounder

Flounder is the term for any one of three families of flatfish in the Atlantic and Pacific oceans; more than two hundred species are represented. Fish referred to as sole in the United States are actually varieties of flounder, as are halibut. The only members of the true sole family found in North American waters are tiny and of no economic importance. But several North American flounder—in particular, lemon sole, gray sole, and rex sole—are similar to the European Dover sole (a true sole) used for classic fillet of sole dishes.

One last point of clarification—Dover sole is also the common name of a species of Pacific flounder found from California to Alaska and widely sold in western America. Having distinguished sole from flounder from halibut, we turn now to individual species.

Winter flounder is the most abundant and popular flatfish in eastern America. This fish is marketed as flounder if weighing three pounds or less, and as lemon sole if weighing more. The meat is very sweet, finely flaked, and, especially in the smaller sizes, fragile in texture. This is fish that people often say doesn't taste like fish.

Delicate texture and flavor have made European Dover sole and North American winter flounder, gray sole, and rex sole central in the seafood creations of chefs. Spices, herbs, sauces, fruits and vegetables, and contrasting seafood is used with these fish to create scores of entrees.

Winter flounder ranges from Newfoundland south to the Chesapeake Bay, in coastal zones and bays as well as in deeper offshore grounds. Fish caught generally range in size from one to five pounds.

Much of this fish's habitat is polluted waters, but it is low in fat, and pollutants in fish concentrate in the fats. Still, a flounder spending half its life in a northern New Jersey bay carries highly undesirable substances. Winter flounder range widely; wherever caught, they spent a good part of life in shallow coastal waters of unknown quality.

Summer flounder, marketed as fluke, is similar in texture and taste to winter flounder, though somewhat larger. It too is a shallow-water species, as is its smaller cousin the southern flounder, caught from North Carolina to Texas.

American plaice, marketed as dab, sand-dab, long rough-dab, and roughback, ranges from Cape Cod to the Grand Banks and across the Atlantic to Europe. This deep-water flounder is found at depths from 120 to 2,000 feet. The usual market fish weighs from two to three pounds. Their small size, deep-water habitat, and a northern range along lightly populated coasts combine to make this fish ideal food. This important commercial species is generally available in the northeastern United States.

Petrale sole, rex sole, butter sole, sand sole, and Dover sole are among the Pacific varieties of flounder, in the order of usual ranking for flavor. All range north as far as Alaska. Pacific Dover sole (as mentioned above, not to be confused with European Dover sole, a true sole) is a deep-water variety.

Pacific flounder caught in waters off northern California, Oregon, Washington, British Columbia, and Alaska have likely lived mostly or entirely in relatively unpolluted waters. Rex, butter, and sand sole are quite small. Dover sole may weigh as much as ten pounds, and petrale sole is somewhat larger.

Steelhead

Steelhead is the oceangoing form of the rainbow trout, returning to rivers to breed. Found seasonally throughout the Pacific Northwest, steelhead is pink, soft, almost salmon-like, and somewhat comparable in flavor. Fillets can be from fish as small as a pound, though fish up to ten or twelve pounds are not uncommon.

Striped Bass

Striped bass are most common from Cape Cod to South Carolina, though they are found north to the Gulf of Saint Lawrence and south to the Gulf of Mexico. Like salmon, stripers live in saltwater but depend on freshwater rivers to reproduce. Most fish now caught along the East Coast have been spawned in tributaries of the Chesapeake Bay and the Hudson River, two bodies of water not particularly clean, especially the latter. Striped bass populations have proven highly resistant to pollution, but flavor suffers noticeably in fish taken in polluted waters; as an oily species they concentrate toxins. Some of the finest stripers are caught in waters off Montauk Point (the eastern tip of Long Island) and the New England coast.

Flavor is also dependent upon how quickly the fish is gutted and iced when caught. Skin is sparkly and silvery if the fish is fresh, becoming more reddish and dull with time. The tastiest stripers weigh no more than five to six pounds. Broiling or poaching suits fillets, and the whole fish is excellent baked in a wine sauce. Striper from clean waters makes fine sushi and sashimi.

Striped bass were transplanted to the Pacific Coast in the late 1800s, and many Oregon and California rivers support substantial populations. Striper is seasonally available commercially in these areas.

Descriptions of North America's eastern waters by early settlers makes apparent the incredible multitude of striped bass, bluefish, mackerel, Atlantic salmon, and other species gracing the coasts in years past. Destruction of coastal breeding areas, and overfishing in North America's waters, particularly by huge Japanese and Russian vessels, have together eliminated or made scarce many species. Pollutants have tainted remaining fish; one had best ask where a fish was caught. Those who value a clean environment and abundant fish and wildlife have so far been unable to restrain forces threatening the destruction of North America's wilderness heritage. Modern life has paradoxes; a man urinating on a public beach may be arrested and jailed, yet he may pour thousands of gallons of toxic chemicals into public waters and go unpunished. The battle will be won or lost in the courts.

Swordfish

Like tuna, swordfish are found around the world in tropical and temperate seas, and those taken off American shores are tastiest in late summer and fall. The meat is firm, with a distinctive flavor, and is excellent for sushi and sashimi.

Swordfish has been shown to concentrate mercury and PCBs, and has the additional problem of being very large; large fish concentrate these toxins in higher concentrations than smaller fish. Nevertheless, occasional broiled or raw swordfish is for me impossible to resist; one hopes that the benefits of this otherwise outstanding food outweigh the liabilities.

Tilefish

This rather ignored species has distinct advantages—habitat and flavor. Requiring very cold water and feeding on bottom-dwelling crustaceans, tilefish live at depths of three hundred to more than one thousand feet, from Nova Scotia to Florida, and also off the Pacific coast. When they do come into shallow water, they feed differently, which apparently results in a harmless but rather bitter flavor. The deep dwellers taste similar to lobster or scallops, sweet and tender; the flesh is firm and makes fine sushi and sashimi.

The common tilefish inhabits more northern Atlantic waters, the blackline tilefish more southern. The Pacific species is called ocean whitefish. Reasonably priced, marketed tilefish are generally six- to eight-pound fish sold as fillets, and make a good choice when seeking a tasty and clean fish.

Tuna

The geography of ancient Europe was much influenced by tuna. In pre-Christian times, crude spruce observation posts built atop coastal cliffs were used to spot tuna migrations from afar; a cry would go up, and fishermen would set to sea to row out and spread their nets. Around these posts grew various cities, all about the Mediterranean and Atlantic coasts.

Every part of the tuna was utilized by ancient fishermen; the roe in particular was long considered a great delicacy. In Mediterranean cultures, specific cuts of the often very large bluefin tuna are known for their superior culinary qualities. Tuna makes excellent sushi and sashimi.

Tuna is quite fatty, but the amount of fat varies greatly by season—they are fattiest and tastiest in late summer and early fall. The meat of different species is classed as white, light, or dark; flavor is strongest in darker species.

Six species come to American markets fresh, frozen, or canned. Most delicately flavored and valuable is albacore, the tuna with the lightest-colored flesh. Found in tropical and temperate waters of both the Atlantic and the Pacific, albacore are caught from several to one hundred miles or so offshore, and typically weigh ten to fifteen pounds. A mainstay of the California canning industry, they seldom are seen fresh in markets.

Blackfin is also a small tuna, typically eight to ten pounds. Like the albacore, the meat is delicately flavored and light in color. Though a favorite of tuna connoisseurs, it too is seldom seen in North American markets. Blackfin is an Atlantic species and ranges from Cape Cod to Brazil.

Yellowfin is the key species for the California canning industry. It is found all around the world in tropical and subtropical waters. Fresh yellowfin steaks are generally cut from ten- to twenty-pound fish; the meat is a little less light than albacore, and very tasty.

Skipjack tuna too is a tropical and semitropical species, with light meat comparable to the yellowfin. The average size is six to eight pounds.

The largest tuna is the bluefin, ranging to more than one thousand pounds, though four to six hundred is considered large today. Meat darkens as the size increases; usually fish over 120 pounds are too dark to be classed as light.

Popular in Europe and Japan, the lighter, smaller fish make excellent sushi and sashimi. Raw bluefin has no strong fish flavor and is very softly textured. Bluefin is found in all temperate and subtropical seas.

Canned tuna is labeled in one of three ways: solid pack or "fancy" (large pieces with no fragments); chunks or "standard" (three pieces of solid meat, filled in with flakes); or salad or "flakes" (crumbs or finely divided meat, packed down solid). Only albacore may be labeled white-meat tuna. Yellowfin, skipjack, and small bluefin are other varieties of U.S. canned tuna; they are labeled light-meat tuna.

Albacore is the smallest of commercially caught tuna and is available canned, packed in water; unfortunately it is salted. Yellowfin tuna is very tasty broiled lightly with a little butter and lemon or used for sushi and sashimi.

Toxic residues make one hesitate to use much tuna; because they are fatty, highly carnivorous, and often grow large, tuna has higher concentrations of mercury and PCBs than most other fish. Tuna has the further disadvantage of not being a cold-water species; the eicosapentaenoic acid (EPA) content is thus considerably lower than that of salmon, mackerel, and several other fatty species that have not been reported to concentrate mercury and PCBs.

Whitebait

As served seasonally in some fine seafood restaurants, whitebait consists of very small specimens (usually less than three inches) of some or all of several species—young silversides, sardines (herring), anchovies, surf smelts, and sand launce—that have been floured and flash-fried. These fish when marketed as whitebait, either fresh or frozen, are sold whole and ungutted. They may be fried quickly in butter or olive oil, or broiled quickly in a hot oven.

These fish are often seen at the edge of the surf and may easily be netted by two people working a short length of fine-meshed net. Silversides and sand launce are especially numerous in New England.

SHELLFISH

Abalone

Of the world's approximately 100 species of abalone, 8 occur along the Pacific coast of North America, mostly in California, which prohibits the canning or shipping of abalone out of state. Vast quantities of this once abundant shellfish were formerly shipped to the Orient.

Relative scarcity, high demand, and succulent, sweet meat make abalone an expensive, but unforgettable entree. White-meat steaks are sliced from flesh that has been pried away from colorful shells. Gentle pounding with a mallet on a wooden board tenderizes the steaks, which are then cooked quickly and lightly. Overcooked, they become tough.

Univalve vegetarian mollusks, West Coast abalone average four pounds; they feed with tiny teeth on seaweed. Because they do not filter water as bivalves do, abalone do not concentrate bacteria in polluted waters and are immune to red tide. They are excellent for sushi and sashimi.

A dried Japanese abalone product, brined, smoked, and dried in the sun, is available in many markets specializing in Oriental foods. Shredded, this is called *kaiho;* powdered, it is called *meiho.*

Clams

Many widely divergent species of clams abound along all American coasts. Both hardshell and softshell clams are found in shallow eastern waters from the Arctic Ocean to Cape Hatteras. Hardshells, or quahogs (pronounced *cohogs*), usually eaten raw on the half shell or in chowder, are classed by size. Smallest is the littleneck (three to four years old, up to two inches across); a bit larger is the cherrystone (about five years old); and larger still (more than three inches), too big to eat on the half-shell and without the delicate flavor of smaller clams, is the chowder clam, often called simply the quahog.

Softshell clams are also found on the coast of the Pacific Northwest, along with razor clams, littlenecks, and butter clams. Pacific littlenecks are unrelated to eastern littlenecks and are not really good raw; usually they are steamed. Butter clams are usually found small, on gravelly intertidal beaches. They look and taste about the same as East Coast littlenecks—tender, succulent, and absolutely marvelous fresh out of the sand.

Softshell clams are called steamers. Boil them in a half inch of water until the shells have opened—just a minute or two. Lemon juice and butter complete the broth.

Razor clams are too tough to be eaten raw, unless they are very small. They are usually steamed.

Live softshell or razor clams constrict their necks when the neck is touched; hardshells whose shells are open will close tightly. Throw away any dead ones. Clams will live at forty degrees in a refrigerator for several days, but they lose some freshness and flavor. If bought shucked in a container (preferably glass), the liquid should be clear, the clams plump. Like fresh clams in the shell, they are best eaten within forty-eight hours. If they are a little old, rinse them with cold water before eating; this also freshens up jarred oysters.

Bivalves are safest and tastiest in months with an "r" in them. Toxic plankton overgrowths such as red tide are most likely during warm months of May through August (no "r"). September through April are all "r" months, and generally safe. Bivalves taste best during these times, and some enthusiasts eat them several times a week.

Abstaining in the warmer months seems to make clams, oysters, and mussels taste better than ever by September. Fresh raw shellfish of good quality is among the most strengthening of foods. Shellfish is one of the best sources of vitamin D.

Crab

The many varieties of crabs inhabiting our coastal zones differ markedly in habitats. Some species live in shallow water just offshore and in bays and estuaries; others live far offshore, at depths well beyond one thousand feet.

The blue crab is the most common crab on the East Coast. Warmer months find it in shallow waters from New England to Florida. Females are full of eggs much of this time; she-crab soup is made from their meat and roe.

The jonah crab of the Northeast is generally a deep-water species. Though in some areas it appears in shallows, and even in intertidal zones in the spring, generally the jonah stays in open waters, often at great depths. Typically five or six inches across the shell, the jonah crab has appeared commercially with the development of deep-water crabbing operations now harvesting the Continental Shelf. The red crab, too, usually lives at great depths on the outer shelf, though it may be found in waters as shallow as 150 feet. Once taken only during deep-water lobstering, the red and the jonah have assumed greater commercial importance with the development of specialized traps. Both are delicious and are often compared to the king crab.

The king crab of the northern Pacific is usually called the Alaska king crab. They average ten pounds but, as with all crabs, the yield of meat is only about 25 percent. The most important other Pacific coast species is the Dungeness crab, found from Alaska to southern California. Like the jonah, it is a type of rock crab, spending most of the year at considerable depths and venturing into shallow waters and intertidal zones seasonally. Dungeness crabs are delicious and are popular on the West Coast.

The snow crab is worthy of mention because it is widely available canned and lives at depths beyond one thousand feet. Also known as the tanner crab, it is a northern Pacific species and lives along the Continental Shelf. Most taken are found in king crab traps off the coast of Alaska.

The lady crab is the little crab felt nipping at one's feet and seen scampering in shallow water on Atlantic beaches. Rarely more than three inches across the shell, they are tasty and easily netted. Many a fine meal has been made of whitebait and lady crabs cooked over an open fire on the beach.

The oyster crab is found living within some oysters. Seldom more than an inch across the shell, they are collected by some oyster wholesalers during shucking operations for sale to the few retailers who carry them. Seldom seen, oyster crabs are softshelled and, like the lady crab, need not be dressed; cook them as they are, or use them in crab soup.

A crab periodically sheds its shell as it grows; until the soft covering underneath toughens, we have a softshell crab. Usually crabs are captured a few days before shedding and marketed afterward at a premium. Softshell blue crab is the common commercial species.

Lobster

Lobster species are found in oceans all over the world. Maine is the traditional home of the American lobster, though it is found as far south as North Carolina. Although still most abundant in the cold waters off the Maine and eastern Canadian coasts, the catch in Maine has declined over the years.

Maine (American) lobster usually weigh from one to five pounds, but may grow to fifty. Their usual habitat is the ocean bottom at depths of ten to two hundred feet, though they have been captured at depths up to six hundred feet one hundred miles offshore. Lobsters are omnivores, eating slow-moving, bottom-dwelling sea-animal life and seaweed. Their range is very limited, and they feed mostly in warmer months.

Beware the lobster's claws! The two are different. On is larger and for crushing, the other is a lighter biting claw, which the lobster can be very quick with. Bands seen around the claws in lobster tanks prevent cannibalism.

When picking out a live lobster, select a lively one, for a listless lobster may have been captive quite some time. Lobsters lose weight in captivity, which one may notice when cracking a lobster open after cooking. Select from a busy market with a rapid turnover. When buying precooked lobster, if in doubt about freshness, extend the tail out straight; if it snaps back to a curled position when released, the lobster was alive until cooked.

Females are preferred by those who enjoy the roe, called coral, which cooks to a bright red. Females have a broader abdomen than males of the same size, and the first pair of tail appendages are reduced in size.

Surprisingly, the size of a lobster gives no indication of tenderness and even the largest lobsters may be tender. But as with all seafood, younger and smaller individuals accumulate the smallest amount of pollutants in any given environment. Lobsters from one to one and a half pounds are called quarters and are adequate for most appetites, though some people prefer a large (one and a half to two and a half pounds). Jumbos are more than two and a half pounds, while chickens weigh less than a pound and are often missing one claw.

Nearly all of a lobster is edible. The green pasty material inside the body cavity is called tomalley and is the lobster's liver. Rich but not quite as sweet as the firm white meat of the claws, tail, body, and legs, it is quite delicious in its own right. Roe or coral of the female also has a unique taste. The shells, like those of all crustaceans, are rich in carotene (giving them their color), protein, and calcium. Shells may be used in making a stock that lends a distinct flavor to a soup or sauce.

Lobster is most easily cooked by boiling or steaming. Plunge headfirst into actively boiling water, cover, and keep heat on high to return the water to a boil; this will take a few minutes. Begin timing when the water has returned to a boil. When cooking more than one lobster, per animal, allow seven minutes for the first pound and three minutes more for each additional pound.

Steaming causes less loss of nutrients than boiling does. To steam a lobster, boil an inch or two of water; then place the lobster in the pot and keep the pot covered. A perforated plate may be used in the bottom to keep the lobster above water. When steam reappears, begin timing as above.

Lobster is also wonderful baked. Stuffings are made with tomalley and coral; other ingredients may include crab meat. The claws are cracked; the lobster is split, stuffed, and then baked.

From North Carolina through Florida, and around the Gulf, the spiny lobster (also called rock lobster or sometimes crawfish, not to be confused with crayfish) makes its home. This lobster has no claws. Related species are found in many parts of the world; the South African lobster tails seen on many menus are from one such species.

Several other members of the lobster family have in recent years made an appearance in American markets. Collectively called lobsterettes, or sometimes langoustines or Danish lobsters, they are similar to the American lobster but smaller and very brightly colored. Their meat is mostly in the tail, and they live in deep water at depths from six hundred to more than six thousand feet, making them less proximal to coastal pollutants.

Mussels

Mussels have never enjoyed in America the popularity they do in Europe, though they taste much like steamers and are considerably less expensive. Found from Canada to North Carolina clinging to rocks and seawalls in intertidal zones, mussels are most numerous in New England and can be gathered on many beaches. The blue or edible mussel is the most common species (not all saltwater mussels are edible); it is also found on the Pacific coast, along with the California mussel.

Rich in nutrients, mussels (like clams and oysters) are tastiest and least susceptible to toxic algae growths in fall, winter, and early spring. After spawning in late spring, they become watery and lose some of their flavor.

Unlike steamers, live mussels may open up when removed from the refrigerator and exposed to a temperature change but this does not mean they are dead. Try to slide the two halves of the shell laterally across one another; a live mussel holds quite rigidly. If the shells move much, the mussel is dead. Cook mussels similarly to steamers. Discard any that do not open in cooking, for they may have been dead beforehand.

Octopus

The octopus is a predator living largely on shellfish; this makes its flesh very tasty. Octopuses are caught off both coasts, generally about a mile offshore in one hundred to two hundred feet of water. The usual size is one to three pounds.

Most of the demand for octopus in the United States is from people of Mediterranean or Oriental origin. Scarcer than squid, octopus is also considerably more expensive. It is considered a great delicacy by those who enjoy it. Cooked octopus is very popular at sushi bars.

Oysters

Oysters grow best in bays and river mouths where the salinity of seawater has been diluted. Vegetarians, they feed on tiny unicellular plants filtered from the gallon of water their bodies process each hour. The flavor and color of oysters reflect the type and quality of these plants; these influences are in turn determined by the quality and temperature of the water, salinity and proximity to freshwater, nutrients available, and a host of other immeasurable contributory elements.

Cultivation of oysters has been successfully accomplished since Roman times, and among the finest oysters are cultivars from Cape Cod Bay in New England and Tomales Bay in California. Cultivars begin growth when oyster larvae catch on scallop shells that are threaded on strings suspended from racks; they grow until harvesting, far from the bottom and safe from predators.

Natural oyster beds are found in intertidal zones. The Atlantic coast, particularly the Chesapeake Bay with its thousands of rivers, bays, and streams, is the home of the most common North American oyster. Among its many names are the bluepoint, the Chincoteague, the Apalachicola, and the Cape Cod. Best known of Pacific coast oysters is the Olympia, bred in the brackish waters of the Puget Sound near the capital of Washington. Other oysters are native to the Gulf Coast.

Oysters spawn during the warm months, and during that time produce excessive glycogen (the form in which glucose is stored in muscles), causing a milky look and poor taste. In northern areas oysters are best in fall, winter, and early spring; in the south, they taste best only in winter.

Oysters vary greatly in size; the smaller have the finest flavor. Shells should be tightly closed, and there should be no hint of strong odor. If not very fresh, oysters do not taste quite right. If purchased already shucked, the container should be glass so one can see if the liquid is clear. If it is cloudy or milky, the oysters are not completely fresh. This liquid, which runs off the half-shell when oysters are shucked, is excellent to drink or use in oyster cookery. Particularly along the Gulf Coast, oysters are a popular item in many gourmet dishes.

Scallops

Of hundreds of species throughout the world, only a few types of scallops are sold commercially. Only the adductor muscle of the scallop is consumed in North America, though the scallop is edible. The two species most often seen are the bay scallop and the sea scallop, both East Coast natives. Several others are found on the West Coast, but except in Alaska, not in sufficient quantities to be of much commercial importance.

The bay scallop is a shallow-water species found from Virginia to the Gulf of Mexico. The adductor muscle—what we call a scallop—is rarely more than an inch across. The sea scallop is much larger, up to about four inches across, and is taken from waters as deep as one thousand feet off the coast, from New Jersey to northeastern Canada. Maine is the center of the sea scallop trade. Another deep-water species is the calico, taken off Florida's east coast.

Scallops are perhaps the sweetest of all seafood and are outstanding lightly broiled, or sautéed in butter and herbs. Distributors sometimes soak scallops in fresh water for a few hours to increase bulk, much to the detriment of their flavor. Color is the clue; this process whitens them, and fresh scallops should be beige or cream colored. Excellent when raw in sushi or as sashimi, scallops need only minimal cooking for, like all fish, they turn tough when overcooked. Quick broiling in a hot oven or sautéing in a hot skillet seals in the juices.

Shrimp

Like shellfish, shrimp are a wonderful source of vitamin D. The ubiquitous shrimp cocktail has made shrimp the seafood of greatest commercial importance. Hundreds of freshwater and saltwater species exist. Several very similar species are taken in waters off the southeastern coast of the United States and in the Gulf of Mexico, and several others are taken off the Pacific coast, mainly in Alaskan waters.

Though the word "prawn" is used to describe any large shrimps, prawn actually indicates a freshwater species, whereas "shrimp" means a saltwater species. Shrimp are classed by size; so-called prawns or jumbo shrimp are generally considered to number fifteen or fewer to a pound.

Fresh shrimp should be firm and clean smelling, with no offensive odor. Shrimp taken offshore may smell and taste of iodine because the organisms they feed on in waters of normal ocean salinity tend to concentrate iodine, making them a rich source of this nutrient. In the less saline water of bays, shrimp feed on organisms less rich in iodine and rarely concentrate sufficient iodine for that odor and taste to be noticeable. However, sulfites are often sprinkled on shrimp and other fish as a preservative, and sodium bisulfate in particular causes an iodine taste or magnifies one that may be present. So while offshore shrimp may be more desirable in areas where bay waters are of questionable cleanliness, one may not know if any iodine taste is natural or chemically induced.

As always, the best safeguard is dealing with merchants is to be aware of the source of the seafood as well as how it's been handled. Small or medium-sized fresh shrimp are often available whole—complete with shell, tail, head, and roe—quite reasonably priced. When very fresh, they may be sautéed in a hot skillet in a quarter inch of wine, butter, and their own juices, then served over brown rice or vegetables. Though not suited to everyone's taste, the entire shrimp is edible and this is indeed a sweet and succulent dish. Nutrients minimally supplied by the meat alone are richly supplied by the organs, roe, and head.

When estimating how much shrimp to purchase, consider that two-fifths of the weight is lost in shelling and deveining. Steamed shrimp compared to boiled are equally firm but more tender, and flavor is not lost into the cooking water as it is when shrimp are boiled.

Squid

This ten-armed mollusk exists in scores of varieties, ranging in size from one inch to sixty feet, and is found in oceans throughout the world. Important in the cuisine of many countries, especially in the Mediterranean and the Orient, squid is firm, tender when not over-cooked, and gently flavored. Squid is a highly nutritious and tasty food, though rarely used simply because of its unfamiliarity.

As usually marketed, squid weigh a few ounces each. The white firm flesh turns yellow in cooking. More than three-quarters of the total weight of the animal is edible; even the ink is used in many European dishes. Ink, incidentally, is discharged as the squid propels itself away from predators, jetting water out of a funnel in its body. The ink leaves a cloud, and perhaps an image of itself to serve as a decoy, behind which the squid rapidly disappears.

FRESHWATER FISH

The problems of the oceans discussed earlier under the heading "Water Pollution" are being compounded in rivers, lakes, and streams by the increasing acidity of rainwater in many parts of the country. Sulfur dioxide emissions from coal combustion at power plants, and nitrogen oxides from automobile exhaust and various industrial sources, are converted into sulfuric rain and affect the acidity of freshwater ecosystems.

As a result, freshwater fish even in relatively unpolluted areas in the eastern part of the country have been affected. In areas of concentrated population, freshwater fish have long been of questionable value because of pollution problems. Still, particularly in the West, there are vast unspoiled areas with high mountain lakes, free-running streams, and good fishing.

While freshwater fish do not contain the high amounts of EPA found in many saltwater species, they provide excellent nutrition, and are available commercially in some parts of the country. Most of us have a limited selection of freshwater fish, in particular, fish from a clean environment. Comments here will be limited to bass, trout, and whitefish.

Bass

Freshwater black bass are unrelated to black sea bass and striped bass. Members of the sunfish family, they have meat that is lean and white. Not sold commercially, largemouth and smallmouth bass are popular game fish, and those under two pounds are firm and sweet, much tastier than larger ones. Bass survive and reproduce in many polluted waters; the taste depends on the quality of the water and deteriorates markedly in less than clean waters.

Trout

A popular game fish, trout is found on many restaurant menus and in most seafood markets. But trout on the menu or in the market must by law be hatchery raised, unless it is lake trout or steelhead. Trout caught by fishermen in more populated parts of the country are also hatchery raised; wild trout are found primarily in lakes, rivers, and streams of the Rocky Mountains.

The meat of hatchery-raised trout is white; its flavor, even if from the better hatcheries, does not compare with that of the red to pink or orange flesh of wild trout. Carotenoids are found in crayfish, shrimp, and other crustaceans. Wild steelhead and rainbow trout of the American West feed upon them, causing the red tinge of their flesh. Wild brook trout, native to eastern North America and transplanted throughout the rest of the continent, has more of a yellow to orange flesh.

Wild brook, rainbow, and cutthroat trout of the West are, at their best, comparable to the androminous steelhead trout discussed earlier. Lake trout is larger, usually ten to twenty pounds, and much oiler than other trout species. Quality varies greatly; in the Great Lakes they feed mainly on alewives, hence the flavor suffers. Quality of hatchery-raised trout also varies greatly; some are quite tasty. Others are mealy and without flavor.

OTHER FISHY CONCERNS

Sushi and Sashimi

Sashimi is the Japanese word for raw fish, carefully cut, eaten with tamari and wasabi (grated horseradish root). Sufficiently fresh fish is delicate in taste and firm in texture; the aroma has a hint of sweet freshness. The finest quality sashimi is made from fresh fish no more than a day out of the water.

Raw fish was central in the diets of traditional seacoast cultures everywhere; each culture had special ways of preparing species important to it. Special techniques of cutting different species of fish for sashimi prepare each type of fish in the best form for enjoyment raw. While the home chef does not have the training and knowledge of the skilled Japanese sashimi artist, the application of a few principles pertaining to the cutting of raw fish enables one to enjoy raw many fish that are commonly cooked. Parts of fish to be broiled or otherwise cooked may be prepared to eat as sushi or sashimi prior to the main course.

Very firm fish such as tuna, swordfish, shark, squid, octopus, tilefish, and abalone are usually cut into cubes. Those a little less firm, like striped bass, cod, and red snapper, are cut into paper-thin slices. A variety of cuts are used on fish of more delicate texture to produce slices about one-quarter inch thick.

Sushi refers to raw fish that is consumed together with rice, the seaweed nori, and sometimes other vegetables. While the finer points of sushi and sashimi are best accomplished by one with the skill and time to be creative, the incorporation of raw fish into the diet may be simple; one need not feel bound by the conventions of sashimi. Lemon juice and other ingredients are useful in marinating raw fish.

Parasites occasionally infect saltwater fish, but are reported (by A. J. McClane in *The Encyclopedia of Fish Cookery*) to be harmless varieties that do not infect humans. In the years since the book was published in the 1970s, a few cases of problems have been reported to be caused by ingestion of parasite-infested sushi and sashimi, but the severity and incidence of these isolated cases has been blown all out of proportion. Freshwater fish, however, may harbor various disease-causing parasites and should never be eaten raw or undercooked.

If one has or can develop a taste for raw fish and shellfish, including sushi and sashimi in the diet may be a major step in developing a primal diet.

Smoked and Salted Fish

Substances in smoked and grilled foods have been found to cause cancer in test animals, and some investigators have linked the use of smoked and salted fish and meat products to increased incidence of stomach cancer. And yet, traditional cultures often preserved fish and meats with smoking and salting, and among these people cancer of all forms was rare. Modern medicine blames skin cancer on the sun's rays, yet contemporary primitive people exposed daily to the sun apparently get no skin cancer.

A plausible explanation is that the degree of susceptibility to all carcinogens is largely determined by the quality of the entire diet. Many substances in the environment and in food that can cause cancer in individuals with insufficient immunity may not cause cancer in those on more adequate diets. This has been demonstrated in dietary experiments with animals, and surveys designed to examine human susceptibility to lung cancer have recently shown that smokers eating more green vegetables have a significantly lower incidence of lung cancer than smokers eating fewer green vegetables. The emphasis on carcinogenic effects of the use of smoked fish may thus be misplaced. Ancestral humans, and later our more immediate ancestors, cooked and smoked fish and game over open fires for perhaps four hundred thousand years.

Many kinds of fresh smoked fish are available regionally; salmon and cod almost universally so. A wide variety of smoked fish and shellfish—herring, mussels, clams, sardines, and many others—are available canned, usually packed in oil. Many influences affect the smoking of fish: the lengths of time at which various temperatures are maintained, kinds of wood used, and amounts of salt employed. Salt is applied first, either as a brine solution of a specific strength or by direct application. Salt removes fluids from the flesh by osmosis. Bacteria are inhibited by lack of water; the fluids drained are replaced by salt to a certain extent. Smoke adds flavor by dehydrating the fish further, and firms the flesh by strengthening connective tissues. If temperatures are kept low enough to prevent coagulation of all protein in the tissues, the flesh becomes firm yet remains somewhat moist.

Hot-smoking and cold-smoking are the two extremes of this process. In the former, the temperature range is from 120 to 180 degrees Fahrenheit, and the smoking time is from six to twelve hours. Considerable coagulation of protein occurs during curing; still, the product remains firm. Without refrigeration, hot-smoked fish keeps only a few days.

Hot-smoking and barbecuing are somewhat similar, but in barbecuing, the fish is placed closer to the heat and cooked slowly at about two hundred degrees Fahrenheit. A smoked flavor is imparted, but the fish crumbles easily and will not keep, for it has not been cured.

Cold-smoking is the traditional method that was used by coastal and northern Indians to preserve vast quantities of fish and meat for winter use. The fish is not cooked, for the temperature of the fish as it is dried is kept around eighty degrees Fahrenheit and the flesh is cured through drying. Protein coagulation is minimal; the fish is essentially preserved raw. This method requires minimal brining and at least two days of smoking, though the fish may be smoked for two or three weeks to make a product that will keep a long time. These methods can produce a superior product that is moist, not too salty, firm, and easily sliced.

Variations on cold-smoking are used by commercial smokehouses in the Pacific Northwest, and in England and Scotland, to produce superior smoked salmon. For salmon smoked in the British Isles, "Scotch smoked salmon" refers to Atlantic salmon, while "smoked salmon" refers to coho and chinook imported fresh from Washington and Alaska. By the time these fish are smoked and returned to America for sale, they may have logged more air miles than ever they did ocean miles. Perhaps this is why they cost upward of twenty dollars a pound.

Roe

Roe were very important foods in coastal traditional cultures. Roe are egg masses in the ovaries of female fish. The ovaries appear as elongated sacs, usually a shade of yellow or orange, with visible round clear eggs (roe) covered by a membrane. In the mature male fish, gonads are long white sacs, small, and white with sperm. Both male gonads and ovaries with their eggs were considered important foods by primitive cultures, and Weston Price reported they were eaten raw. As I have indicated, dried salmon eggs were an important food for coastal North American Indians, especially for the women and children. The men believed that eating the gonads raw increased virility. Even today this "white roe" is a great delicacy in many cuisines around the world.

Most modern palates prefer roe slightly cooked; some simple methods include poaching in water with lemon juice and butter, quick broiling for a minute or so, and sautéing in butter. Types of fish with edible roe sometimes available commercially include salmon, flounder, cod, haddock, halibut, tuna, mackerel, dolphin, herring, and shad. The roe of most fish are edible, though those of some species (none described in this book) are toxic.

Stocks

From both a culinary and a nutritional standpoint, the fish head is the key to good fish stock. The brain is very fatty, full of the fatty acids EPA and DHA, and the gelatin-like texture of the head makes for stock that may be frozen. The head may be poached or used in soups or fish stews. The bones also contribute nutritionally to a stock, as well as enhancing the flavor of it. Adding a little vinegar to the simmering pot helps leach calcium from the bones.

Preservatives

In some places regulations have been adopted concerning the use of preservatives, particularly sulfites, on fresh vegetables. Sulfites are commonly used to keep greens and other raw vegetables looking fresh at restaurant salad bars. The move for regulations governing their use began when they were found to cause severe allergic reactions in susceptible individuals, which occasionally included asthmatic attacks and anaphylactic shock, in several cases resulting in death.

Still, preservatives may be used on fresh fish. Sodium tripolyphosphate, for one, is commonly used. Sulfites are sometimes sprinkled on clams, lobsters, crabs, scallops, and especially shrimp. Sodium benzoates, known to cause adverse reactions in sensitive individuals, are commonly used to kill bacteria. Polytrisorbates are commonly used to control yeasts and molds, and polyphosphates are used to control the moisture content of fish.

These substances are seldom used when fish is sold locally, but are often used when fish is shipped any great distance. Some fish retailers display signs stating that their fish has not been treated with any of these chemicals; this assures that whatever fish is not locally caught has been efficiently and rapidly shipped, and that what appears fresh truly is.

APPENDIX 3

UNDERSTANDING LABORATORY TESTS

Laboratory tests are a useful tool for gathering information, but too often may fail to indicate problems in areas where attention is needed. A broad range of relative wellness exists between optimal health and overt illness; tests do little to indicate where in that range one lies. An awareness of the limitations of laboratory tests allows their use within the broader framework established by the medical history and the physical exam. Results of laboratory tests and special diagnostic procedures seldom surprise the discerning physician; rather, they usually confirm what was suspected after the history and physical.

Discussions of some routine blood and urine tests follow. The objective is to provide a simple and clear understanding of their purpose and meaning. Following this we will detail normal components of the blood and discuss how they may be impacted by disease.

COMPLETE BLOOD COUNT

The complete blood count (CBC) and an analysis of the urine (urinalysis) are basic screening tests routinely done to check for abnormalities. The CBC determines the number of red and white blood cells per milliliter of blood. Red blood cells (RBCs), with their hemoglobin, carry oxygen to all tissues of the body. White blood cells (WBCs) are part of the immune system; among other things, they attack bacteria and other foreign invaders. A significant increase in the WBC count usually indicates inflammation or infection.

Anemia is defined as the failure of the blood to deliver adequate oxygen to the tissues. The RBC count may be depressed in anemia, but in some types of anemia it never becomes depressed. Tests for hematocrit and for hemoglobin, also part of the CBC, are used to screen for anemia. The hematocrit test measures the percentage of the blood volume made up by RBCs. The hemoglobin test measures the amount of hemoglobin carried by the RBCs, thus determining the oxygen-carrying capacity of the blood. Both hematocrit and hemoglobin may also be normal in early stages of anemia.

On the other hand, the RBC count, hematocrit, and hemoglobin may all be below normal in a person with no signs or symptoms of anemia, and in good health. This is typical in those getting a great deal of endurance exercise—running, swimming, bicycling, cross-country skiing, or walking. Endurance exercise can cause the body's total volume of blood to increase dramatically, reportedly up to 30 percent over time. With this increase, there are fewer RBCs per unit of volume. Still, because of the increased volume, the overall capacity of the blood to deliver oxygen to the tissues is increased. The three tests may be low simply because the blood volume has increased.

True anemia occasionally occurs in such individuals and may be difficult to diagnose. If suspected, anemia can be confirmed by further tests involving levels of iron and iron-carrying molecules in the blood.

The CBC also may include a differential, the description of a blood smear made on a glass slide that is examined microscopically. The relative number of different types of white blood cells is determined, both white and red blood cells are examined for abnormalities, and the number of platelets is estimated. Leukemia, bone-marrow failure, adverse drug reactions, various types of anemia, inflammation, and the presence of malarial parasites are some of the many problems detectable by the CBC.

URINALYSIS

Urine is routinely tested in several ways and examined under a microscope. Specific gravity (density) is a measure of the number of particles suspended in the urine, and indicates the ability of the kidneys to concentrate urine adequately. Sediments are concentrated by centrifuging a small sample of the urine specimen. They are then examined microscopically for presence of cells indicating problems of the kidneys, bladder, and associated anatomy.

Other tests are performed by dipping a paper strip into a sample of the urine. Small squares on the strip have been treated chemically to react individually to glucose (the form of sugar in the blood), protein, blood, and several other substances that may be found in the urine. Reactions cause color changes of the small squares that are read by the physician or medical technologist performing the test, giving approximate levels of the various substances. Abnormalities—for example, the presence of blood, sugar, or proteins—may be followed up by more quantitative tests. Abnormalities may also arouse suspicion about certain problems and indicate need for other tests and diagnostic procedures.

ERYTHROCYTE SEDIMENTATION RATE (ESR)

Erythrocytes are red blood cells. The ESR measures the extent to which erythocytes settle toward the bottom of a thin glass tube in one hour, which is a function of the relative amounts of proteins, antibodies, and other substances in the blood. In health, they settle very little. This is a nonspecific screening test, frequently done. The result is elevated in many diseases, and also, often, in a normal pregnancy.

The ESR is commonly used as a relative measure of the activity of autoimmune diseases in which the body reacts adversely to its own tissues, such as rheumatoid arthritis and lupus. In general, the more severe the problem, the greater the elevation.

The normal sedimentation range is up to ten millimeters per hour in men and twenty in women. In very healthy individuals, the ESR may approach zero. Although the blood may be thin due to endurance exercise, in an individual with proper diet the red blood cells scarcely settle at all in the test. Readings consistently between zero and one are commonly seen over the years in such individuals.

BLOOD-CHEMISTRY TESTS

Many substances normally found in the blood may become elevated or depressed in disease. Some are nutrients used by cells throughout the body; their levels may give indications about grossly inadequate nutrition. Others are byproducts of the metabolism of certain specific cells and, if elevated, give indications about disease in the organs in which those cells predominate.

This section doesn't attempt to discuss all routine blood-chemistry tests. Rather, salient points, as well as a few more subtle points, about tests of concern to many individuals are explained.

Evaluating Cholesterol
Cholesterol is found throughout the body and is used in a wide variety of normal metabolic reactions. The human body makes, on the average, about three times as much cholesterol each day as the average diet contains. Cholesterol is as normal to human metabolism as any other nutrient found in foods. It is a constituent of all animal foods, and while cholesterol is found in the plaque that may build up in the arteries (including those to the heart, the coronary arteries) of some individuals developing heart disease, there is overwhelming evidence that dietary cholesterol is not the cause.

Many foods recommended in previous chapters are rich in

cholesterol: liver and other organs, eggs, shellfish, dairy products, and meat. Evidence was presented demonstrating that these foods should be an important part of a healthy primal diet.

The laboratory result most frequently discussed in association with cholesterol is the serum cholesterol (serum is the fluid portion of the blood remaining after the red blood cells and clotting factors have been removed). Ironically, in my opinion, the only reason to measure cholesterol is to determine whether or not it's too low. You read correctly. So-called high blood cholesterol is not a problem. It does serve as an excuse to prescribe some twenty billion dollars a year of cholesterol-lowering, highly toxic drugs.

Levels of cholesterol well over 200 mg per deciliter that were considered normal years ago are now classified as abnormally high. As the upper limit of normal has dropped, sales of cholesterol-lowering drugs have soared—circumstantial evidence of influence by drug companies on laboratory standards. There is no proof, but this reminds me of what Ralph Waldo Emerson once said when asked about circumstantial evidence that milk supplies were being watered down with water from the Charles River by milk distributors in nineteenth-century Boston. "Some circumstantial evidence is quite strong," Emerson commented, "as when there is a trout in the milk."

Low blood cholesterol is a different matter. It may indicate a plethora of problems caused primarily by a poor diet that lacks adequate quality animal foods.

Evaluating Triglycerides

Serum triglycerides are blood fats that are proving to be increasingly significant; they are the body's chief storage form of fat. Dietary fats break down in the intestines, pass through the intestinal wall, and are reassembled as triglycerides as they are absorbed into the blood. These triglyceride molecules in the blood then transport fats throughout the body.

Because dietary carbohydrates are converted into substances that can be made into triglycerides in the liver, carbohydrate consumption can greatly increase serum triglyceride levels. This is especially true of simple carbohydrates such as refined sugar (sucrose), refined (white) flour, concentrated fructose (as in fruit juices or fructose that has been added to processed foods), and dried fruits.

All of these substances are absorbed and enter the blood very quickly. As a result, a more rapid rate of conversion to triglycerides occurs than when the complex carbohydrates of vegetables or whole grains are consumed. Alcohol also causes a rapid elevation of metabolites (substances formed in the body from precursors) in the blood, which are converted by the liver into triglycerides.

In recent years, research has indicated that elevated serum triglycerides are statistically correlated with heart disease. These metabolic pathways for dietary fats, carbohydrates, and alcohol indicate why so many Americans have high triglyceride levels. Overconsumption of alcohol and refined foods obviously contributes to this, but other foods commonly consumed and considered nutritious are also contributing factors. Fruit juice, as mentioned, is an example. Furthermore, fruit juice provides calories, without bulk to slow down digestion. Instead of consuming fruit juice, one is better off obtaining one's vitamin C from fresh raw vegetables, fruits, raw dairy, and lightly cooked meat (raw milk and raw meat both contain significant amounts of vitamin C).

Fasting Glucose

Fasting blood glucose is the sugar level in the blood after a twelve-hour fast. It is measured in a standard chemistry screen that screens for diabetes. The results, as in the case of serum triglyceride levels, are influenced by the amount of refined flour, sugar, and other sweeteners, fruit, fruit juice, and alcohol in the diet.

Normal values for any given laboratory tend to be based on averages for the population it serves, however, the upper limit of normal for the fasting blood-glucose test has risen considerably over the years. Levels formerly considered indicative of possible or probable diabetes now often fall within the normal range. It should also be noted that the upper limit of the test can vary from lab to lab.

Regardless of a laboratory's upper limit of normal, a result falling within the range of 100 to 130 should be considered borderline. If falling within this range, the test should be repeated—confirmation of elevation calls for further evaluation. A glucose-tolerance test is often done in borderline cases to determine if the individual is indeed diabetic.

A blood test called glycohemoglobin is also helpful (see below). Since the late 1970s it has been routinely used to determine the average blood sugar in diabetics, and it may be used as an additional screening test when screening a potential diabetic.

Glucose-Tolerance Test

The glucose-tolerance test (GTT) is routinely used in diagnosing diabetes and hypoglycemia. However, in my opinion, use of the GTT is unnecessary in most cases, since either diabetes or hypoglycemia may be diagnosed from symptoms, physical findings, and other laboratory tests. With the GTT, after a twelve-hour fast, a sample of blood is taken to determine the fasting-glucose level. The individual then drinks a standardized sugar solution, and blood-sugar levels are measured for up to six hours. Many people subjected to this test become acutely ill and may feel poorly for as long as a few days.

A two-hour post-prandial blood-glucose determination is more useful. In this case, the individual comes to the laboratory for a blood glucose test two hours after completing a carbohydrate-rich meal. Although this test will also make many individuals feel poorly, approaching the diagnosis in this manner at least avoids putting the individual through the metabolic insult of the glucose tolerance test.

Evaluating Glycohemoglobin

Glycohemoglobin molecules form in the blood when glucose and hemoglobin combine. A normal number form when the average blood-sugar (glucose) level is normal. If glycohemoglobin is high, the average blood-sugar level is also correspondingly high. Thus a physician may periodically determine if a diabetic is adequately controlling his or her blood sugar. The test may also be routinely used in the initial evaluation of older individuals, or others in whom diabetes or borderline diabetes is suspected.

The glycohemoglobin test is of limited use in diagnosing hypoglycemia (low blood sugar); results are consistent in nonreactive hypoglycemia but inconsistent in reactive hypoglycemia. For both types, symptoms occur when blood sugar is low, but blood sugar in reactive hypoglycemia (hypoglycemia occurring in response to food) varies widely and may indeed at times be high.

As a result, average blood sugar and glycohemoglobin may be high, low, or average. In chronic, nonreactive hypoglycemia, blood sugar is nearly always low, and glycohemoglobin is thus low.

THYROID-HORMONE TESTING

A determination of thyroid-hormone levels is commonly ordered along with a CBC and a chemistry screen, particularly if the physician suspects under- or overactivity of the thyroid gland. The routine tests are called T_3 and T_4 (triiodothyronine and thyroxine), and while they may confirm a condition of myxedema (grossly underactive thyroid function) or thyrotoxicosis (grossly overactive thyroid function), these tests often show normal values in people suffering from chronic low-thyroid function.

T_3 and T_4 replaced the basal metabolism rate test in the 1950s as the standard laboratory procedure for evaluating thyroid function. Since then, researchers and clinicians have often emphasized in the medical literature that these tests may fail to adequately determine thyroid status and that the physician must primarily consider symptoms, signs, history, and physical findings (rather than laboratory results).

In my experience, hundreds of people in whom T_3 and T_4 tested normal suffered from conditions related to a chronically underactive thyroid gland. Though this is not the prevailing view of thyroid problems, it is an important one, well expressed by Dr. Broda Barnes in his 1975 book *Hypothyroidism: The Unsuspected Illness.* (Barnes's work, and the evaluation and treatment of thyroid problems, were discussed in chapter 9.)

MOVEMENT, GAMES, AND SPORTS

Throughout our time on the planet, human beings have been hunters, food-gatherers, and eventually, agriculturists. Traditionally, people have spent each day working at physical tasks, walking, and sometimes running. Entertainment as well revolved around vigorous exercise, primarily in games and dance. Physical activity is as natural to us as breathing.

These things are missing from most of our lives today. Instead, we exercise for its own sake, if at all. And yet, the intense use of one's body in sport, game, or dance may give great satisfaction. So too may the simpler pleasure of a walk. Many of us allow little time for these things. Periodically, we may strive for regularity in our exercise in an attempt to "get in shape." We may take an occasional walk or a run after work, or perhaps play a weekend round of golf, but everyday pressures on our time seem to preclude doing more.

Exercise that is enjoyed may most easily become a habit. Children may play until exhausted; time is suspended, and all life centers on the action of the play itself. Adults too may enjoy and benefit from vigorous physical play. The development of skills makes an activity fun, and commitment and practice lead to enjoyment. The play of games and the often solitary enjoyment of activities such as walking may work well together for those who make the time for both.

WALKING AND RUNNING

Walking and running require no team, partner, appointment, or court. The setting is outdoors and, for walking, street clothes are appropriate. A pair of shoes is the only equipment needed.

Regular walking keeps one fit for occasional running, and occasional running keeps one fit for occasional racing—as well as for most other sports.

People often ask if running is good for you. This depends on the individual. Approached reasonably and adapted to personal needs, running may be both fun and of lasting value.

However, all exercise initially fatigues muscles, tendons, and joints; when we stop, we are weaker than when we started. As the body recovers during the ensuing period of rest, strength returns. Given sufficient rest, the body's natural response to exercise is to become stronger. This is the physiological basis for increasing strength and endurance. Thus a runner or walker becomes progressively weaker if he or she attempts so much at each session that the body cannot fully recover by the next session. Injuries eventually and inevitably result. In the excitement of getting involved, most of us begin in just that way.

For most people, the surest and safest way to become involved in running is to begin by walking. If interested in becoming a fit walker and runner, follow this plan: Begin with two daily walks of five to fifteen minutes each, depending on previous exercise levels. This is more exercise than it appears. The great marathoner Bill Rodgers wrote that even a trained runner can never increase the total workload by more than 10 percent in one week without risking injury. For most people, adding five to fifteen minutes of walking twice a day to the total current amount of steady daily walking represents at least a 10 percent increase. So ease into this. Don't push the pace, and if you are ever stiff, sore, or just plain tired, skip a day and consider that too much may have been attempted.

Once ten to thirty minutes a day becomes effortless, with no stiffness or soreness, add five minutes a day to the total each week, building up to thirty minutes twice a day. The pace should keep you just short of breathing hard, with the pulse in the 90- to 120-beats-per-minute range. Even the athletic individual is wise not to push harder than this in the beginning, for if one has not recently walked or run regularly, the muscles and joints easily become sore in the beginning.

Most people start out moving faster, but for shorter periods of time—running a mile or two in ten or twenty minutes is typical. This may be quite easily done, but the risk of injury is usually high. The heart and cardiovascular system can in most people take more strain than the joints. A preliminary walking program strengthens and trains the muscles, tendons, and joints to stand the strain of regular running. This beginning period builds a foundation for enjoying injury-free running. The body adapts slowly but very surely. As soon as an hour a day of walking becomes easy, some light jogging may easily be intermixed. A gradual buildup to thirty to sixty minutes of jogging on some days may follow.

A principle well known among runners is that of hard days and easy days. The body does not fully recover from a taxing effort in twenty-four hours. Days when one puts in extra effort (in distance or speed) are best followed with a day of easy or no effort. And very hard efforts may require more than one subsequent easy day. A hard-easy pattern is more natural, more interesting, and more fun than doing the same thing every day, and more rapid conditioning results.

Hard running that leaves one out of breath (anaerobic running) is best avoided the first few months. Such running rapidly conditions the heart for faster running, but the musculoskeletal system at this early stage is rarely able to handle the strain. Injuries usually result.

For the Serious Runner

The challenge of competitive running is to discover what a concerted effort of body and mind can accomplish. Most people who race compete primarily against themselves; the other runners serve to spur one on to the exhilaration of one's own best effort. It is a unique satisfaction.

The individual interested in becoming a runner capable of covering several miles quickly may have difficulty proceeding slowly in the early stages. The adult previously involved in other sports, and with the cardiovascular fitness to run at a rapid pace, finds this especially true. Distance running is unlike most other sports, however, in that continual stress is placed on the muscles and joints. Both the accomplished runner and the person seeking to become one should understand that musculoskeletal fitness lags behind cardiovascular fitness during the first few years of running

Most runners are thus capable of routinely running a given distance much faster than the muscles and joints can regularly stand. This is why so many runners hurt so often. The sports-medicine business has grown by treating injured runners with surgery, special shoes, physiotherapy, and a host of other methods, mostly because people insist on running too much too soon. We are built to run, indeed to run very fast, but not to run very fast continuously. The adaptations the body must make to do so without injury take time.

Many champion runners have never hurt themselves running, so we know it's possible to reach one's potential without creating injuries. Indeed, development proceeds most rapidly when the demands placed on the body are the maximum possible but remain shy of causing injury. Running that becomes a natural and balanced part of life will not cause injuries, especially if one eats a primal diet. Poor nutrition makes runners more susceptible to injuries.

HOW SPORTS CAN HELP YOU

We balk at the salaries of today's professional athletes. But pay is determined by supply and demand; we collectively place a premium on their skills. Can we help but envy a bit the man or woman paid handsomely to play a game? Most of all, we may admire the winners, those who through some combination of gifts and hard work have become what we sometimes would like to be—rich, famous, admired, and successful.

Those of us with an interest in sports occasionally live vicariously through athletes. Their victories and defeats are to an extent ours as well. They know intimately the excitement of physical competition, the fear of injury, the thrill of winning.

For most of us, these things are a more subtle part of our lives; we miss the directness of sport. We compete instead for jobs, money, spouses, cars, prestige, houses . . . but inside we miss the more elemental competition of the athlete, the warrior, the primitive hunter.

Playing at a sport need not become all of these things. But personal sports and competition may fill a real and natural need. If we ourselves compete more in sports that we enjoy, we might have less need to compete so viciously (as we sometimes do) economically, and less need for millions-of-dollars-a-year heroes.

Athletic events may have marvelous moments. The way a person wins or loses may tell us a great deal about him or her. The way some teams work together like a family—or a tribe—calls to mind a not-so-distant past when survival depended on such cooperative but exhilarating effort. In our serious approach to the business of life, we often forget to laugh and have fun. Playing helps keep the child inside us alive.

SPORTS, FITNESS, AND RECOVERY FROM INJURIES

Ever since I can remember, I played baseball, basketball, or tennis. I loved baseball as a kid and played until I was fifteen. I played basketball until I was thirty-five or so. Since then, I've played tennis.

The basis for playing sports well is discipline in three specific areas—nutrition, fitness, and practice. Discipline in nutrition means carefully following the dietary principles I've written about on our website and in my books. The human body is built from the foods we eat. You can build a healthy, strong body and mind capable of optimal performance by eating only the best foods. Discipline in fitness requires both understanding and dedication. It's critical to understand, as mentioned earlier, that cardiovascular and musculoskeletal fitness often operate somewhat independently. The cardiovascular system strengthens quite rapidly and often outpaces the musculoskeletal system. The musculoskeletal system is much slower to strengthen. The joints and muscles often can't take the workout that the heart can take. Injuries result.

Recovery from injury, as well as recovery from surgery, is tremendously helped by using bovine tracheal cartilage (BTC) as a food supplement (see chapters 9 and 15 to learn more about BTC). Here is one very personal example.

On September 15, 2014, my wife, Elly, and I were in the water at the beach in Ponte Verda, Florida, when Elly was bitten on the right foot by a shark. The tendons to the four small toes of her foot were severed. That night she was in surgery for nearly two hours, receiving over 75 stitches to repair the tendons and close the wound. She was in bed and then on crutches for six weeks.

In addition to the bedrest and crutches, we started Elly on BTC, 12 daily, the day after the surgery. She began physical therapy once she was off the crutches, including a regimen of gradually walking more and more. Elly is a talented and dedicated tennis player, and we weren't sure how long it would be before she would be able to play again. In December, just three months post shark bite and surgery, she began playing doubles. By January 15, she was playing singles, fully recovered just four months after the tendons were severed. This is a remarkable recovery. Credit a highly skilled surgeon, our nutrition, and bovine tracheal cartilage.

Rest after any injury or surgery is critical. Too often, we begin stressing the injured area again far too soon. Healing takes time, even under ideal conditions of rest and superior nutrition. Begin movement again with slow walking, just 50 or 100 feet at a time initially. Good judgment is required. If it hurts at all, don't do it. Allow the injured tissues to heal. A sprain or severe strain, even when ligaments are not torn, may take weeks or months to heal completely. A gradual resumption of activities allows the healing to take place while slowly building the body back to full strength.

I can't emphasize enough the value of walking in building the basic musculoskeletal fitness needed to avoid injury, facilitate practice, and play an active sport like tennis well. The older you get, the truer this is.

Cardiovascular and musculoskeletal fitness form the physical basis for the disciplined practice necessary for good performance. Disciplined practice means regularly working on the basics using the techniques taught by an expert coach. Before you do things your way, learn the right way first. Later, make it your own. Whatever your age and whatever your sport, there is no substitute for a good teacher and a disciplined approach to nutrition, fitness, and practice.

GREATNESS IN LIFE AND IN SPORT

Have you ever thought of someone you knew personally as "a great person?" I'll bet most of us have, and not because that person had fame or fortune. He (when I use "he" in this section, I mean "he or she") might have been a parent or other relative, a teacher or coach, a friend or co-worker. He was there when he said he would be, and he did what he said he'd do—always, and to the best of his ability. He had time and kindness for all the people in his life. When he made mistakes, he owned up to them, and learned from them. He stood firmly for what he believed in, but he respected those who respectfully disagreed with him.

Anyone can choose to live that way. Being a great person, not in the conventional sense of measuring greatness by worldly accomplishments, fame, and fortune, but rather in the sense of character—is a choice anyone can make. Greatness is a matter of character. Choose to live by ethical principles and you will become a great person. The people in your life will see this. Rewards will be yours in more ways than you might imagine.

Greatness in sport usually is measured by more conventional parameters—titles and trophies, records, championships. Such greatness is no easy task, and we rightly admire great athletic achievements.

We recognize the dedication and discipline required, the thousands of hours of practice and hard work that even the most gifted individuals must endure to bring their gifts to world-class fruition, to greatness. Often there are elements of physical courage in the face of danger and pain that make the greatest athletes excel as they do.

None of this makes a great athlete a great person. We know this is true at an intellectual level, as time and again we see the disconnect between sport and life when athletic heroes very publicly reveal their character shortcomings in various ways. But there is always a sense of disappointment when that happens. The letdown is strongest for kids—"How could my hero do that?" But when this happens, we're all disappointed to some degree. We want our great athletes—and our great artists, musicians, actors, writers, politicians—to be great *people*. Like that special parent, teacher, or friend was.

So how does a great athlete transcend his or her sport to become a great person? The same way you or I can be great, by making that choice. Some athletes do this. If you watch for it, you'll see it: the great athlete who is also a great person.

Several years ago, I clipped a small, very unusual photograph out of a newspaper. Then twenty-four-year-old tennis player Rafael Nadal had won his fifth French Open title a short time before. In the photo, he is surrounded and being carried aloft by the grounds crew staff, ten or twelve older men smiling excitedly, flashing victory signs, and congratulating Nadal. The trophy had been presented, the awards ceremony was over, the TV cameras turned off. But a photographer had captured this moment wherein the grounds crew spontaneously embraced the young champion and he responded graciously in turn.

A ferocious competitor on the court, Nadal has long had a reputation as a kind, humble, and sweet young man liked by everyone with whom he has come in contact. This picture says everything you need to know about how a great athlete may transcend his or her sport to become a great person. When the grounds crew loves you, you know you're doing something right.

BIBLIOGRAPHY

Abelson, P. "Oil Spills." *Science* 195 (1977): 137.

Ahmed, A. "PCB's in the Environment." *Environment* 18, no. 6 (1976).

Alcoholics Anonymous. *Alcoholics Anonymous.* New York: Alcoholics Anonymous.

———. *Pass It On: The Story of Bill Wilson and How the A.A. Message Reached the World.* New York: Alcoholics Anonymous World Services, Inc., 1984. Originally published by Princeton University Press in 1953.

Allen, C. E., and M. A. Mackey. "Compositional Characteristics and the Potential for Change in Foods of Animal Origin." In D. C. Beitz and R. G. Hansen, eds., *Animal Products in Human Nutrition.* New York: Academic Press, 1982.

Angel, J. L. "Paleoecology, Paleodemography, and Health." In S. Polgar, ed., *Population, Ecology, and Social Evolution.* The Hague: Mouton, 1975.

Ashley-Montagu, F. M. "The Socio-Biology of Man." *Scientific Monthly,* June 1940.

Atkins, Robert, and Ruth West Herwood. *Dr. Atkins' Diet Revolution.* New York: Bantam Books, 1972.

Bang, H. O., et al. "Plasma Lipids and Lipoproteins in Greenlandic West Coast Eskimos." *Acta Medica Scandinavia* 192, nos. 1 and 2 (1972): 85–94.

———. "The Composition of the Eskimo Food in North Western Greenland." *American Journal of Clinical Nutrition* 33, no. 12 (1980): 2657–61.

Barnes, Broda, and Lawrence Galton. *Hypothyroidism: The Unsuspected Illness.* New York: Thomas Y. Crowell Co., 1976.

Baynes, C. F., and R. Wilhelm, trans. *I Ching* or *Book of Changes.* Princeton, N.J.: Princeton University Press, 1967.

Berkow, Robert, ed. *The Merck Manual.* Rahway, N.J.: Merck, 1982.

Bland, Jeffrey. "Lecture on Calcium Metabolism, May 12, 1979." In Ronald F. Schmid, ed., *Lectures of Dr. Jeffrey Bland: Nutrition, Exercise, and Health.* Portland, Ore.: The National College of Naturopathic Medicine, 1980.

————. *Historical Use of, Biological Basis For, and Preparation of Glandular-Based Food Supplements.* Tacoma, Wash.: Self-published, 1979.

Blumer, M. "Scientific Aspects of the Oil Spills Problem." Paper presented to the Oil Spills Conference Committee on Challenges of Modern Society, NATO. Brussels, 1970.

Blumer, M., et al. "A Small Oil Spill." Contribution no. 2630 of the Woods Hole Oceanographic Institution. *Environment* 13, no. 2 (1971): 2–12.

Brehm, Wayne. "Potential Dangers of Viosterol During Pregnancy With Observations of Calcification of the Placenta." *Ohio State Medical Journal,* 33, no. 9 (September 1937): 990–94.

Bronowski, Jacob. *The Ascent of Man.* Boston: Little Brown & Co., 1974.

Bronsgeest-Schoute, H., et al. "The Effect of Various Intakes of Omega-3 Fatty Acids on the Blood Lipid Composition in Healthy Human Subjects." *American Journal of Clinical Nutrition* 34 (1981): 1752–57.

Bunn, H. T. "Archaeological Evidence for Meat-Eating by Plio-Pleistocene Hominids from Koobi Fora and Olduvai Gorge." *Nature* 291 (1981): 574–77.

Byerly, T. C. "Effects of Agricultural Practices on Foods of Animal Origin." In R. S. Harris and E. Karmis, eds., *Nutritional Evaluation of Food Processing.* Westport, Conn.: Avi, 1975.

California Certified Organic Farmers. "Improve Your Life For Good" (pamphlet). Santa Cruz, Calif., 1985.

California Legislative Counsel's Digest. Chapter 914, Assembly Bill No. 443. "California Organic Foods Act of 1982."

Cavalli-Sforza, L. L. "Human Evolution and Nutrition." In D. N. Walcher and N. Kretchmer, eds., *Food, Nutrition, and Evolution: Food As an Environmental Factor in the Genesis of Human Variability.* New York: Masson, 1981.

Clark, John. *Hunza, Lost Kingdom of the Himalayas.* New York: Funk and Wagnalls, 1956.

Cohen, M. N. *The Food Crisis in Prehistory: Overpopulation and Origins of Agriculture.* New Haven, Conn.: Yale University Press, 1977.

Coleman Natural Beef, Inc. "Coleman Certified Chemical-Free Meats From the Colorado Rockies." Collection of letters from government officials, veterinarians, and feed suppliers, dated 1983–1986, verifying Coleman meats are completely chemical free and organically grown, as verified by USDA.

Connor, W., et al. "A Comparison of Dietary Polyunsaturated Omega-6 and Omega-3 Fatty Acids in Humans: Effects upon Plasma Lipids, Lipoproteins and Sterol Balance." *Arteriosclerosis* 1 (1981): 363.

Connor, W., et al. "Dietary Deprivation of Linolenic Acid in Rhesus Monkeys: Effects on Plasma and Tissue Fatty Acid Composition and on Visual Function." *Transactions of the Association of American Physicians* 97 (1984): 1–9.

Crawford, M. A. "Fatty-Acid Ratios in Free-Living and Domestic Animals." *Lancet* 1 (1968): 1329–33.

Culp, B. R., et al. "The Effect of Dietary Supplementation of Fish Oil on Experimental Myocardial Infarction." *Prostaglandins* 20 (1980): 1021.

Czap, A. I. "Take Two Tablets of BHT and Call Me in the Morning." *Townsend Letter for Doctors.* Issue no. 16, June 1984.

———. "Are Vitamin Companies Solvent: A Non-Pecuniary Review." *Townsend Letter for Doctors,* Issue no. 17, July 1984.

Dadd, Debra. *Nontoxic and Natural.* Los Angeles: Jeremy P. Tarcher, Inc., 1984.

Darwin, Charles. *On the Origin of Species: A Facsimile of the First Edition.* Cambridge, Mass.: Harvard University Press, 1975.

———. *The Illustrated Origin of Species.* Introduced and abridged by R. E. Leakey. New York: Hill & Wang, 1979.

Davies, David. *The Centenarians of the Andes.* Garden City, N.Y.: Anchor, 1975.

Degowin, E., and R. Degowin. *Bedside Diagnostic Examination.* New York: Macmillan Co., 1981.

Detrick, Mia. *Sushi.* San Francisco: Chronicle Books, 1982.

Dong, Collin H., and Jane Banks. *New Hope for the Arthritic.* New York: Ballantine Books, 1975.

"Dream Meat." *The Cook's Magazine: The Magazine of Cooking in America.* May–June 1984.

Dyerberg, J., et al. "Eicosapentaenoic Acid and Prevention of Thrombosis and Atherosclerosis." *Lancet* 2 (1978): 117.

Eaton, S. B., and M. Konner. "Paleolithic Nutrition." *New England Journal of Medicine* 312 (January 1985): 283–89.

Enos, W. F., et al. "Coronary Disease Among United States Soldiers Killed in Action in Korea." *Journal of the American Medical Association* 152, no. 1 (1953): 90–93.

Exler, I., and J. Weihrauch. "Finfish: Comprehensive Evaluation of Fatty Acids in Foods." *Journal of the American Dietetic Association* 69 (1976): 243.

Fehily, A., et al. "The Effect of Fatty Fish on Plasma Lipid and Lipoprotein Concentrations." *American Journal of Clinical Nutrition* 38 (1983): 349.

Foley, R. "A Reconsideration of the Role of Predation on Large Mammals in Tropical Hunter-Gatherer Adaptation." *Man* 17 (1982): 393–402.

Frank, Benjamin S., and Philip Miele. *Dr. Frank's No-Aging Diet.* New York: Dell, 1976.

Fredericks, Carlton. *Look Younger, Feel Healthier.* New York: Simon and Schuster, 1972.

Gaulin, S., and M. Konner. "On the Natural Diet of Primates, Including Humans." In R. Wurtman and J. Wurtman, eds., *Nutrition and the Brain,* vol. 1. New York: Raven Press, 1977.

Gerber, W. "Coastal Conservation." *Editorial Res. Rep.* 1 (1970): 141–49.

Gerson, Max. *A Cancer Therapy: Results of Fifty Cases.* Del Mar, Calif.: Totality Books, 1958. Reprint Bonita, Calif.: The Gerson Institute, 1986.

Goodnight, S., Jr. "The Effects of Dietary Omega-3 Fatty Acids Upon Platelet Composition and Function in Man: A Prospective, Controlled Study." *Blood* 58, no. 5 (1981): 880–85.

Goodnight, S., Jr., et al. "Polyunsaturated Fatty Acids, Hyperlipidemia, and Thrombosis." *Arteriosclerosis* 2, no. 2 (1982): 87–113.

Goto, M., and K. Higuchi. "The Symptomatology of Yusho (Chlorobiphenyls Poisoning) in Dermatology." *Fukuoka Acta Med.* 60, no. 6 (1969): 409–31.

Grant, N. "Mercury in Man." *Environment* 13 (1971).

Gribbin, John, and Jeremy Cherfas. *The Monkey Puzzle: Reshaping the Evolutionary Tree.* New York: Pantheon, 1982.

Hammond, H. "Mercury in the Environment: Natural and Human Factors." *Science* 171, no. 3973 (1971): 788–89.

Harris, W., et al. "The Comparative Reductions of the Plasma Lipids and Lipoproteins by Dietary Polyunsaturated Fats: Salmon Oil versus Vegetable Oil." *Metabolism* 32, no. 2 (1983): 179–84.

Harris, W., et al. "The Mechanism of the Hypotriglyceridemic Effect of Dietary Omega-3 Fatty Acids in Man." *Clinical Research* 32 (1984): 560 (abstract).

Harrower, Henry. *An Endocrine Handbook*. Glendale, Calif.: The Harrower Laboratory, 1939.

————. *Practical Organotherapy: The Internal Secretions in General Practice*. Glendale, Calif.: The Harrower Laboratory, 1922.

Haught, S. J. *Has Dr. Max Gerson a True Cancer Cure?* North Hollywood, Calif.: London Press, 1962. Reprinted as *Cancer? Think Curable! The Gerson Therapy*. Bonita, Calif.: The Gerson Institute, 1983.

Hayden, B. "Subsistence and Ecological Adaptations of Modern Hunter-Gatherers." In R. Harding and G. Teleki, eds., *Omnivorous Primates: Gathering and Hunting in Human Evolution*. New York: Columbia University Press, 1981.

Hemmings, W. A., and E. W. Williams. "Transport of Large Breakdown Products of Dietary Protein Through the Gut Wall." *Gut* 19 (1978): 715–23.

Hippocrates. *Hippocratic Writings*. Edited by G. Lloyd, translated by J. Chadwick and W. Mann. Cambridge, England: Penguin Books, 1978.

Hirai, Aizan, et al. "Eicosapentaenoic Acid and Platelet Function in Japanese." *Lancet* 2, no. 8204 (1980): 1132–33.

Holman, R. "Significance of Essential Fatty Acids in Human Nutrition." In R. Paoletti, et al., eds., *Lipids,* vol. 1. New York: Raven Press, 1976.

Hooten, Ernest A. *Apes, Man and Morons*. New York: Putnam, 1937.

————. *Up from the Apes*. New York: Macmillan Co., 1946.

Hornstra, G., et al. "Fish Oils, Prostaglandins, and Arterial Thrombosis." *Lancet* 11, no. 2 (1979).

Howells, W. W. *Evolution of the Genus Homo*. Reading, Penn.: Addison-Wesley, 1973.

Humane Farming Association. "Consumer Alert: The Dangers of Factory Farming" (pamphlet). San Francisco, Calif.: 1985.

Iritani, N., et al. "Reduction of Lipogenic Enzymes by Shellfish Triglycerides in Rat Liver." *Journal of Nutrition* 110, no. 8 (1980): 1664–70.

Jakubowski, J. A., and N. G. Ardlie. "Modification of Human Platelet Function by a Diet Enriched in Saturated Fat or Polyunsaturated Fat." *Atherosclerosis* 31, no. 3 (1978): 335–44.

Jensen, S. "The PCB Story." *Ambio* 1, no. 4 (1972): 123–31.

Kay, R. "Diets of Early Miocene African Hominoids." *Nature* 268 (1977): 628–30.

Keys, A. *Seven Countries: A Multivariate Analysis of Death and Coronary Heart Disease.* Cambridge, Mass.: Harvard University Press, 1980.

Kinderlehrer, Jane. "Liver May Hold the Secret of Cancer Prevention." *Cancer Control Journal* 3, nos. 1–2 (1975).

Krebs, C., and K. Burns. "Long-Term Effects of an Oil Spill on Populations of the Salt-Marsh Crab Uca Pugnax." *Science* 197, no. 4302 (1977): 484–87.

Kromhout, D., et al. "The Inverse Relation Between Fish Consumption and 20-Year Mortality from Coronary Heart Disease." *New England Journal of Medicine* 312, no. 19 (1985): 1205–9.

Kuratsume, M., et al. "Yusho, a Poisoning Caused by Rice Oil Contaminated With Polychlorinated Biphenyls." *HSHMA Health Rep.* 86, no. 12 (1971): 1083–91.

Kushi, Michio, and Alex Jack. *The Cancer Prevention Diet.* New York: St. Martin's Press, 1983.

Kushi, Michio. *The Macrobiotic Approach to Cancer.* Wayne, N.J.: Avery Publishing, 1981.

Leaf, Alexander. "Every Day Is a Gift When You Are Over 100." *National Geographic,* January 1973.

Leakey, Richard E., and Roger Lewis. *Origins: The Emergence and Evolution of Our Species and Its Possible Future.* New York: E. P. Dutton, 1977.

Lee, R. "What Hunters Do For a Living, or, How to Make Out On Scarce Resources." In R. Lee and I. De Vore, eds., *Man the Hunter.* Chicago: Aldine, 1968.

Lee, R., and I. DeVore, eds. *Kalahari Hunter-Gatherers: Studies of the Kung San and Their Neighbors.* Cambridge, Mass.: Harvard University Press, 1976.

Lieb, Clarence W. "The Effects of an Exclusive Long Continued Meat Diet, Based on the History, Experience, and Clinical Survey of Vilhjalmur Stefansson, Arctic Explorer." *Journal of the American Medical Association* 87, no. 1 (1926): 25–26.

Lopez, Barry. *Of Wolves and Men.* New York: Charles Scribner's Sons, 1978.

Lossonczy, T., et al. "The Effect of a Fish Diet on Serum Lipids in Healthy Human Subjects." *American Journal of Clinical Nutrition* 31, no. 8 (1978): 1340–46.

MacNeish, R. "A Summary of the Subsistence." In D. Byers, ed., *The Prehistory of the Tehuacan Valley*, vol. 1. Austin: University of Texas Press, 1967.

Maugh, T. "Polychlorinated Biphenyls: Still Prevalent, But Less of a Problem." *Science* 178, no. 4059 (1972): 388.

McCarrison, Robert. "Faulty Food in Relation to Gastro-Intestinal Disorder." *Journal of the American Medical Association* 78 (1922): 1.

———. *Studies in Deficiency Diseases*. London: Oxford Medical Publications, Henry Frowde and Hodder & Stoughton, 1945.

———. *Nutrition and Health*. London: Faber and Faber, 1953.

McClane, A. *The Encyclopedia of Fish Cookery*. New York: Holt, Rinehart & Winston, 1977.

Moncada, S., and J. L. Amezcua. "Prostaglandins, Thromboxane A2 Interactions and Thrombosis." *Haemostasis* 8 (1979): 252–265.

Moodie, P. *Aboriginal Health*. Canberra: Australian National University Press, 1973.

Moss, Ralph, and H. Leon Abrams, Jr. *Your Body Is Your Best Doctor*. New Canaan, Conn.: Keats Publishing Co., 1972. Originally titled *Health Versus Disease*.

Moss, Ralph. *The Cancer Syndrome*. New York: Grove Press, 1980.

Neuringer, M., et al. "Dietary Omega-3 Fatty Acid Deficiency and Visual Loss in Infant Rhesus Monkeys." *Journal of Clinical Investigation* 73, no. 1 (1984): 272–76.

Nickens, P. "Stature Reduction as an Adaptive Response to Food Production in Mesoamerica." *Journal of Archaeological Science* 3 (1976): 31–41.

Omae, Kinjiro, and Yuzuto Tachibana. *The Book of Sushi*. New York: Kodansha International Ltd., 1981.

Oregon Homegrown Meats. "Fat Content and Lean Yield by Boneless Primal Cut." Comparison of grass-fed and grain-fed beef by Oregon State University scientists, in private correspondence from Oregon Homegrown Meats. Eugene, Oregon, March 1, 1986.

Page, Melvin. *Degeneration-Regeneration*. Page Foundation, 1949.

Passwater, Richard A. *EPA: Marine Lipids*. New Canaan, Conn.: Keats Publishing, 1982.

———. *Cancer and Its Nutritional Therapies*. New Canaan, Conn.: Keats Publishing Co., 1978.

————. *Supernutrition.* New York: Dial Press, 1975.

Pearson, Durk, and Sandy Shaw. *Life Extension: A Practical Scientific Approach.* New York: Warner Books, 1982.

Phillipson, B., et al. "Reduction of Plasma Lipids, Lipoproteins, and Apoproteins by Dietary Fish Oils in Patients with Hypertriglycidemia." *New England Journal of Medicine* 312, no. 19 (1985): 1210–16.

Pimentel, D. "Effects of Pollutants on Living Organisms Other Than Man." In *Restoring the Quality of Our Environment.* Report of the Environmental Pollution Panel, President's Science Advisory Committee, Appendix Y10. Washington, D.C.: U.S. Government Printing Office, November 1965.

Pottenger, Elaine, and Robert Pottenger, Jr., eds. *Pottenger's Cats: A Study in Nutrition.* La Mesa, Calif.: The Price-Pottenger Nutrition Foundation, 1983. The edited writings of Francis Pottenger.

Pottenger, Francis M., Jr. "Clinical Evidences of the Value of Raw Milk." *Certified Milk,* July 1938.

————. "The Importance of a Vital, High Protein Diet in the Treatment of Tuberculosis and Allied Conditions." *Bulletin of the American Academy of Tuberculosis Physicians,* July 1941.

————. "Heat Labile Factors Necessary for the Proper Growth and Development of Cats." *Journal of Laboratory and Clinical Medicine,* December 1939.

————. "Hydrophilic Colloidal Diet." *American Journal of Digestive Diseases* 5, no. 2 (April 1938).

————. "Nutritional Aspects of the Orthodontic Problem." *The Angel Orthodontist* 12, no. 4 (October 1942).

————. "The Clinical Significance of the Osseous System." *Transactions of the American Therapeutic Society,* 1940.

————. "The Therapeutic Value of a Thermolabile Factor Found in Fats, Particularly the Lecithins, in Dermatoses." *Transactions of the American Therapeutic Society,* 1943. *Southern Medical Journal,* April 1944.

Pottenger, Francis M., Jr., and Bernard Krohn. "Influence of Breast Feeding on Facial Development." *Archives of Pediatrics,* October 1950.

————. "Reduction of Hypercholesterolemia by High-fat Diet Plus Soybean Phospholipids." *American Journal of Digestive Diseases,* April 1953.

Pottenger, Francis M., Jr., and D. Simonsen. "Deficient Calcification Produced by Diet: Experimental and Clinical Considerations." *Transactions of the American Therapeutic Society*, 1939.

———. "The Influence of Heat Labile Factors on Nutrition in Oral Development and Health." *Journal of Southern California State Dental Association*, November 1939.

Pottenger, Francis M., Jr., and F. M. Pottenger, Sr. "Adequate Diet in Tuberculosis." *American Review of Tuberculosis* 54, no. 3 (September 1946).

———. "Applied Nutrition—President's Address." *Journal of Applied Nutrition* 18, nos 1–4 (1965).

———. "Essentiality of Fats in Nutrition." *Journal of Applied Nutrition* 9, no. 2 (Autumn 1956).

Pottenger, Francis M., Jr., and F. M. Pottenger, Sr. "Milk—The Importance of Its Source." *Modern Nutrition*, November 1961.

———. "The Effect of Heat-Processed Foods and Metabolized Vitamin D Milk on the Dentofacial Structures of Experimental Animals." *Journal of Orthodontics and Oral Surgery* 32, no. 8 (August 1946).

———. "The Effects of Disturbed Nutrition on Dento-Facial Structures." *Southern California State Dental Journal*, February 1952.

———. "The Responsibility of the Pediatrician in the Orthodontic Problem." *California Medicine* 65, no. 4 (October 1946).

———. "The Use of Copper, Cobalt, Manganese, and Iodine in the Treatment of Undulant Fever." *Annals of Western Medicine and Surgery* 3, no. 9 (1949): 309–13.

———. "Therapeutic Effect of Lamb Fat in the Dietary." *Journal of Applied Nutrition* 10, no. 2 (Spring 1957).

Pottenger, Francis M., Jr., I. Allison, and W. Albrecht. "Brucella Infections." *Merck Report*, July 1949.

Potts, R., and P. Shipman. "Cutmarks Made by Stone Tools on Bones From Olduvai Gorge, Tanzania." *Nature* 291 (1981): 577–80.

Price, Weston. "Acid-Base Balance of Diets Which Produce Immunity to Dental Caries Among the South Sea Islanders and Other Primitive Races." *Dental Cosmos* 77 (1935): 842.

———. "Changes in Facial and Dental Arch Form and Caries Immunity in

Native Groups in Australia and New Zealand Following the Adoption of Modernized Foods." An address to the Connecticut State Dental Association, at Hartford, May 12, 1937.

———. "Eskimo and Indian Field Studies in Alaska and Canada." *Journal of the American Dental Association* 23, no. 3 (1936): 417–37.

———. "New Light on Some Relationships between Soil Mineral Deficiencies, Low Vitamin Foods, and Some Degenerative Diseases Including Dental Caries with Practical Progress in Their Control." *Oral Health,* August 1932.

———. "Studies of Relationships between Nutritional Deficiencies and (a) Facial and Dental Arch Deformities and (b) Loss of Immunity to Dental Caries Among South Sea Islanders and Florida Indians." *Dental Cosmos* 77 (1935): 1033–45.

———. "The Experimental Basis for a New Theory of Dental Caries, with Chemical Procedures for Determining Immunity and Susceptibility." *Dental Cosmos* (December 1932): 1139.

———. *Nutrition and Physical Degeneration.* La Mesa, Calif.: The Price-Pottenger Nutrition Foundation, 1945 (originally published by the American Academy of Applied Nutrition, Los Angeles, 1939).

———. "Field Studies Among Primitive Races in Australia and New Zealand." *New Zealand Dental Journal* 34 (1938): 76–86.

———. "New Light on the Cause of Tooth Decay in Man from Field Studies of Primitive Districts Providing Immunity." *Australian Journal of Dentistry,* December 1, 1933.

———. "Why Dental Caries with Modern Civilizations?" Parts 1–4, "Field Studies"; Part 5, "An Interpretation"; Part 6, "Practical Procedures for the Nutritional Control of Dental Caries." *Dental Digest,* March-August 1933.

Pritikin, Nathan, and Patrick McGrady, Jr. *The Pritikin Program for Diet and Exercise.* New York: Grosset & Dunlap, 1979.

Rendel, J. "The Time Scale of Genetic Change." In S. Boyden, ed. *The Impact of Civilization on the Biology of Man.* Canberra: Australian National University Press, 1970.

Rodale, J. I. *Organic Gardening.* Garden City, N.Y.: Hanover House, 1959.

Rodgers, Bill. *Marathoning.* New York: Simon & Schuster, 1982.

Sanders, T. A., and K. M. Younger. "The Effect of Dietary Supplements of Omega-3 Polyunsaturated Fatty Acids on the Fatty Acid Composition of Platelets and Plasma Choline Phosphoglycerides." *British Journal of Nutrition* 45 (1981): 613.

Sanders, T., et al. "Cod-Liver Oil, Platelet Fatty Acids, and Bleeding Time." *Lancet* 1, no. 8179, (1980): 1189.

Sattilaro, Anthony, and Tom Monte. *Recalled by Life: The Story of My Recovery from Cancer.* Boston: Houghton-Mifflin, 1982.

Schachter, Michael, and David Shienken. *Food, Mind and Mood.* New York: Warner Books, 1980.

Schaefer, O. "Medical Observations and Problems in the Canadian Arctic." *Canadian Medical Association Journal* 81 (1959): 386–93.

Schell, Orville. *Modern Meat: Antibiotics, Hormones, and the Pharmaceutical Farm.* New York: Random House, 1984.

Schoeninger, M. "Diet and the Evolution of Modern Human Form in the Middle East." *American Journal of Physical Anthropology* 58, no. 1 (1982): 37–52.

Seton, Ernest Thompson. *The Gospel of the Red Man.* (out of print)

Shelton, Herbert. *Fasting for Renewal of Life.* Tampa, Fl.: Natural Hygiene, 1974.

Shute, Wilfrid E., and H. Taub. *Vitamin E for Ailing and Healthy Hearts.* New York: Pyramid, 1972.

Siess, W., et al. "Platelet-Membrane Fatty Acids, Platelet Aggregation, and Thromboxane Formation During A Mackerel Diet." *Lancet* 1, no. 8166 (1980): 441–44.

Squire, Mark. "How Natural are Natural Vitamins." Fairfax, Calif.: Good Earth Natural Foods, 1977.

——. "Organically Grown: A Consumer's Guide to Sustainable Agriculture" (pamphlet). Fairfax, Calif.: Good Earth Natural Foods, 1984.

Stallings, D., and F. Mayer, Jr. "Toxicities of PCB's to Fish and Environmental Residues." *Environmental Health Perspectives* 1 (1972): 159–64.

Stefansson, Vilhjalmur. "Adventures in Diet." *Harper's Monthly Magazine.* Part 1, November 1935. Part 2, December 1935. Part 3, January 1936.

——. "Food of the Ancient and Modern Stone Age Man." *Journal of the American Dietetic Association* 13, no. 2 (July 1937): 102–29.

——. *My Life with the Eskimo.* New York: Macmillan Co., 1951.

——. *The Fat of the Land.* New York: Macmillan Co., 1957.

Stini, W. "Body Composition and Nutrient Reserves in Evolutionary Perspective." In D. Walcher and N. Kretchmer, eds., *Food, Nutrition, and Evolution: Food As an Environmental Factor in the Genesis of Human Variability.* New York: Masson, 1981.

Straus, Charlotte Gerson. "The Gerson Therapy." *Cancer Control Journal* 3, nos. 1–2 (1975).

Tarnower, Herman, and Samm S. Baker. *The Complete Scarsdale Medical Diet.* New York: Bantam Books, 1978.

Taylor, Renée. *Hunza Land: The Fabulous Health and Youth Wonderland of the World.* New York: Award Books, 1964.

Thompson, Kevin. "Chemical-Free Meat: Is It a 'Natural' or Just Another Gimmick?" *Meat Industry,* January 1986.

Thomsen, Robert. *Bill W.* New York: Harper & Row, 1975.

Trowell, H. "Hypertension, Obesity, Diabetes Mellitus and Coronary Heart Disease." In H. Trowell and D. Burkitt, eds., *Western Diseases: Their Emergence and Prevention.* Cambridge, Mass.: Harvard University Press, 1981.

Truswell, A., and J. Hansen. "Medical Research Among the !Kung." In R. Lee and I. DeVore, eds. *Kalahari Hunter-Gatherers.* Cambridge, Mass.: Harvard University Press, 1976.

Velican, D., and C. Velican. "Atherosclerotic Involvement of the Coronary Arteries of Adolescents and Young Adults." *Atherosclerosis* 36 (1980): 449–60.

Walker, A., et al. "A Possible Case of Hypervitaminosis A in Homo Erectus." *Nature* 296 (1982): 248–50.

Walker, N. W. *Fresh Vegetable and Fruit Juices.* Phoenix, Ariz.: Norwalk Press, 1978. Originally published as *Raw Vegetable Juices* (1936).

Warmbrand, Max. *The Encyclopedia of Health and Nutrition.* New York: Pyramid Books, 1974. Originally published as *The Encyclopedia of Natural Health,* 1962.

Watt, V., and A. Merrill. *Composition of Foods.* Washington, D.C.: U.S. Government Printing Office, 1975. U.S. Department of Agriculture Handbook 8.

Wehmeyer, A., et al. "The Nutrient Composition and Dietary Importance of Some Vegetable Foods Eaten by the !Kung Bushmen." *South African Medical Journal* 43 (1969): 1529–30.

White, Paul Dudley. *Heart Disease.* New York: Macmillan Co., 1943.

INDEX

Numbers in *italics* indicate illustrations

BOOKS OF RELATED INTEREST

Primal Body, Primal Mind
Beyond the Paleo Diet for Total Health and a Longer Life
by Nora T. Gedgaudas, CNS, CNT

Primal Cuisine
Cooking for the Paleo Diet
by Pauli Halstead
Foreword by Nora T. Gedgaudas, CNS, CNT

The Acid–Alkaline Diet for Optimum Health
Restore Your Health by Creating pH Balance in Your Diet
by Christopher Vasey, N.D.

The Slow Down Diet
Eating for Pleasure, Energy, and Weight Loss
by Marc David

Radical Medicine
Cutting-Edge Natural Therapies That Treat the Root Causes of Disease
by Louisa L. Williams, M.S., D.C., N.D.

The Seasonal Detox Diet
Remedies from the Ancient Cookfire
by Carrie L'Esperance

The Whole Food Bible
How to Select & Prepare Safe, Healthful Foods
by Chris Kilham

The Transformational Power of Fasting
The Way to Spiritual, Physical, and Emotional Rejuvenation
by Stephen Harrod Buhner

INNER TRADITIONS • BEAR & COMPANY
P.O. Box 388
Rochester, VT 05767
1-800-246-8648
www.InnerTraditions.com

Or contact your local bookseller